Cardiac Adaptation to
Hemodynamic Overload, Training and Stress

Cardiac Adaptation to Hemodynamic Overload, Training and Stress

Edited by

R. Jacob,

R. W. Gülch,

G. Kissling (Tübingen)

Steinkopff Verlag Darmstadt 1983

CIP-Kurztitelaufnahme der Deutschen Bibliothek

Cardiac adaptation to hemodynamic overload, training and stress / [Internat. Erwin Riesch Symposium]. Ed. by Ruthard Jacob . . .– Darmstadt: Steinkopff, 1983.

ISBN-13: 978-3-642-85328-9 e-ISBN-13: 978-3-642-85326-5
DOI: 10.1007/978-3-642-85326-5

NE: Jacob, Ruthard [Hrsg.]; International Erwin Riesch Symposium <1982, Tübingen>

Herstellung: Ungeheuer+Ulmer KG GmbH+Co, Ludwigsburg

Preface

Cardiac hypertrophy and accompanying phenomena have received increasing attention in recent years – particularly in the basic sciences. The present volume contains the proceedings of the Erwin RIESCH SYMPOSIUM on "CARDIAC ADAPTATION TO HEMODYNAMIC OVERLOAD, TRAINING AND STRESS" held in Tübingen on September 19–22, 1982.

In addition to the topics of the previous symposia (1976 and 1979) concerned with problems of cardiac hypertrophy, the scope of this sequel meeting has been expanded to include related fields. The intention was to consider numerous related features and problems of chronic reactions of the heart (and vascular system) to abnormal hemodynamic loading, as well as alterations due to maturation, aging, training, neuroendocrine status and stress. Special attention has been paid to cardiac reactions at the level of contractile proteins.

The results are considered primarily in light of long-term adaptation of the heart. Of course, research at the forefront of current knowledge need not always lead to congruent conclusions. Neither can the individual contributions always agree with the viewpoint of the editors. However, the broad array of individual approaches employed by biochemists, biologists, pathologists, physiologists, pharmacologists and clinical cardiologists will certainly help to provide a more balanced interpretation of the results in individual fields, stimulate reexamination of established concepts and provide direction for future research.

R. Jacob
R. W. Gülch
G. Kissling

Contents

Preface V

Editorial

Chronic reactions of myocardium at the myofibrillar level. Reflexions on "adaptation" and "disease" based on the biology of long-term cardiac overload
R. Jacob 3

Fundamental biochemical processes – Control of myocardial cell growth and gene expression

Molecular dynamics of contraction – relaxation
J. Gergely 27

Effects of activity on some physiological properties of skeletal muscles
G. Vrbová 33

Relationship between the synthesis rates and mRNA levels af the α and β cardiac myosin heavy chains in normal and thyrotoxic rabbits
A. W. Everett, A. M. Sinha, M. Rabinowitz, and R. Zak 39

Dissociation between factors resulting in hypertrophy and changes in myosin isoenzyme population of the pressure-loaded rat heart
H. Rupp, N. Popova, and R. Jacob 46

Dissociation of hypertrophy and altered function in senescent rat myocardium
E. G. Lakatta 53

Differential effect of thyroid hormones on catecholamine enzymes and myosin isoenzymes in ventricles and atria of the rat heart
A. R. Bukhari and H. Rupp 59

The adrenals in experimental cardiac hypertrophy
F. Kölbel, V. Schreiber, J. Stepan, T. Pribyl, and I. Gregorova 65

Myocardial nucleus in growing and hypertrophied heart
F. Cluzeaud, J. Perennec, E. de Amaral, M. Willemin, and P. Y. Hatt 69

A pathomorphological study on the diabetogenic drug induced heart disease in the rat
S. Onishi, H. Nunotani, and Y. Tochino 70

The role of cyclic nucleotides in the pathogenesis of myocardial hypertrophy
N. Popova, B. Bozhkov, R. Kolarova, and I. Petkova 78

The role of cytoplasmic factors in RNA synthesis activation during hyperfunction of heart and liver
F. S. Meerson and M. P. Javich 83

New trends in biology of cardiac overload: plasma membranes, enzymes, cytoskeleton proteins and in vitro traduction of RNA
P. Mansier, K. Schwartz, L. Lelievre, J. M. Moalic, D. Charlemagne, J. L. Samuel, L. Rappaport, and B. Swynghedauw 94

Structural changes of contractile proteins

Adaptive changes in cardiac isomyosins as visualized by immunofluorescence
S. Schiaffino, L. Gorza, S. Sartore, C. Valfré, and P. Pauletto 101

Myosin isoenzymic distribution in hypertrophied rat and human hearts
J. J. Mercadier, A. M. Lompré, P. Bouveret, J. L. Samuel, L. Rappaport, B. Swynghedauw, and K. Schwartz 104

Thyroxine-induced molecular alteration of heavy and 27,000-dalton light chains of rabbit ventricular myosin. Reconstitution of heavy and light chain molecules of subfragment-1 isozymes of cardiac myosin
S. Ueda and Y. Yazaki 113

Structural variants of heavy and light chains of atrial and ventricular myosins in hypertrophied human hearts
C. R. Tuchschmid, T. Srihari, H. O. Hirzel, and M. C. Schaub 123

Myosin isozymes in normal and pathological human cardiac muscle
F. A. Sreter, K. Mabuchi, E. Somogyi, and P. Sotonyi 129

Structural and enzymatic alterations of cardiac contractile proteins under chronic pressure overload
M. Nagano, N. Takeda, H. Maeno, K. Noma, and T. Ohkubo 134

The phosphorylation of cardiac contractile proteins
P. J. England, D. Mills, S. A. Jeacocke, and H. T. Pask 139

Morphological and functional aspects of adaptation or damage

Isoenzyme contribution to economy of contraction and relaxation in normal and hypertrophied hearts
N. R. Alpert, L. A. Mulieri, and R. Z. Litten 147

Heat liberation in experimentally induced tetanic contractions of myocardium from normal and Goldblatt rats
Ch. Holubarsch, R. P. Goulette, L. A. Mulieri, and N. R. Alpert 158

Energetics of the rat heart in chronic pressure overload
G. Kissling, L. Malloy, and H. Rupp 167

Alterations in electrical properties of rat myocardium accompanying different models of cardiac hypertrophy
R. W. Gülch and J. Mohrmann 174

Calcium binding and Na–Ca exchange in cardiac sarcolemma in experimental hypertension
M. Kawamura, S. Watari, T. Nagata, T. Iimura, T. Ohkubo, M. Kawanishi, and M. Nagano 182

Cardiac muscle function during the development of hypertrophy in pigs due to pressure overload
P. K. Singal, K. S. Dhillon, V. Panagia, and N. S. Dhalla 189

Biochemical and mechanical correlates at peak systole in myopathic Syrian Hamster
J. Wikman-Coffelt, R. Sievers, R. J. Coffelt, and W. W. Parmley 197

Buffer capacity of the myocardium after swimming training
G. Kissling and A. Beyer 204

Coronary circulation, ischemia, adenine nucleotide content in cardiac overload

Coronary reserve in spontaneously hypertensive rats: the effect of blood pressure, hypertrophy and long-term vasodilator therapy
M. Klepzig and B. E. Strauer 213

Effect of aortic constriction on rat heart function and mortality
H.-G. Zimmer 220

Metabolic effects of low-flow ischemia on the perfused hypertrophied rat heart: a phosphorus (^{31}P) nuclear magnetic resonance (NMR) study
N. Lavanchy, J. Martin, J. Aussedat, A. Ray, and A. Rossi 228

Myocardial mechanics of infarcted and hypertrophied non-infarcted myocardium following experimental coronary artery occlusion
O. H. L. Bing, W. W. Brooks, Ch. H. Conrad, K. B. Weinstein, J. Spadaro, and P. Radvany 235

The interference of respiratory chain function with lipid metabolism in the left ventricular myocardium of rats with compensated chronical volume overload
J. Moravec and J. Nzonzi 245

Neuroendocrine, cardiac and vascular alterations in hypertension and stress – Pathogenesis, and effects of interventions

Cardiovascular abnormalities in spontaneously hypertensive rats. Causes or consequences of the increased blood pressure?
M. J. Mulvany, E. Mikkelsen, O. Lederballe Pedersen, N. Nyborg, and L. T. Jespersen 253

Mechanisms of heart sarcolplasmic reticulum damage under stress
Yu. V. Arkhipenko, V. E. Kagan, and F. Z. Meerson 258

Changes of heart catecholamine levels, metabolism and adrenergic receptors in actually and repeatedly stressed rats
R. Kvetňanský and T. Torda 265

Modulation of catecholamine synthesizing and degrading enzymes by swimming and emotional excitation in the rat
H. Rupp, A. R. Bukhari, and R. Jacob 267

Blood pressure and cardiac myosin heterogeneity in the rat as influenced by swimming and emotional excitation
H. Rupp, H.-R. Felbier, and R. Jacob 274

Calcium-Antagonism: A new therapeutic access to hypertensive heart disease
W. Motz and B. E. Strauer 282

Magnesium as the physiologic calcium antagonist: its vascular effects and therapeutic use
H. Nguyen Duong and K. Brecht 288

Reactions at the tissue level

Effects of hemodynamic load on myocardial fibre orientation
B. Korecky and K. Rakusan 297

Biochemical characteristics and cellular mechanisms of fibrotic processes
J. Rauterberg, B. Voss, and G. Pott 304

Cardiovascular aging
J. Lindner and P. Schmiegelow 314

Connective tissue alterations in coronary arteries of spontaneously hypertensive rats (SHR); electron microscopic and morphometrical investigation
H. Ziegler, H. Schmiebusch, M. Heisterkamp, and J. Staubesand 330

Myocardial mass and collagen content in Crotalaria spectabilis-induced pulmonary hypertension of young and adult rats
I. Medugorac and R. Jacob 341

Heterogeneity of collagen in the normal and hypertrophied left ventricle of the rat
I. Medugorac and R. Jacob 349

Determination of left ventricular diastolic wall stress and elasticity in situ. A methodological investigation
Ch. Brilla, R. Jacob, and G. Kissling 354

The influence of antihypertensive treatment on left ventricular compliance and myocardial stiffness
W. Motz, R. Ippisch, G. Ringsgwandl, and B. E. Strauer 364

Acknowledgements 369

Authors' Index 370

Subject Index 371

Editorial

Cardiac Adaptation to Hemodynamic Overload, Training and Stress
Dr. D. Steinkopff Verlag 3–24 (1983)

The use of ambiguous and poorly defined terms tends to obscure ignorance and impede progress
R. F. Rushmer (1963)

Chronic reactions of myocardium at the myofibrillar level Reflections on "adaptation" and "disease" based on the biology of long-term cardiac overload*)**)

R. Jacob

Physiologisches Institut (II), University of Tübingen (FRG)

Summary

A brief review of the current state of knowledge on long-term reactions of myocardium at the level of the myosin molecule is presented followed by functional interpretation of these alterations. Fundamental questions of "adaptation", including the conceptual separation of "adaptational" and "disease" or "pathological processes", are discussed primarily in light of chronic myofibrillar reactions. It is shown that the decrease in myofibrillar ATPase activity and maximum unloaded shortening velocity under chronic cardiac pressure load in the rat heart model is compatible with an adaptional interpretation. However, the terms "adaptive" and "pathologic" need not be mutually exclusive. Consideration of long-term reactions of the myofibrillar apparatus, during maturation and aging, physical training and general stress reveals that it is not yet possible to definitively delineate adaptive processes at the myofibrillar level which can be attributed solely to changes in mechanical load.

With regard to human myocardium, further investigation will be required to determine the extent of possible changes in functional parameters attributable to variation of the myosin molecule, including the light chains.

Key words: adaptation, myosin isoenzymes, myofibrillar function, pressure overload, training, stress, endocrine status, transmitters

Introduction

In recent decades, experimental cardiology has primarily dealt with cardiac reactions to interventions in short-term experiments – not least because of the relative ease with which publishable results can be obtained under such conditions. Research of long-term reactions of the heart not only tries the patience of the investigator but also poses considerable difficulties of interpretation.

A fundamental question is whether the individual phenotypical alterations should be classified as having essentially beneficial or detrimental consequences; alternative classifications attempt to distinguish between

*) Dedicated to Prof. Dr. E. Bauereisen, Würzburg, in honour of his 70th birthday

**) Supported by the Deutsche Forschungsgemeinschaft (Ja 172/12)

"adaptive processes" and "cellular damage" – or between "physiologic" and "pathologic" alterations (2, 3, 5, 6, 54–59, 90–92, 157).

Chronic cardiac pressure overload leads to alterations at many levels of the organ: i.e., the whole ventricle, as reflected by mass increase and changes in configuration; the tissue level, such as an increase in connective tissue and decrease in catecholamine concentration; as well as the cellular and subcellular level involving practically all cell components and organelles (for references see 2, 14, 19, 20, 41, 57, 90, 91, 93, 103, 104, 108, 109). In the compensatory stage of pressure-induced cardiac hypertrophy of the rat, for example, prolongation of the action potential is observed (40) as well as decrease in the transport capacity of the sarcoplasmic reticulum (42), increase in the ratio of myofibrils to mitochondria (155) and decrease in myofibrillar ATPase activity (for ref. see 4, 56, 126) – a change which is accompanied by decreased unloaded myofibrillar shortening velocity (31, 88).

Particularly the functional interpretation of the last of the above alterations is controversial. Are the changes in biochemical structure at the myofibrillar level adaptive in nature (5, 6, 51, 57–59, 62, 80, 145) or do they represent a biochemical "defect", i.e., a sign of "wear and tear" due to disturbance of protein synthesis and/or degradation (37, 46, 90, 91, 143)? Does decreased myofibrillar ATPase activity and shortening velocity thereby permit differentation of "physiological" and "pathological" hypertrophy even in the stage of compensatory cardiac hypertrophy (157)? In light of the great significance generally attributed to unloaded shortening velocity in evaluation of myocardial "contractility" (13, 53, 56, 114, 135), the above question is not purely academic and is worthy of being the primary subject of the following discourse. Because of numerous tangential features and related problems it will be necessary to consider not only myocardial reactions to hemodynamic overload, but also alterations due to maturation, aging, training, stress, and altered neuroendocrine status.

Variability of myosin structure

Although our discussion will be focussed primarily on general questions of physiology and pathophysiology, some essential biochemical, mechanical and energetical findings seem to be worthy of introductory consideration. Details of biological processes in early stages of cardiac hypertrophy, including contractile protein changes, have been reported in several informative reviews (4, 21, 34, 41, 90, 92, 108, 109, 126, 141, 163, 164).

Cardiac myosin isoenzymes

Chronic reactions at the myofibrillar level have been discovered in the form of structural modifications of the myosin molecule. Enzymatic, electrophoretic, immunochemical and histochemical procedures, as well as peptide mapping, indicate that mammalian ventricular myocardium contains distinct variants of myosin with different ATPase activities, which differ in the biochemical structure of their heavy chains (23, 24, 27, 49, 67, 105, 124, 127, 154, 163). The differences in enzyme activity can be related to the existence of two different heavy chains, HC_α and HC_β. These molecular subunits may occur in the form of two different homodimers (VM-1 and VM-3; VM = ventricular myosin) or a heterodimer (VM-2) (fig. 1).

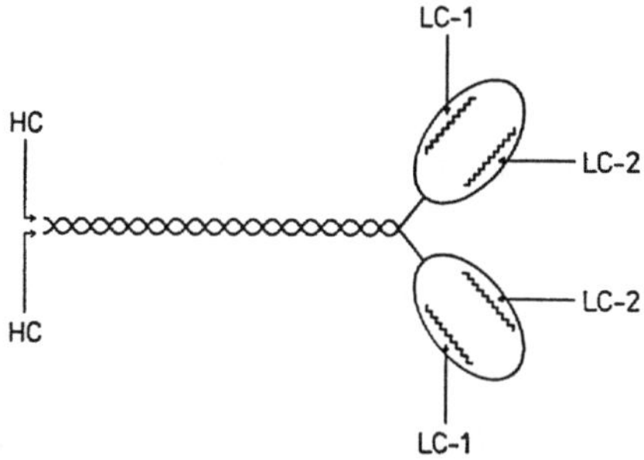

Fig. 1. Schematic of the quaternary structure of ventricular myosin. The isoenzymes which can be separated by pyrophosphate gel electrophoresis are constituted as follows:
VM-1: $HC_\alpha HC_\alpha \cdot (LC\text{-}1)_2 \cdot (LC\text{-}2)_2$
VM-2: $HC_\alpha HC_\beta \cdot (LC\text{-}1)_2 \cdot (LC\text{-}2)_2$
VM-3: $HC_\beta HC_\beta \cdot (LC\text{-}1)_2 \cdot (LC\text{-}2)_2$
Abbreviations: VM = ventricular myosin; HC = heavy chains; LC = light chains.

Thus, in the model of rat ventricular myocardium, 3 isoenzymes of myosin can be demonstrated by pyrophosphate gel electrophoresis according to Hoh (48) and d'Albis (27), i.e., under non-denaturating conditions.

The isoenzyme pattern is influenced by ontogenetic development and maturation, endocrine status, and loading conditions of the heart.

Apparently, different isoenzymes of myosin can coexist within a given myocardial cell. The fetal form is indistinguishable from the isoenzyme VM-3 of adult animals (96). In the 4–5-week-old rat, a fairly homogenous VM-1 pattern is present. A limited redistribution occurs during the maturational period, although VM-1 still predominates over VM-3 and the heterodimer VM-2, whereas other species such as the rabbit and pig return to a substantially VM-3 pattern after several weeks of age.

In adult rats, a shift towards VM-1 can be induced by application of thyroid hormones, small doses of isoproterenol, and prolonged swimming training. In contrast, redistribution in favour of VM-3 is observed under chronically increased pressure load; after hypophysectomy, adrenalectomy, thyreostatic treatment, or application of 6-hydroxydopamine; and in the diabetic rat (30, 38, 48, 51, 55, 58, 59, 77 (rabbit), 78, 79, 80, 96, 97, 117, 119–122, 127, 161, 163).

Gene expression

The differences in the polypeptide composition of the heavy chains can be attributed to an expression of different myosin genes occurring at specific developmental stages, or as a result of changes in loading or neuroendocrine conditions. In fact, hybridization and nucleotide sequence analysis have shown that two different HC-genes coding for proteins of different length are expressed in ventricles of adult rats (83). The level of expression of fetal and adult HC genes varies throughout the life span of the animal and can also be modulated in a reversible fashion by the factors mentioned above.

Apparently, pretranslational processes play a major role in regulating the expression of cardiac myosin heavy chains α and β (33). The conceivable involvement of posttranscriptional mechanisms, however, does not yet appear to be fully clarified.

Functional significance of the myosin isoenzyme pattern

The isoenzyme pattern has been shown to exert substantial influence on myofibrillar function. Prevalence of VM-1, the isoenzyme with the highest electrophoretic mobility, is expressed in high myofibrillar ATPase activity and unloaded shortening velocity, whereas a redistribution in favour of VM-3 causes a reduction of both parameters.

In propylthiouracil-treated rats (with fairly homogenous VM-3 pattern) myofibrillar ATPase activity is ca. 35 % lower than in 4–5-week-old rats (with fairly homogenous VM-1 pattern) (105, 121). The well-known relation between myofibrillar (or myosin) ATPase activity and shortening velocity (4, 11, 29, 44, 56, 88) can be reduced to the underlying relationship between myosin isoenzyme pattern and maximum unloaded shortening velocity (31, 55, 58, 130). The magnitude of change in the maximum unloaded shortening velocity of native and chemically skinned myocardial preparations, accompanying extreme changes in myosin isoenzyme pattern, was found by our group to be ca. 40 % (31). Probably due to additional, nonmyofibrillar factors, other authors reported substantially higher differences (130).

In chronically pressure-loaded myocardium; ATPase activity, isoenzyme pattern of myosin, and shortening velocity are changed in a manner typical of slowly working myocardium, shortening velocity of fibrotic preparations being distinctly more reduced. Dose-response curves did not indicate concomitant changes in calcium sensitivity and cooperativity (31).

Isometric myofibrillar force development of skinned rat myocardium with predominance of VM-3, however, is only insignificantly diminished (31, 88), heat release (5, 6, 51, 78) and O_2 consumption (63, 64) per unit muscle mass and stress are significantly reduced. This means that economy of tension development is increased, which may be due to prolonged on-time of the cross bridges during slow cross-bridge cycling (5, 6).

In native myocardium and the whole heart, a number of other factors are superimposed on the functional alterations of the myofibrillar apparatus (action potential and excitation-contraction coupling, O_2 and substrate supply, nonmuscular tissue content – action potential conduction, hypertrophy, ventricular geometry) (4, 36, 54, 55, 57, 59). For example, peak isometric tension, and even the maximum rate of tension development, in the early stage of Goldblatt hypertension is significantly increased compared with age-matched controls – despite significant redistribution of the isoenzyme pattern in favour of VM-3. The situation in the whole heart is, of course, even more complex. Work and power capacity of the pressure-hypertrophied ventricle is generally increased – despite transformation in favour of a more slowly functioning myofibrillar apparatus. Thus the significance of the isoenzyme pattern for cardiac pumping function seems to be frequently rather overestimated than underestimated (55).

Species differences, human myocardium

The peptide patterns of ventricular and atrial myosin indicate differences in the primary structure of the respective myosin heavy chains. There are also differences in the respective light chains and ATPase activity (10, 26, 106, 148, 162, 163).

A point which is worthy of special consideration is the species dependence of the ATPase activity, the essential features of which were reviewed earlier by Scheuer and Bhan (126). With regard to myosin isoenzymes, the general theme appears to be the same in all mammals examined to date; the ventricle contains several variants of myosin composed of HC_α and HC_β. The relative proportion of the isoenzymes VM-1 and VM-3, however, differs widely between various animal species. Whereas in small mammals, such as the rat or rabbit, both isoenzymes occur in appreciable amounts (depending on the stage of development) – in other, mostly larger animals, VM-3 greatly predominates, that is to say, only small amounts or traces of VM-1 are present. The functional significance of alterations in isoenzyme pattern due to alterations in endocrine status, or hemodynamic load, is unclear in man or those species in which VM-1 only accounts for a small proportion of cardiac myosin.

Human ventricular myosin reveals primarily an isoenzyme which comigrates with VM-3 of the rat and only little myosin of higher mobility which may correspond to VM-1 (96, 156). We are thus confronted with the question of how alterations of cardiac myofibrillar ATPase activity in human beings can occur on a magnitude reported by Alpert and Gordon (3), Gordon and Brown (37), Leclercq and Swynghedauw (74) and Peters et al. (102). Alterations in the isoenzyme pattern of myosin due to changes in heavy chain composition do not seem to play an essential role in patients with cardiac hypertrophy due to hemodynamic overload (96, 137, 148, 156) although immunocytochemistry with specific antibodies indicated that an isoenzyme considered to be VM-1 disappears in hypertrophied hearts of hypertensive patients as well as in papillary muscles of patients with mitral stenosis (128). In obstructive hypertrophic cardiomyopathy, indications of alterations at the level of the myosin molecule have not been forthcoming (86, 129).

Although a number of authors reject the notion of an age-dependent change in ATPase activity in man (37, 84), the data of Gordon and Brown (37) may provide indications of age dependence in human beings. Fetal cardiac myosin appears to possess low ATPase activity (129). According to Cummins (26) a portion of light chains later accounted for by VLC-1 is taken up by FLC-1 in fetal human myosin. After reaching a maximum in early childhood, ATPase activity appears to decrease with increasing age (10, 37, fig. 3, 74). Banerjee and Wiener (10) have found the actin-activated ATPase activity to be reduced approx. 40 % and the alkali sensitivity increased with aging; whereas pyrophosphate gel electrophoresis, Ca^{2+} and K^{+}(EDTA)-activated ATPase, and one-dimensional peptide mapping remained unchanged.

Important problems of methodology also remain to be clarified. A current discussion involves the question of the suitability of conventional in vitro methods for measuring differences in myofibrillar ATPase activity. According to Mornet et al. (98) the ATPase activity measured by conventional means is only a fraction of the actual ATPase hydrolysis which occurs in stimulated intact muscles. Scheuer and Bhan (126) had already commented in detail on the potential for discrepancies – in the quantitative amount and even the direction of changes in ATPase activity – depending on whether myofibrils or purified myosin are examined, as well as the respective mode of activation. A better approximation of natural conditions may perhaps be achieved by merely measuring initial ATP-splitting and not that under steady-state conditions. Furthermore, when covalent crosslinking is performed between myosin S-1 and F-actin, this results in highly increased ATPase activity (98, 142).

Significance of myosin light chains

It is improbable that the increase in ATPase activity of the failing human heart reported by Nebel and Bing (99) is indeed a phenomenon generally common to cardiac insufficiency in man. It is also quite difficult to imagine that myofibrillar ATPase activity in man could be absolutely rigid despite the substantial changes demonstrated in response to pressure-induced hypertrophy in numerous species including small and large mammals: cats, dogs, guinea pigs, rabbits, calves (for references see 126).

At the present time, one cannot definitively say how many isoenzymes actually exist in the heart. The homogeneity of the isoenzymes VM-1 and VM-3 is questionable (153). Alterations in myosin molecular structure need not be detectable using pyrophosphate gel electrophoresis. Investigations on hyperthyrotic guinea pigs have revealed that the electrophoretic appearance can be unchanged (24) despite: immunological detection of a change in the proportion of isomyosins, increased Ca^{2+}-activated ATPase activity, and altered amino acid composition (36, 147, 161).

Alterations of light chains seem to contribute to the thyroxine-induced change of ATPase activity in rabbits (149).

In contrast to Klotz et al. (66) – Sreter et al. (137) and Tuchschmid et al. (148) have observed alterations involving the myosin light chains in patients with severe cardiac disease; the functional significance of such changes has not yet been clarified. Normal human ventricular myosin contains two different light chains (fig. 1) which differ from those of porcine myocardium (65) and are not identical with those of atrial myosin. The light chains play a decisive role in transformation of skeletal muscle (152). Although the situation is much different in cardiac muscle, the potential significance of the light chains deserves further attention. The biological role of phosphorylation of these subunits has also not been fully clarified (32).

Characterization of adaptive processes

Discussion of the various alterations at the myofibrillar level with regard to adaptation is based on the premise that one is capable of definitely distinguishing an adaptive response from a nonadaptive alteration. Thus one is confronted with the question of the criteria of adaptive processes. Furthermore, one must ponder the conceptual justification for considering adaptive and pathologic processes as mutually exclusive opposites.

Adaptation, in the present context, can be viewed as a phenotypical reaction of an organism, organ system(s), tissue(s) or cell(s) in response to alterations of the environment or the appearance of special demands, which permits coping with the altered conditions and thereby has a tendency which is conducive to the normal processes of life.

The subject of our considerations is primarily those changes which are limited by the genome and – although generally initiated without delay – are fully manifested within days or weeks. Thus, acute regulatory mechanisms will not be considered. The same applies to genetic alterations appearing over a great number of generations.

In his last work of 1878/79, the great French physiologist Claude Bernard (15) introduced the concept of the internal environment. Despite numerous alterations of the environmental conditions and the demands on the individual organs, the physical properties and chemical composition of "body fluids" and tissues are maintained remarkably constant. This maintenance of constant conditions in the internal environment or, as Walter Cannon (22) formulated, "homeostasis", is one of the essential features of life.

Like acute regulatory mechanisms, long-term adaptive processes enable the organism to stabilize its essential composition and functions, for example: ion concentration and osmotic pressure, but also other parameters such as blood pressure and body temperature. Thus the organism is capable of accepting information from the environment and processing it such that the resulting reactions are appropriate to the given circumstances. Adaptive processes are frequently periodic in nature (45), which may explain differences in the findings of various authors. The altered conditions confronting a given organ may originate within the body – for example, increased pressure load of the heart.

The term "internal environment" originally referred essentially to the extracellular fluid. However, the concept of homeostasis has also been extended to include structural aspects. Thus "disease" has been defined as "existence at the limits of structural and functional adaptation" (75), or, "disturbance of the equilibrium, accompanied by decreased functional capability", i.e., disturbance of the structural and functional homeostasis, due either to extreme stimuli which overtax the physiological adaptive capacity or to insufficiency of the regulatory systems involved (116).

Adaptation to altered demands is only possible within genetically determined limits. The genome codes for macromolecular structure, and thus phenotypical alterations cannot occur beyond these limits. When the details of adaptation at the complex levels of the organism and organs are to be understood, one must analyze alterations down to the levels of cellular organelles and even molecules. The mechanisms constituting the main strategies of biological adaptation involve either an alteration of the types of macromolecules in a given system, a change of their concentrations, or a change in the regulation of their function (47). Enzyme concentration can be regulated at various steps in synthesis or degradation.

The biological basis of long-term adaptation is derived from the fact that the genes of a cell are not equally active at a given time. Genetic information is recalled in accordance with the given physiological requirements. Transcription of a given section of a DNA molecule is induced or blocked by a specific chemical signal depending on whether an inductor or repressor is involved. In principle, control at the gene level can lead to quantitative decrease or increase in enzyme concentration, as well as a change in enzyme type or in the relative proportion of enzyme variants (isoenzymes) which all catalyze the same reaction, although their individual catalytic properties are different. Less is known about regulation of protein synthesis at the level of translation (47, 163).

Some common misunderstandings of the nature of "adaptation"

Constancy of biochemical and ultrastructural composition

There appears to be general agreement on Cannon's concept of homeostasis. As always, however, the problems are in the fine print, particularly when we direct our attention to an overloaded organ itself and the changes at the cellular level.

Functional adaptation requires a material basis. Therefore, homeostasis can neither mean absolutely fixed composition of fluid compartments, nor absolute constancy of biochemical and morphological structure. Thus one is confronted with the question of which material and physical properties of the cell may change without forcing one to assume a disturbance of homeostasis and, indeed, which properties have to change in order to permit adaptation.

If, for example, one acknowledges training-induced increase in muscle mass, and the necessarily accompanying alterations in the physical proportions of the organism as constituting necessary and favourable adaptation – then one also need not see a detrimental development in every deviation in cell composition, such as moderate changes in the amount, composition and distribution of proteins and the proportion of the individual cell organelles observed in various stages of chronic pressure loading.

In the final analysis, we should keep in mind that maintenance of function, that is, coping with imposed demands, is decisive. Prosser (107) distinguishes "homeostatic adaptation" from "homeokinetic adaptation", the latter permitting the constancy of energy production and thereby relative constancy of biological activity even when the internal state varies within certain limits. In the case of the pressure-loaded heart, one must distinguish between homeostasis of the entire organism and preservation of the material composition of the overloaded organ itself. The object of adaptation of the heart should essentially be preservation of the internal environment of the organism as a whole.

Decrease in biological parameters in the framework of adaptive processes

A further trivial misunderstanding one often encounters is the notion that any decrease in biological parameters, for example: a decrease in the number of receptors or transport molecules, or a decrease in the rate of biological processes, such as enzyme activities or shortening velocity, must generally be considered to be detrimental, that is to say, an indication of "damage". Yet skeletal muscle physiology provides a number of examples of a reduction in biochemical and mechanical parameters which can be interpreted as an adaptation to changed loading conditions or stimulation pattern (152). Physical training leads to a change in tone of the vegetative nervous system which may be accompanied by a decrease in the activity of various enzymes such as those of cardiac catecholamine metabolism (118), and this certainly cannot be viewed as "damage" or enzymatic "defect".

Thus the decrease in myofibrillar ATPase activity of the chronically pressure-loaded ventricular myocardium is certainly also worthy of discussion in light of adaptation. This interpretation is supported by detection of more economic development of tension in isolated myocardial preparations (5, 6, 51), as well as the whole ventricle (63, 64).

With regard to the myofibrillar alterations under chronic pressure load, there are three conflicting views. According to a widely acknowledged notion, which we also previously supported, the decrease in myofibrillar ATPase activity and shortening velocity reflects a "biochemical defect" which plays a major role in manifestation of cardiac insufficiency (37, 90, 102, 157). Another view holds the decrease in ATPase activity to be adaptive; cardiac failure would occur when the limits of adaptation, i.e., of isoenzyme redistribution, are reached (80). We now favour a third interpretation assuming an adaptive process which, however, in itself may also have unfavourable effects under certain conditions. Assumption of adaptive transformation towards a slower but more economically working muscle does not exclude that considerable redistribution of the isoenzymes could contribute to manifestation of cardiac insufficiency – although we do not attribute substantial significance to such a conceivable interrelationship (55, 57–59). The adaptive character of the mechanical and energetical alterations under chronic pressure load, including the decrease in unloaded shortening velocity, contradicts a concept of evaluation of cardiac performance, based solely on velocity parameters.

As mentioned above with regard to the pressure-loaded human heart; the potential magnitude, biochemical basis and significance of a decrease in ATPase activity is a subject of dispute. It is conceivable that a decrease in ATPase activity and shortening velocity in human myocardium must be interpreted and evaluated quite differently than in small-animal models. Clarification of the above question as well as the identification of potential changes in the myofibrillar apparatus as a function of age and endocrine status in man is a very urgent problem.

Ambiguity of adaptive alterations

Another misunderstanding which was briefly referred to above is the notion that characterization of a process as adaptive principally excludes unfavourable effects. Krayenbühl (71) used the very instructive symbol of the head of Janus for illustrating the ambiguous effects of the hypertrophy process as a whole. Obviously, this point can be applied equally well to many structural and functional details of the hypertrophied organ or other adaptive alterations. In principle of course, adaptive alterations should tend to be favourable for coping with extraordinary demands; but in the final analysis, they indeed have ambiguous consequences in most cases. This ambiguity is frequently apparent from the onset and applies in a number of respects:

Adaptation necessarily involves narrowing of the remaining adaptive reserve and furthermore, specialization with consequently limited suitability for other demands. A weight lifter or a shot putter is not likely to be a first class sprinter or high jumper. The heart in hypertension is likewise not programmed to generate increased cardiac output at high heart rates. Moreover, an organism is only equipped with a limited number of relatively stereotypic reaction mechanisms. A response which appears to be favourable under certain conditions may be considered detrimental or even pathologic under other conditions, or localization. In light of different functional considerations a given adaptive alteration may be evaluated differently. Increased erythrocyte count in high altitude adaptation increases the oxygen capacity of the blood and permits survival, for example, of the inhabitants of the Andes. Increase in hematocrit, however, simultaneously increases viscosity and therefore vascular resistance. Another example is the possible occurrence of cardiac arrhythmias in intensely trained athletes. In the pressure-loaded left ventricle, the increase in myocardial mass leads to a decrease in coronary reserve and may endanger subendocardial areas of the ventricular wall (50). Marked increase in cell size and overproportional increase of intracellular contractile material content in rat myocardium (20, 109, 155, 160) – while useful in light of force development – may also endanger the myocardial cell from the viewpoint of energetics. Moreover, an adaptive process can be subject to qualitative or quantitative disturbances.

Thus the final consequences of adaptive alteration need not be beneficial to the organism (22, 39, 57, 134, 151). The potential negative effects of connective tissue reactions are particularly noticeable – as already indicated by Cannon with regard to wound healing (22). In the context of the present discussion it should suffice merely to mention the difficulty of distinguishing connective tissue changes induced in the framework of myocardial hypertrophy from those induced by additional factors (hypoxia, edema, vasculopathy, damage due to extreme overload) (12, 19, 52, 57, 76, 90, 93, 94, 95, 110, 138, 146). Thus, one may be confronted with substantial difficulties in distinguishing between cause and effect. Connective tissue reactions which cause a considerable increase in myocardial stiffness and, in turn, may impair diffusion of oxygen, substrates and transmitters should certainly be interpreted as being detrimental. But in no case can a primarily adaptive character be rejected a priori on the basis of negative consequences. The example of connective tissue reactions also shows that even reversibility is not a final criterion of adaptation.

A working hypothesis of cellular reactions to external stimuli or noxa is presented in figure 2 based on the above considerations. In myocardium, clearly regressive alterations may occur in the early phase of acute, extreme overload or in later stages as a result of exhaustion of macromolecular syntheses – often combined with coronary insufficiency. However, one can conceive of two intermediate zones between the favourable effects of physiologic adaptation, on the one hand and degeneration or necrosis, on the other hand. The term "pathologic" is generally applied to degenerative alterations and also to disturbed adaptation – that is to say, primary or secondary failing adaptation or qualitatively incorrect adaptation. In every day speach, however, occasionally even the inherent negative side effects of regular adaptation are called pathologic. The term

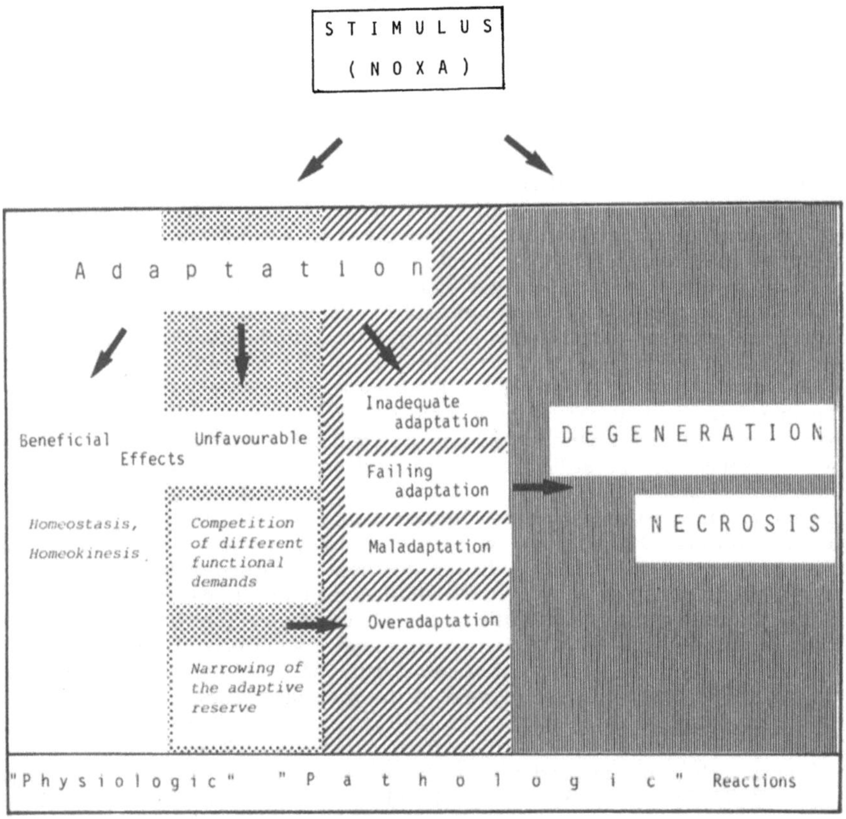

Fig. 2. Cellular reactions to external stimuli or noxa. The notions "adaptive" and "pathologic" are not necessarily mutually exclusive.

"overadaptation" would seem to be most appropriate for a degree of alteration in which the negative consequences of the generally ambiguous adaptive phenomena clearly predominate. Thus, in the final analysis, the question of whether a process is "pathologic" or "adaptive" in character is conceptually false. Characterization of a process as "adaptive" does not rule out "pathologic" consequences.

Although Virchow's cellular pathology has been expanded to a pathology of morphological ultrastructure and molecular structures, and of defective regulation of the body's information and immune systems, it still seems hardly possible to comprehensively define the term "disease", or to exhaustively characterize "pathological processes". Terms like "pathologic" or "adaptive" involve an interpretation. We are generally not aware that such classifications involve a teleological view. Even though we are reluctant to admit it and generally regard a teleologic view as being unscientific, our terms are anthropomorphic in the final analysis (136). One cannot express it more succinctly than E. von Brücke did about a century ago:

> "The relationship between a researcher in the natural sciences and teleology is like that between a lover and his mistress; he can't do without her, but he is not eager to be seen with her in public" (112, 115).

Interpretation of hypertrophy-induced and hypertrophy-accompanying alterations as being adaptive is thus based consciously or unconsciously on the functional appropriateness of the alterations. Comparative physiological and morphological studies (ontogenesis; regeneration; phylogenesis; and hypertrophic alterations of other organs, particularly skeletal muscle – including comparison of different species –) can facilitate an adaptive interpretation. In light of the fact that terms such as "adaptation" or "enzyme defect" actually involve an interpretation, preference should generally be given to neutral expressions such as "reactions", "response", etc. Besides clarification of biochemical mechanisms, however, investigation of the functional consequences for whole heart dynamics remains a preeminent aim of research. Myocardial alterations in the framework of other chronic reactions have to be taken into account, – i.e., changes consistent with or deviating from those occurring under hemodynamic overload – above all the role of neuroendocrine status and transmitters.

Adaptive alterations of the myosin isoenzyme pattern of the pressure-loaded heart in light of other long-term reactions: maturation and aging, physical exercise, stress, and altered neuroendocrine status

For a number of reasons, consideration of other long-term myocardial reactions is essential to the understanding of the structural and functional alterations of the myofibrillar apparatus occurring under hemodynamic overloading.

The postnatal redistribution of the isoenzyme pattern in the rat correlates closely with thyroid hormone levels (58, 121). Conclusions about the myosin isoenzyme pattern are only reasonable when findings are related to a defined, age-specific isoenzyme pattern. One must also assume that the potential reactions of myocardium are generally age-dependent. For example, physical exercise has been observed to lead to paradox changes in creatine kinase activity of senile mice (139).

Age-related alterations in isoenzyme pattern are also important in the interpretation of pressure-induced redistribution of myosin isoenzymes: should the shift towards VM-3 due to chronic pressure load be equated with a premature process of aging? The fact that the decrease in myofibrillar ATPase activity essentially occurs during the maturation period and not in the period of advanced aging (73) contradicts such a notion, at least with regard to the rat.

In hemodynamic overload and physical exercise, the myofibrillar apparatus is certainly also influenced by concomitant reactions of the neuroendocrine status, transmitter release and receptor density. It is not yet clear whether redistribution in favour of VM-3 under pressure loading is related to a decrease in catecholamine content (19) and "down regulation" of β-receptors; the latter may result from continuous activation of the sympatho-adrenergic system (121). Myocardial β-adrenergic receptors are regulated by glucocorticoids, thyroid hormones, and catecholamines (for ref. see 1, 125, 150). Whether simultaneously occurring alterations in the cholinergic system (81) may influence the isoenzyme pattern of myosin has not yet been examined.

The intermittent character of the sympathetic activation and the resulting readjustment of the vegetative nervous system (121) may be involved in the opposite alterations towards a more rapidly working myocardium as a result of chronic swimming training (17, 18, 60, 117, 119–121). An intermittently increased release of thyroid hormones (111) could also play a role.

Endurance training of swimming rats generally induces a significant redistribution in favour of VM-1 (117, 119–121). The lack of such an effect of treadmill running (8) has not yet been sufficiently clarified, although the intensity and frequency of the training program seems to be decisive (Rupp, H., unpublished results). Discrepancies between Ca^{2+}-ATPase activity and responsiveness to catecholamines, on the one hand, and Ca^{2+}, Mg^{2+}-dependent ATPase activities of natural actomyosin, on the other hand, were observed in running-trained rats (113).

In skeletal muscle, adaptation of actomyosin ATPase activity to endurance training differs, depending on the type of muscle fiber. Treadmill running does not cause a change in the ATPase activity of fast twitch white or heart muscle, whereas it does cause a decrease in fast twitch red and an increase in slow twitch red muscles (9). The glycogenolytic capacity and actomyosin ATPase activity appear to be regulated in parallel.

The significance of the pituitary in the framework of the process of hypertrophy has been known for some time (16). Beznak (16) emphasized the necessity of growth hormone, Nicholson et al. (100) the significance of the adrenal cortex, Östman-Smith (100a) of noradrenaline release from cardiac sympathetic nerves, whereas Kölbel (68) reveals indications for the existence of a digoxinlike substance originating in the adrenals. One must postulate, however, that the mechanisms governing cell growth, on the one hand, and myosin isoenzyme pattern and ATPase activity, on the other hand, are different (59, 122). This notion is particularly supported by the fact that substantial increase in myocardial mass can be accompanied by transformation either in the direction of a more slowly working muscle (pressure loading) or a more quickly working muscle (high doses of thyroxine).

The involvement of the pituitary and adrenal glands in physical exercise and hemodynamic overload (28, 68, 100) also reveals interrelationships with the concept of stress.

The problems of defining the term "stress", and thereby the conflicting views of stress, can only be mentioned briefly in the framework of the present discourse. Selye also did not place equal emphasis on certain aspects of the stress concept in the course of his work, for example: the conceptual separation of "stressor" and "stress", the specificity of the reaction, and the relative significance of the adrenal medullary system (132–134). Selye's classical division of the so-called adaptation syndrome into 3 stages: the "initial alarm syndrome", the " stage of resistance", and the "stage of exhaustion" need not necessarily be recognizable, depending on the inducing conditions – a situation similar to Meerson's 3 stages of hemodynamic overload (90). Selye concentrated his attention on the pituitary-adrenocortical system. In recent years, however, the overriding significance of psychoemotional factors already mentioned by Cannon (22) in initiating the stress reaction and the role of the sympathoadrenergic medullary system (and thereby catecholamines) in coping with increased demands have received increasing recognition (35, 43, 69, 72, 87, 140). Sympathetic nervous system activity is frequently used as the simplest parameter of stress. The adrenocortical system is activated as a secondary reaction (whereby other hormones such as glucagon, growth hormone, and prolactin as well as endogenous opiates are also involved) (for ref., see 140). Both systems are integrated by the hypothalamus. Biosynthesis of catecholamines is controlled both by the pituitary gland and the adrenal cortex (7).

The nonspecific element emphasized by Selye appears to be an expression of the same general psychological reaction in many stress experiments (87).

However, different effects on endocrine status are reported depending on the pattern of the psychological reaction; release of catecholamines seems to correlate more with activity and aggressive and flight reactions – whereas ACTH and cortisol correlate more with anxiety, loss of control, hopelessness, submissiveness, and depression. In any case, psychological aspects of the stressful situation are important in determining the effects on physiological function (for ref. see 25, 43, 72, 82).

It is not the aim of the present discourse to add another definition of stress to the long list which has already been created (70, 87, 132–134, 151). As is the case with other hardly definable terms (e.g., "contractility"), it would rather appear helpful to avoid usage of unclear labels and to describe precisely what is meant in each individual situation. In any case, it does not appear to be useful to collect every slight psychophysical reaction to every given, ever so slight, stimulus under the term "stress". If one is neither willing nor able to avoid this term, then it should at least be reserved for a state of the organism induced by stimuli which endanger the organism's integrity. Thus one should not attribute a stressful character to physical exercise in general, but rather only to exercise involving extraordinary loading.

The relation of the stress topic to myofibrillar alterations is derived from the assumption that the plasma concentrations of catecholamines, as well as the time pattern and intensity of transmitter release, have an effect on turnover of the myosin isoenzymes. In contrast to swimming training, experimentally induced emotional excitation ("emotional stress") did not lead to a redistribution in favour of VM-1; indeed, the opposite, an increase in VM-3, was the case in spontaneously hypertensive rats, possibly as a result of long-term activation of the sympathetic nervous system (119). One also cannot exclude that psychologic factors may play a role in the above-mentioned differences in the response of the organism to voluntary and forced treadmill running.

Thus a number of problems remains to be solved with regard to the type, regulation, and functional interpretation of alterations at the myofibrillar level. In particular, the interrelationships of these alterations with the overriding regulatory systems during physical training and hemodynamic overload need further clarification in order to distinguish between the significance of changes in mechanical load alone, as opposed to the influence of neuroendocrine factors.

Acknowledgement

The author is obliged to Dr. R. H. Zak, Chicago, for providing an outline of the discussion on myosin isoenzymes at the Erwin Riesch Symposium in Tübingen, 1982.

References

1. Abrass, B., J. Scarpace: Glucocorticoid regulation of myocardial β-adrenergic receptors. Endocrinology **108,** 977–980 (1981).
2. Alpert, N. R. (ed.): Cardiac hypertrophy. Academic Press (New York and London 1971).
3. Alpert, N. R., M. S. Gordon: Myofibrillar adenosine triphosphatase activity in congestive heart failure. Amer. J. Physiol. **202,** 940–946 (1962).
4. Alpert, N. R., B. Hamrell, W. Halpern: Mechanical and biochemical correlates of cardiac hypertrophy. Circulat. Res. **34/35** (Suppl. II), 71–82 (1974).
5. Alpert, N. R., L. A. Mulieri: The utilization of energy by the myocardium hypertrophied secondary to pressure overload. 153–163. In: Strauer, B. E. (ed.). The heart in hypertension. Internat. Boehringer Mannheim Symposia, Springer (Berlin–Heidelberg–New York 1981).
6. Alpert, N. R., L. A. Mulieri: Increased myothermal economy of isometric force generation in compensated cardiac hypertrophy induced by pulmonary artery constriction in the rabbit. Circulat. Res. **50,** 491–500 (1982).
7. Axelrod, J.: Catecholamines and stress: A brief informal history. In: Catecholamines and stress: Recent Advances, Usdin, E., R. Kvetnanský, I. J. Kopin (eds.), 3–5. Elsevier North Holland, Inc. (Amsterdam 1980).
8. Baldwin, K. M., S. B. Ernst, R. E. Herrick, A. M. MacIntosh: Effects of physical training and thyroxine on rodent cardiac functional and biochemical properties. Pflügers Arch. **391,** 190–194 (1981).
9. Baldwin, K. M., W. W. Winder, J. O. Hollozky: Adaptation of actomyosin ATPase in different types of muscle to endurance exercise. Amer. J. Physiol. **229,** 422–426 (1975).
10. Banerjee, S. K., J. Wiener: Effects of aging on atrial and ventricular human myosin. Basic Res. Cardiol. (1983, in press).
11. Bárány, M.: ATPase activity of myosin correlated with speed of muscle shortening. J. Gen. Physiol. (No. 6, part 2) **50,** 197–216 (1967).
12. Bartosova, D., M. Chvapil, B. Korecky, O. Poupa, K. Rakusan, Z. Turek, M. Vizel: The growth of the muscular and collagenous parts of rat heart in various forms of cardiomegaly. J. Physiol. **200,** 285–295 (1969).
13. Bauereisen, E.: Kontraktilität. Begriffsbestimmung und Bewertung. 401–409. In: Das chronisch kranke Herz (Ed. H. Roskamm, H. Reindell), F. K. Schattauer (Stuttgart–New York 1972).

14. Beneke, G., R. Rohrbach, C. P. Adler. W. Sandritter: Störungen des Wachstums. 8582. In: Sandritter, W., Beneke, G. (eds.), Allgem. Pathologie. F. K. Schattauer (Stuttgart–New York 1974).
15. Bernard, Cl.: Leçons sur les phénomènes de la vie communs aux animaux et aux végétaux. 165. Paris, 1878/79 (zit. Rotschuh, K. E., Geschichte der Physiologie, Springer (Berlin–Göttingen–Heidelberg 1953).
16. Beznak, M.: Hormonal influences in regulation of cardiac performance. Circulat. Res. **14/15,** Suppl. II, 141–162 (1964).
17. Bhan, A. K., J. Scheuer: Effects of physical training on cardiac actomyosin adenosine triphosphatase activity. Amer. J. Physiol. **223,** 1486–1490 (1972).
18. Bhan, A. K., J. Scheuer: Effects of physical training on cardiac myosin ATPase activity. Amer. J. Physiol. **228,** 1178–1182 (1975).
19. Borchard, F.: Differences between transmitter depletion in human heart hypertrophy and experimental cardiac hypertrophy in Goldblatt rats. Basic Res. Cardiol. **75,** 118–125 (1980).
20. Büchner, F., S. Onishi: Cardiac hypertrophy and cardiac failure in electron microscopy. Urban & Schwarzenberg (München–Berlin–Wien 1970).
21. Caldarera, C. M., C. Guarnieri, C. C. O. R. Ferrari, A. Casti: Early biochemical events of myocardial hypertrophy. Internat. Soc. Heart Res., Europ. Section, Dijon 139–147 (1979).
22. Cannon, W. B.: Der Weg eines Forschers. Hermann Rinn Verlag (München 1945).
23. Chizzonite, R. A., A. W. Everett, W. A. Clark, S. Jakovcic, M. Rabinowitz, R. Zak: Isolation and characterization of two molecular variants of myosin heavy-chain from rabbit ventricle. Change in their content during normal growth and after treatment with thyroid hormone. J. Biol. Chem. **257,** 2056–2065 (1982).
24. Clark, W. A., R. A. Chizzonite, A. W. Everett, M. Rabinowitz, R. Zak: Species correlations between cardiac isomyosins. J. Biol. Chem. **257,** 5449–5454 (1982).
25. Conner, R. L., J. Vernikos-Danellis, S. Levine: Stress, fighting and neuroendocrine function. Nature **234,** 564–566 (1971).
26. Cummins, P.: Transition in human atrial and ventricular myosin light chain isoenzymes in response to cardiac-pressure-overload-induced hypertrophy. Biochem. J. **205,** 195–204 (1982).
27. d'Albis, A., C. Pantaloni, J.-J. Bechat: An electrophoretic study of native myosin isoenzymes and of their subunits content. Europ. J. Biochem. **99,** 261 (1979).
28. Dawson, C. A., S. M. Horvath: Swimming in small laboratory animals. Medicine and Science in Sports **2,** 51–78 (1970).
29. Delcayre, C., B. Swynghedauw: A comparative study of heart myosin. ATPase and light subunits from different species. Pflügers Arch. **355,** 39–47 (1975).
30. Dillmann, W. H.: Diabetes mellitus induces changes in cardiac myosin of the rat. Diabetes **29,** 579–582 (1980).
31. Ebrecht, G., H. Rupp, R. Jacob: Alterations of mechanical parameters in chemically skinned preparations of rat myocardium as a function of isoenzyme pattern of myosin. Basic Res. Cardiol. **77,** 220–234 (1982).
32. England, P. J., D. Mills, S. A. Jeacocke, H. T. Pask: The phosphorylation of cardiac contractile proteins. This issue, p. 139–143.
33. Everett, A. W., A. M. Sinha, M. Rabinowitz, R. Zak: Relationship between the synthesis rates and mRNA levels of the α and β cardiac myosin heavy chains in normal and thyrotoxic rabbits. This issue, p. 39–45.
34. Fanburg, B. L.: Experimental cardiac hypertrophy. New Engl. J. Med. **282,** 723–732 (1970).
35. Frankenhaeuser, M.: The role of peripheral catecholamines in adaptation to understimulation and overstimulation. 172–191. In: Psychopathology of Human Adaptation. Serban, G. (Ed.), Plenum Press (New York–London 1976).

36. Goodkind, M. J., G. E. Dambach, P. T. Thyrum, R. J. Luchi: Effect of thyroxine on ventricular myocardial contractility and ATPase activity in guinea pigs. Amer. J. Physiol. **226,** 66–72 (1974).
37. Gordon, M. S., A. L. Brown: Myofibrillar adenosine triphosphatase activity of human heart tissue in congestive failure: Effects of ouabain and calcium. Circulat. Res. **18,** 534–542 (1966).
38. Gorza, L., P. Pauletto, A. L. Pessina, S. Sartore, S. Schiaffino: Isomyosin distribution in normal and pressure overload rat ventricular myocardium. An immunohistochemical study. Circulat. Res. **49,** 1003–1009 (1981).
39. Gross, R.: Gesundheit und Krankheit in ihren verschiedenen Aspekten. Dtsch. Ärztebl. Ärztl. Mitt. **77,** 1397–1406 (1980).
40. Gülch, R. W.: The effect of elevated chronic loading on the action potential of mammalian myocardium. J. Molec. Cell. Cardiol. **12,** 415–420 (1980).
41. Hatt, P. Y., P. Jouannot, J. Moravec, B. Swynghedauw: Current trends in heart hypertrophy. Basic Res. Cardiol. **69,** 479–483 (1974).
42. Heilmann, C., T. Lindl, W. Müller, D. Pette: Characterization of cardiac microsomes from spontaneously hypertonic rats. Basic Res. Cardiol. **75,** 92–96 (1980).
43. Henry, J. P.: Present concept of stress theory. In: Kvetnanský/Kopin. Catecholamines and stress. Recent Advances 557–571 (1980).
44. Henry, D., G. G. Ahumada, W. F. Friedman, B. E. Sobel: Simultaneously measured isometric tension and ATP hydrolysis in glycerinated fibres from normal and hypertrophied rabbit hearts. Circulat. Res. **31,** 740–749 (1972).
45. Hildebrandt, G.: The time structure of adaptive processes. 24–39. In: Biological adaptation. Hildebrandt, G., H. Hensel (Eds.) Georg Thieme (Stuttgart–New York 1982).
46. Hoar, P. F., K. T. Shiverik, B. B. Hamrell, N. R. Alpert: The ATPase activity and Ca^{2+} affinity of myosin B from hypertrophied nonfailing cat hearts. 333–344. In: Alpert, N. R. (Ed.). Cardiac Hypertrophy. Academic Press (New York and London 1971).
47. Hochachka, P. W., G. N. Somero: Strategien biochemischer Anpassung. Georg Thieme (Stuttgart–New York 1980).
48. Hoh, J. F. Y., P. A. McGrath, P. T. Hale: Electrophoretic analysis of multiple forms of rat cardiac myosin: Effects of hypophysectomy and thyroxine replacement. J. Molec. Cell. Cardiol. **10,** 1053–1076 (1978).
49. Hoh, J. F. Y., G. P. S. Yeoh, M. A. W. Thomas, L. Higginbottom: Structural differences in the heavy chains of rat ventricular myosin isoenzymes. FEBS Lett. **97,** 330–334 (1979).
50. Holtz, J., W. v. Restorff, P. Bard, E. Bassenge: Transmural distribution of myocardial blood flow and of coronary reserve in canine left ventricular hypertrophy. Basic Res. Cardiol. **72,** 286–292 (1977).
51. Holubarsch, Ch., R. Goulette, R. Z. Litten, L. A. Mulieri, N. R. Alpert: Myokardiale Energetik und Myosin-Isoenzym-Muster der Ratte. Z. Kardiol. (Abstr.) **72,** Suppl. 1, 56/198 (1983).
52. Holubarsch, Ch., Th. Holubarsch, R. Jacob, I. Medugorac, K.-U. Thiedemann: Passive elastic properties of myocardium in different models and stages of hypertrophy: A study comparing mechanical, chemical, and morphometric parameters. Cardiovasc. Res. **7,** 323–336 (1983).
53. Hugenholtz, P. G , R. C. Ellison, C. W. Urschel, I. Mirsky, E. Sonnenblick: Myocardial force-velocity relationship in clinical heart disease. Circulation **41,** 191–202 (1970).
54. Jacob, R., G. Ebrecht, A. Kämmereit, I. Medugorac, M. F. Wendt-Gallitelli: Myocardial function in different models of cardiac hypertrophy. An attempt at correlating mechanical, biochemical and morphological parameters. Basic Res. Cardiol. **72,** 160–167 (1977).

55. Jacob, R., G. Ebrecht, Ch. Holubarsch, H. Rupp, G. Kissling: Mechanics and energetics in cardiac hypertrophy as related to the isoenzyme pattern of myosin. In: Alpert, N. R. (Ed.). Biology of myocardial hypertrophy and failure. Raven Press (1983, in press).
56. Jacob, R., A. Kämmereit, I. Medugorac, M. F. Wendt-Gallitelli: Maximalgeschwindigkeit der lastfreien Verkürzung (V_{max}), myokardiale Leistungsfähigkeit und „Kontraktilitätsindizes“ beim hypertrophierten Myokard. Z. Kardiol. **65,** 392–400 (1976).
57. Jacob, R., G. Kissling, G. Ebrecht, Ch. Holubarsch, I. Medugorac, H. Rupp: Adaptive and pathological alterations in experimental cardiac hypertrophy. Advanc. Myocardiol. **4,** 55–77 (1983).
58. Jacob, R., H. Rupp, G. Ebrecht, R. W. Gülch, G. Kissling: Chronic reactions of myocardium at the myofibrillar level. The functional significance of the isoenzyme pattern of myosin. Proc. Japan. Soc. Cardiac Metabolism **4,** 1–28 (1981).
59. Jacob, R., H. Rupp, G. Ebrecht, Ch. Holubarsch, G. Kissling: Das Isoenzymmuster von Myosin und seine Bedeutung für Mechanik und Energetik des Myokards. Z. Kardiol. **71,** 553–565 (1982).
60. Kämmereit, A., I. Medugorac, E. Steil, R. Jacob: Mechanics of the isolated ventricular myocardium of rats conditioned by physical training. Basic Res. Cardiol. **70,** 495–507 (1975).
61. Katagiri, T., E. Morkin: Studies on the substructure of myosin in cardiac hypertrophy. Characterization of light chains. Biochim. Biophys. Acta **342,** 262–274 (1974).
62. Katz, A. M.: Biochemical "defect" in the hypertrophied and failing heart. Circulation **47,** 1076–1097 (1973).
63. Kissling, G., L. Malloy, H. Rupp: Energetics of the heart in chronic pressure overload. This issue, p. 166–172.
64. Kissling, G., H. Rupp, L. Malloy, R. Jacob: Alterations in cardiac oxygen consumption under chronic pressure overload. Significance of the isoenzyme pattern of myosin. Basic Res. Cardiol. **77,** 255–269 (1982).
65. Klotz, C., M. C. Aumont, J. J. Leger, B. Swynghedauw: Human cardiac myosin ATPase and light subunits: a comparative study. Biochim. Biophys. Acta **386,** 461–469 (1975).
66. Klotz, C., J. J. Leger, M. Elzinga: Comparative sequence of myosin light chains from normal and hypertrophied human hearts. Circulat. Res. **50,** 201–209 (1982).
67. Klotz, C., B. Swynghedauw, H. Mendes, F. Marotte, J. J. Leger: Evidence for new forms of cardiac myosin heavy chains in mechanical heart overloading and in ageing. Europ. J. Biochem. **115,** 415–421 (1981).
68. Kölbel, F., V. Schreiber, T. Pribyl: Reflexions on what makes heart grow. In: Advances in Myocardiology **4,** eds. N. Dhalla, E. Chazow, Plenum Publ. (New York 1983).
69. Kopin, I. J., R. McCarty, T. Torda, I. Yamaguchi: Catecholamines in plasma and responses to stress. In: Catecholamines and Stress: Recent Advances, Usdin, E., R. Kvetnanský, I. J. Kopin (eds.), 197–204. Elsevier North Holland, Inc. (Amsterdam 1980).
70. Koslowski, S.: Panel discussion on stress theory. In: Catecholamines and Stress: Recent Advances, Usdin, E., R. Kvetnanský, I. J. Kopin (eds.), 583–586. Elsevier North Holland, Inc. (Amsterdam 1980).
71. Krayenbühl, H. P.: Effects of hypertrophy on contractile function in man, 92–97. In: Jacob, R. The hypertrophied heart. Dr. Steinkopff (Darmstadt 1977).
72. Kvetnanský, R.: Recent progress in catecholamines under stress. In: Catecholamines and Stress: Recent Advances, Usdin, E., R. Kvetnanský, I. J. Kopin (eds.), 7–18. Elsevier North Holland, Inc. (Amsterdam 1980).
73. Lakatta, E. G., C. P. Yın: Myocardial agıng. Functional alterations and related cellular mechanisms. Amer. J. Physiol. (Heart Circ. Physiol.) **11,** H927–H941 (1982).

74. Leclercq, J. F., B. Swynghedauw: Myofibrillar ATPase, DNA and hydroxyproline content of human hypertrophied heart. Europ. J. Clin. Invest. **6,** 27–33 (1976).

75. Lenz, F.: Über die Begriffe Krankheit, Gesundheit und Norm. In: Bauer, Fischer, Lenz: Menschliche Erblichkeitslehre, 3. Aufl. Bd. I (München 1927).

76. Lindner, J., P. Schmiegelow: Cardiovascular aging. This issue, p. 314–329.

77. Litten, R. Z., B. J. Martin, R. B. Low, N. R. Alpert: Altered myosin isoenzyme patterns from pressure-overloaded and thyroxic hypertrophied rabbit hearts. Circ. Res. **50,** 856–864 (1982).

78. Loiselle, D. S., J. R. Wendt, J. F. Y. Hoh: Energetic consequences of thyroid-modulated shifts in ventricular isomyosin distribution in the rat. J. Muscle Res. Cell. Motility **3,** 5–23 (1982).

79. Lompré, A. M., J. J. Mercadier, C. Wisnewsky, P. Bouveret, C. Panalonio, A. d'Albis, K. Schwartz: Species and age-dependent distribution of mammalian cardiac myosin isoenzymes. J. Muscle Res. Cell. Motility **1,** 479 (1980).

80. Lompré, A. M., K. Schwartz, A. d'Albis, G. Lacombe, N. van Thiem, B. Swynghedauw: Myosin isoenzyme redistribution in chronic heart overload. Nature **282,** 105–107 (1979).

81. Lund, D. D., P. G. Schmid, U. J. Johannsen, R. Roskoski, Jr.: Biochemical indices of cholinergic and adrenergic autonomic innervation in dog heart: Disparate alterations in chronic right heart failure. J. Molec. Cell. Cardiol. **14,** 419–425 (1982).

82. Lundberg, U.: Catecholamine and cortisol excretion under psychologically different laboratory conditions, 455–460. In: Kvetnanský/Kopin (Eds.). Catecholamines and Stress: Recent Advances (1980).

83. Mahdavi, V., M. Periosamy, B. Nadal-Ginard: Molecular characterization of two myosin heavy chain genes expressed in the adult heart. Nature **297,** 659–664 (1982).

84. Malhotra, A., A. Bhan, J. Scheuer: Biochemical characteristics of human cardiac myosin. J. Molec. Cell. Cardiol. **9,** 73–80 (1977).

85. Mansier, P., K. Schwartz, L. Lelievre, J. M. Moalic, D. Charlemagne, J. L. Samuel, L. Rappaport, B. Swynghedauw: New trends in biology of cardiac overload: Plasma membranes enzymes, cytoskeleton proteins and introduction of RNA. This issue, p. 94–98.

86. Maron, B. J., V. J. Ferrans, R. S. Adelstein: Isolation and characterization of myosin from subjects with asymmetric septal hypertrophy. Circulat. Res. **40,** 468–473 (1977).

87. Mason, J. W.: A historical view of the stress field. J. Hum. Stress **1,** 6–12 (1975).

88. Maughan, D., E. Low, R. Litten, J. Brayden, N. R. Alpert: Calcium-activated muscle from hypertrophied rabbit hearts. Circulat. Res. **44,** 279–287 (1979).

89. McGrath, J. C.: Vascular adrenergic receptors, 97–106. In: Vanhoutte, P. M., and I. Leusen (Eds.). Vasodilatation. Raven Press (New York 1981).

90. Meerson, F. S.: Hyperfunktion, Hypertrophie und Insuffizienz des Herzens. VEB Verlag Volk und Gesundheit (Berlin 1969).

91. Meerson, F. S.: Insufficiency of hypertrophied heart. Basic Res. Cardiol. **71,** 343–354 (1976).

92. Meerson, F. S., A. M. Breger: The common mechanism of the heart's adaptation and deadaptation: Hypertrophy and atrophy of the heart muscle. Basic Res. Cardiol. **72,** 228–234 (1977).

93. Meessen, H.: Structural basis of myocardial hypertrophy. Brit. Heart J. **33,** Suppl. 94 (1971).

94. Medugorac, I.: Collagen content in different areas of normal and hypertrophied rat myocardium. Cardiovasc. Res. **14,** 551–554 (1980).

95. Medugorac, I., R. Jacob: Characterisation of left ventricular collagen in the rat. Cardiovasc. Res. **17,** 15–21 (1983).
96. Mercadier, J. J., A. M. Lompré, P. Bouvernet, J. L. Samuel, L. Rappaport, B. Swynghedauw, K. Schwartz: Myosin isoenzymic distribution in hypertrophied rat and human heart. This issue, p. 104–112.
97. Mercadier, J. J., A. M. Lompré, C. Wisnewsky, J. L. Samuel, J. Bercovici, B. Swynghedauw, K. Schwartz: Myosin isoenzymic changes in several models of rat cardiac hypertrophy. Circulat. Res. **49,** 525–532 (1981).
98. Mornet, D., R. Bertrand, P. Pantel, E. Audemard, R. Kassab: Structure of the actin-myosin interface. Nature **292,** 301–306 (1981).
99. Nebel, M. L., R. J. Bing: Contractile proteins of normal and failing human hearts. Arch. Internat. Med. **111,** 190–195 (1963).
100. Nichols, J. R., R. L. Clancy, N. C. Gonzalez: Role of adrenals on development of pressure-induced myocardial hypertrophy. Amer. J. Physiol. **244** (Heart Circ. Physiol. 13), H234–H238 (1983).
100a. Östman-Smith, I.: Adaptive changes in the sympathetic nervous system and some effector organs of the rat following long term exercise or cold acclimation and the role of cardiac sympathetic nerves in the genesis of compensatory cardiac hypertrophy. Acta Physiol. Scand. Suppl. **477,** 1–118 (1979).
101. Parizkova, J., R. Kvetnanský: Catecholamine metabolism and compositional growth in exercised and hypokinetic male rats. In: Catecholamines and Stress: Recent Advances, Usdin, E., R. Kvetnanský, I. J. Kopin (eds.), 355–358. Elsevier North Holland, Inc. (Amsterdam 1980).
102. Peters, T. J., G. Wells, C. M. Oakley, I. A. B. Brooksby, B. S. Jenkins, M. M. Webb-People, D. J. Coltart: Enzymic analysis of endomyocardial biopsy specimens from patients with cardiomyopathies. Brit. Heart J. **39,** 1333–1339 (1977).
103. Poche, R.: Morphologische Grundlagen der Herzhypertrophie und Herzinsuffizienz. In: Roskamm, H., H. Reindell: Das chronisch kranke Herz, 77–100. F. K. Schattauer (Stuttgart–New York 1973).
104. Poche, R.: Strukturelle Veränderungen des druck- und volumenüberlasteten Herzens. In: Roskamm, H., H. Reindell: Herzkrankheiten. Springer (Berlin–Heidelberg–New York 1982).
105. Pope, B., J. F. Y. Hoh, A. Weeds: The ATPase activity of rat cardiac myosin isoenzymes. FEBS Lett. **118,** 205–208 (1980).
106. Price, K. M., W. A. Littler, P. Cummins: Human atrial and ventricular myosin light-chain subunits in the adult and during development. Biochem. J. **191,** 571–580 (1980).
107. Prosser, C. L.: Theory of adaptation. In: Hildebrandt, G., H. Hensel: Biological adaptation, 2–22. Georg Thieme (Stuttgart–New York 1982).
108. Rabinowitz, M., K. G. Nair, R. Zak: Cellular and subcellular basis of cardiac hypertrophy. Med. Clin. **54,** 211–219 (1970).
109. Rabinowitz, M., R. Zak: Mitochondria and cardiac hypertrophy. Circulat. Res. **36,** 367–376 (1975).
110. Rauterberg, J., B. Voss, G. Pott: Biochemical characteristics and cellular mechanisms of fibrotic processes. This issue, p. 304–313.
111. Refsum, H. E., S. B. Strömme: Serum thyroxine, triiodothyronine and thyroid stimulating hormone after prolonged heavy exercise. Scand. J. Clin. Lab. Invest. **39,** 455–459 (1979).
112. Remmer, H.: Entwicklung des Problems „Teleologische Aspekte der Biotransformation“. In: Gerok, W., K. Sickinger. Drugs and the liver, 29–37. F. K. Schattauer (Stuttgart–New York 1975).
113. Resink, T. J., W. Gevers, T. D. Noakes, L. H. Opie: Increased cardiac myosin ATPase activity as a biochemical adaptation to running training: Enhanced response to catecholamines and a role for myosin phosphorylation. J. Molec. Cell. Cardiol. **13,** 679–694 (1981).

114. Ross, J., K. L. Peterson: On the assessment of cardiac inotropic state. Circulation **47,** 435–438 (1973).
115. Rotschuh, K. E.: Geschichte der Physiologie. In: Trendelenburg, W., E. Schütz. Lehrbuch der Physiologie. Springer (Berlin–Göttingen–Heidelberg 1953).
116. Rotter, W., J. Peiffer: Krankheit, Ätiologie, Pathogenese, Resistenz, Disposition und Tod, 2–19. In: Rotter, W. Lehrbuch der Pathologie, Schattauer (Stuttgart 1978).
117. Rupp, H.: The adaptive changes in the isoenzyme pattern of myosin from hypertrophied rat myocardium as a result of pressure overload and physical training. Basic Res. Cardiol. **76,** 79–88 (1981).
118. Rupp, H., A. R. Bukhari, R. Jacob: Modulation of catecholamine synthetizing and degrading enzymes by swimming and emotional excitation. This issue, p. 267–273.
119. Rupp, H., H. R. Felbier, R. Jacob: Blood pressure and cardiac myosin heterogeneity in the rat as influenced by swimming and emotional excitation. This issue, p. 274–281.
120. Rupp, H., R. Jacob: Response of blood pressure and cardiac myosin polymorphism to swimming training in the spontaneously hypertensive rat. Canad. J. Physiol. Pharmacol. **60,** 1098–1103 (1982).
121. Rupp, H., G. Kissling, R. Jacob: The hormonal and hemodynamic determinants of polymorphic myosin. In: Perspectives in Cardiovascular Research, Vol. 7, Myocardial Hypertrophy and Failure, Alpert, N. R. (ed.), 373–383. Raven Press (New York 1983).
122. Rupp, H., N. Popova, R. Jacob: Dissociation between factors resulting in hypertrophy and changes in myosin isoenzyme population of the pressure-loaded rat heart. This issue, p. 46–52.
123. Rushmer, R. F.: Some axioms, popular notions, and misconceptions regarding cardiovascular control. Circulation **27,** 118–141 (1963).
124. Sartore, S., L. Gorza, S. Pierobon Bormioli, L. Dalla Libera, S. Schiaffino: Myosin types and fiber types in cardiac muscle. J. Cell. Biol. **88,** 226–233 (1981).
125. Scarpace, P., I. B. Abrass: Thyroid hormone regulation of rat heart, lymphocyte, and lung β-adrenergic receptors. Endocrinology **108,** 1007–1011 (1981).
126. Scheuer, J., A. K. Bhan: Cardiac contractile proteins. Adenosine triphosphatase activity and physiological function. Circulat. Res. **45,** 1–12 (1979).
127. Schiaffino, S., L. Gorza, S. Pierobon-Bormioli, S. Sartore: Myosin polymorphism, cellular heterogeneity and plasticity of cardiac muscle, 559–568. In: Plasticity of the muscle, Pette, D. (Ed.). Walter de Gruyter (Berlin–New York 1980).
128. Schiaffino, S., L. Gorza, S. Sartore, C. Valfré, P. Paulette: Adaptive changes in cardiac isomyosins as visualized by immunofluorescence. This issue, p. 101–103.
129. Schier, J. J., R. S. Adelstein: Structural and enzymatic comparison of human cardiac muscle myosins isolated from infants, adults and patients with hypertrophic cardiomyopathy. J. Clin. Invest. **69,** 816–825 (1982).
130. Schwartz, K., Y. Lecarpentier, J. L. Martin, A. M. Lompré, J. J. Mercadier, B. Swynghedauw: Myosin isoenzyme distribution correlates with speed of myocardial contraction. J. Molec. Cell. Cardiol. **13,** 1071–1075 (1981).
131. Schwartz, K., A. M. Lompré, P. Bouveret, C. Wisnewsky, R. G. Whalen: Comparisons of rat cardiac myosins at fetal stages, in young animals, and in hypothyroid adults. J. Biol. Chem. **257,** 14412–14418 (1982).
132. Selye, H.: Stress beherrscht unser Leben. Econ-Verlag (Düsseldorf 1957).
133. Selye, H.: Confusion and controversy in the stress field. J. Human Stress **1,** 37–44 (1975).
134. Selye, H.: The nature of stress and its relation to cardiovascular disease. In: Bourne, G. H. "Hearts and heart-like organs", 289–332. Vol. 2. Physiology. Academic Press (1980).

135. Sonnenblick, E. H.: Contractility of cardiac muscle. Circulat. Res. **27,** 479–481 (1970).
136. Spaemann, R., R. Löw: Die Frage wozu? Geschichte und Wiederentdeckung des teleologischen Denkens. R. Piper & Co. Verlag (München–Zürich 1981).
137. Sreter, F. A., K. Mabuchi, E. Somogyi, P. Sotonyi: Myosin isoenzymes in normal and pathological human heart muscle. This issue, p. 129–133.
138. Staubesand, J.: Hämodynamische Fehlbelastung – Risikofaktor für die Gefäßwand. In: Ergebnisse der Angiologie, Bd. 20, Hgg. N. Klüken, I. Brändle, R. Stemmer. Schattauer (Stuttgart–New York 1980).
139. Steinhagen-Thiessen, E., A. Reznik, H. Hilz: Negative adaptation to physical training in senile mice. Mechanisms of Ageing and Development **12,** 231–236 (1980).
140. Sudakow, K. V.: Systems approach to the problem of emotional stress. In: Kvetnanský/Kopin. Catecholamines and stress, 579–586. Recent Advances (1980).
141. Swynghedauw, B.: Protein and nucleic acid metabolism in cardiac overload. A review. 151–158. Internat. Soc. Heart Res., Europ. Section (Dijon 1979).
142. Swynghedauw, B.: Discussion contribution. Erwin-Riesch-Symposium (Tübingen 1982).
143. Swynghedauw, B., J. J. Leger: A new myosin molecule in heart overloading. A stimulating working hypothesis, 69. Internat. Study Group Cardiac Metabolism, Europ. Section (Brüssel 1975).
144. Swynghedauw, B., J. J. Leger, K. Schwartz: The myosin isoenzyme hypothesis in chronic heart overloading. J. Molec. Cell. Cardiol. **8,** 915–924 (1976).
145. Swynghedauw, B., K. Schwartz, J. J. Leger: Cardiac myosin. Phylogenic and pathological changes. Basic Res. Cardiol. **72,** 254–260 (1977).
146. Thiedemann, K.-U., Ch. Holubarsch, I. Medugorac, R. Jacob: Connective tissue content and myocardial stiffness in pressure-induced cardiac hypertrophy. Basic Res. Cardiol. **78,** 140–155 (1983).
147. Thyrum, P. T., E. M. Kritchner, R. J. Luchi: Effect of L-thyroxine on the primary structure of cardiac myosin. Biochim. Biophys. Acta **197,** 335–336 (1970).
148. Tuchschmid, C. R., T. Srihari, H. O. Hirzel, M. C. Schaub: Structural variants of heavy and light chains of atrial and ventricular myosin in hypertrophied human hearts. This issue, p. 123–128.
149. Ueda, S., Y. Yazaki: Thyroxine-induced molecular alteration of heavy and 27,000-dalton light chains of rabbit ventricular myosin. Reconstitution of heavy and light chain molecules of subfragment-1 isoenzymes of cardiac myosin. This issue, p. 113–122.
150. U'Prichard, D. C., R. Kvetnanský: Central and peripheral adrenergic receptors in acute and repeated immobilization stress, 299–308. In: Kvetnanský/Kopin (Eds.) Catecholamines and Stress: Recent Advances (1980).
151. Vigas, M.: Contribution to the understanding of the stress concept. In: Catecholamines and Stress: Recent Advances, Usdin, E., R. Kvetnanský, I. J. Kopin (eds.), 573–578. Elsevier North Holland, Inc. (Amsterdam 1980).
152. Vrbova, G.: Effects of activity on some physiological properties of skeletal muscle. This issue, p. 33–38.
153. Watras, J.: Changes in rat cardiac myosin during development and in culture. J. Molec. Cell. Cardiol. **13,** 1011–1021 (1981).
154. Weisberg, A., S. Winegrad, M. Tucker, G. McClellan: Histochemical detection of specific isozymes of myosin in rat ventricular cells. Circulat. Res. **51,** 802–809 (1982).
155. Wendt-Gallitelli, M. F., G. Ebrecht, R. Jacob: Morphological alterations and their functional interpretation in the hypertrophied myocardium of Goldblatt hypertensive rats. J. Molec. Cell. Cardiol. **11,** 275–287 (1979).

156. Wiegand, V., E. Stroh, H. Hennekes, H. Kreuzer: Myosinisoenzyme im normalen und hypertrophierten menschlichen Myokard. Z. Kardiol. **71** (Abstr.) 212 (1982).
157. Wikman-Coffelt, J., W. W. Parmley, D. T. Mason: The cardiac hypertrophy process: Analyses of factors determining pathological vs physiological development. Circulat. Res. **45,** 679–707 (1979).
158. Williams, R. S., T. Bishop: Heterogeneity of adrenergic and cholinergic receptor alterations induced by prolonged physical training in the rat. Circulation **64,** Suppl. IV, 285 (1981).
159. Winegrad, S., G. McClellan, R. Horowitz, M. Tucker, L. E. Lin, A. Weisberg: Regulation of cardiac contractile proteins by phosphorylation. Fed. Proc. **42,** 33–38 (1983).
160. Wollenberger, A., W. Schultze: Über das Volumenverhältnis von Mitochondrien zu Myofibrillen in chronisch überlasteten hypertrophierten Herzen. Naturwissenschaften **49,** 161–162 (1962).
161. Yazaki, Y., M. S. Raben: Effect of the thyroid state on the enzymatic characteristics of cardiac myosin. Circulat. Res. **36,** 208–215 (1975).
162. Yazaki, Y., S. Ueda, R. Nagai, K. Shimada: Cardiac atrial myosin adenosine triphosphatase of animals and humans. Circulat. Res. **45,** 522–527 (1979).
163. Zak, R.: Contractile function as a determinant of muscle growth. Cell. Motility **1,** 1–33 (1981).
164. Zimmer, H.-G., E. Gerlach: Some metabolic features of the development of experimentally induced cardiac hypertrophy. Europ. Heart J. **3,** 83–92 (1982).

Author's address:

Prof. Dr. R. Jacob, Physiologisches Institut, Lehrstuhl II der Universität, Gmelinstraße 5, 7400 Tübingen, FRG

Fundamental biochemical processes – Control of myocardial cell growth and gene expression

Cardiac Adaptation to Hemodynamic Overload, Training and Stress
Dr. D. Steinkopff Verlag 27–32 (1983)

Molecular dynamics of contraction–relaxation*)

J. Gergely

Department of Muscle Research, Boston Biomedical Research Institute; Department of Neurology, Massachusetts General Hospital; and Department of Biological Chemistry, Harvard Medical School, Boston, Massachusetts (U.S.A.)

Summary

Recent findings bearing on the molecular mechanism of muscle contraction and relaxation are assessed. Among the questions considered are the segmental flexibility of myosin; the motion of crossbridges and the relation to force generation and elasticity; the validity of the steric blocking mechanism of regulation; and the identity of the elementary step controlled by Ca^{2+}.

Key words: actin-myosin interaction, crossbridge, myosin flexibility, myosin motion, steric blocking, Ca^{2+} regulation, thin filament, tropomyosin, troponin, ATPase, kinetics, force generation, elasticity

Introduction

The purpose of this brief review is to discuss recent variations on the main theme of muscle contraction and its regulation. Following the discoveries in the 1950's by H. E. Huxley and J. Hanson and A. F. Huxley and R. Niedergerke, the mechanism of muscle contraction based on the relative sliding past each other of two sets of filaments, built chiefly of myosin and actin, respectively, has been generally accepted, and many of the molecular details of the underlying mechanism are beyond question. Thus the projections (crossbridges) found in early electron micrographs on the thick filaments have been identified with the globular heads of the twoheaded myosin molecules whose double helical tail portion constitutes the core of the thick filaments. In active muscle, these myosin heads participate in cycles of attachment to, and detachment from, actin which is accompanied by the hydrolysis of ATP. After a cycle is complete, the myosin head is able to attach to another actin molecule in the thin filament and thereby propel the two filaments past each other (1, 2).

Segmental flexibility in myosin

It has been widely thought that this cycle of attachment and detachment requires flexibility in the myosin molecule so that the myosin heads once

*) The preparation of this manuscript and work in the author's laboratory is supported by grants from NIH (HL-5949), the National Science Foundation and the Muscular Dystrophy Associations of America, Inc.

attached to actin can change the angle between the segment connecting them with the core of the thick filament as well as changing the tilt with respect to the actin filament. Flexibility could be demonstrated by use of polarization fluorescence of small molecules attached to the myosin heads (3) as well as probes possessing magnetic properties (spin labels) whose behavior can be characterized by electron spin resonance spectroscopy (4) in regions of the myosin molecule between the rodlike portion forming the core of the thick filament and the connecting link and between the link and the head, referred to as hinges. A corollary of this picture is that in resting muscle myosin heads are detached from actin and the process of activation initiated by the nerve impulse causes their attachment. This view appears well supported by the conventional interpretation of x-ray diffraction diagrams of live muscle (for a recent summary, see 5). Motion of the crossbridges in situ is supported by time-resolved x-ray studies made possible by powerful new techniques utilizing synchrotron radiation and sophisticated electronic devices (5–7) and by analysis of fluctuation of fluorescence polarization (8). The conventional view is that each myosin head is attached to one actin monomer. Recent work by Kassab's group (9), however, has produced evidence indicating that each myosin head combines with two actins and each actin is bound to two myosin heads. The full import of these findings has not yet been incorporated into detailed molecular schemes that might serve as molecular models of contraction (for a structural interpretation, see ref. 10).

Relation of chemical and mechanical states

Ever since the discovery of Engelhardt and Lyubimova (11) that what they had considered myosin – actually it was actomyosin – is an enzyme catalyzing the hydrolysis of ATP, the close connection between contraction and ATP hydrolysis has been at the heart of any attempt to explain the process of conversion of chemical energy residing in ATP to mechanical work performed by the muscle. During the past ten years or so, detailed schemes have been developed chiefly based on the work of Lymn and Taylor and of Trentham and his colleagues (see ref. 12 for background) showing that the cleavage of ATP catalyzed by myosin results in a tightly bound myosin-ADP-phosphate complex whose breakdown is accelerated by actin during the process of the interaction of the two proteins. The precise details of this mechanism are still being studied, and various efforts are being made to identify chemical intermediates with mechanically distinct states of the crossbridges. In the original Lymn-Taylor-Trentham scheme, the chemical cleavage of ATP occurred on a detached myosin head, and the cycle was completed after the attachment of the head to actin accompanied by the rapid release of the products. Evidence has recently been put forward suggesting that the cleavage itself may occur on myosin attached to actin, which in turn may be in rapid equilibrium with myosin carrying the products (13). If this view gains general acceptance, based on corroborative experiments by other workers, the precise assignment of a chemical state to a given mechanical state may be more difficult than it appeared in previous models.

Force generation and elasticity

The most widely held view is that myosin heads attach to actin in such a way that the long axis of the pear-shaped myosin head forms a 90° angle with the actin filament axis and that tilting to an angle of 45° before detachment is an essential step in tension development or shortening (1, 2, 14). On this view, the change in angle at constant length leads to tension development by stretching some elastic element within the crossbridge. In many models this elastic element is placed in the connecting link between the myosin head and the core, although a leafspring-like torsional elasticity may reside in the junction of myosin and actin of somewhere else in the myosin structure (14). A different model that does not require the tilting of the head has been proposed by Harrington and his colleagues in which the tension-generating element is presumed to be at the junction of the myosin head and the connecting link. The basis of tension development is seen in a transformation of an α-helical structure into a form which tends to assume a coiled form and whose equilibrium length is shorter than that of the helix. Certain experiments showing the temperature-dependent changes in the α-helix content of a portion of the myosin molecule (15) corresponding to the connecting link (subfragment 2) as well as changes in the proteolytic sensitivity of the myosin molecule in a region corresponding to that of the hinge have been taken as strong evidence for the model (16). Evidence derived from experiments on fibers labelled at specific sulfhydryl groups of the myosin head with a spin label has also been taken to indicate that myosin heads do not change their angle with respect to actin on stretching (17). Similarly, x-ray results of Naylor and Podolsky (18) on stretched fibers failed to reveal indications of a changed myosin head attitude. Clearly, caution is necessary in applying these results on muscle in the rigor state in attempts to derive information regarding the active state. More recent results suggest that also in fibers in a state corresponding to activity in muscle, viz. in the presence of MgATP and Ca^{2+}, myosin heads do behave as though they were either detached or were in a state corresponding to rigor making a 45° angle with the filament axis (19). While these results may indeed be used to argue against movement of myosin heads on actin, it has been pointed out that there may be flexibility within the head while the region containing label is rigidly attached to actin.

Ca^{2+}-dependent thin filament regulation

It is now well established that the regulation of the activity of the actin-myosin system depends on small amounts of Ca^{2+} (20). This holds for all types of muscle, but details of the mechanism differ from muscle type to muscle type. The remainder of this discussion is focussed on vertebrate striated muscle, which includes cardiac muscle in which Ca^{2+} released from the sarcoplasmic reticulum in the excitation-contraction coupling process combines with the Ca-binding subunit TnC of the troponin complex. The latter contains two other subunits, troponin T and troponin I, and is in turn attached to tropomyosin which forms part of the thin filament. X-ray and electron microscope studies have shown that Ca-binding to troponin is accompanied by a movement of tropomyosin toward the central groove of the actin filament (for background, see ref. 20,

21). The subject was also discussed in the previous Symposium held under the auspices of the Erwin Riesch Foundation (22), and I shall only deal with some recent developments, which again point to the need of more research before we can say that the intimate details of the process are well understood. It has been widely held that the Ca^{2+}-induced movement of tropomyosin frees those sites on actin at which the myosin heads bind so that in a sense a competition between tropomyosin and myosin for the same site on actin is resolved in favour of myosin by Ca^{2+} bound to troponin. This model which has been referred to as the steric blocking model is based on a three-dimensional reconstruction of the thin filament structure from electron microscope and x-ray data (see 21, 23). Recent work by O'Brien (24) and his colleagues has raised questions concerning the details of this interpretation, and they have pointed out that tropomyosin may not be in a position where it can actually block the binding of myosin. It should be noted that a simple steric blocking model has never really been held in the sense that activation by Ca^{2+} is nothing but the reversal of the inhibition by tropomyosin since it was recognized in the early 1970's that the activity of actomyosin in the presence of tropomyosin, troponin and Ca^{2+} is higher than that of pure actomyosin, and that such increase in activity can be induced by tropomyosin alone in the absence of troponin. These observations led to the concept of potentiation emphasized by A. Weber and her colleagues (21, 23). Taylor et al. (25) have recently proposed a reconstruction of the thin filament structure that would be consistent with steric blocking, and the already mentioned double-actin attachment by each myosin head has recently been considered in conjunction with thin filament structure (9). A final evaluation of the impact of both new proposals concerning myosin attachment as well as the interpretation of thin filament structure (24, 25) may have to await further experimental data.

Binding vs kinetic control

What may be a more serious challenge to certain accepted views on myosin-actin interaction and its regulation comes from some experiments suggesting that the classical concept concerning what is controlled by Ca^{2+} has to be changed. The generally held view is that Ca^{2+} controls the attachment of myosin to actin in the sense that the attachment requires Ca^{2+}, and detachment occurs on removal of Ca^{2+}, in vitro by chelators and in vivo by the pumping action of the sarcoplasmic reticulum. Recent evidence suggests that at least at low ionic strength activation of ATPase can occur without changes in the state of attachment of myosin to actin (26). Observations showing that even in the presence of Ca^{2+} and in the presence of tropomyosin and troponin at low myosin-head to actin ratios the ATPase activity is low also support the view that Ca^{2+} does not fully activate the system (23, 27). They raise questions concerning the precise relationship of the changes in thin filament structure revealed by x-ray diffraction and electron microscopy and the activation of the actin-myosin system. Chalovich and Eisenberg (26) suggest that what is controlled is not the attachment of myosin to actin but a step in the kinetic scheme of ATP hydrolysis catalyzed by actomyosin; specifically, the release of phosphate from the actomyosin ADP. P complex would be slow in the absence of

Ca^{2+} and accelerated in its presence. According to such a scheme, there would be no change in the total attachment of myosin to actin but rather in the distribution of myosin among the various attached states. On this view, relaxation would not be accompanied by the detachment of myosin heads but a shift from a form in which the heads are tightly bound to one in which binding is looser and the process of attachment and detachment in equilibrium proceeds on a faster time scale. Recent experiments (28) indicating that in relaxed muscle there is stiffness, proportional to the degree of overlap between thick and thin filaments, provided sufficiently rapid stretches are applied, lend support to this view.

The concept of cooperativity has played an important role in attempts to understand the interaction of actin and myosin and the regulatory role of Ca^{2+}. In earlier schemes invoking cooperativity, the interactions among actins spanned by the same tropomyosin molecule, which extends over a domain of seven actins, have been stressed (21). More recently, interactions among tropomyosin molecules within a thin filament and the possibility of cooperativity over stretches of several tropomyosin molecules has been considered. Such interactions are particularly helpful in interpreting the high cooperativity that has been reported for the binding of myosin to actin in a state corresponding to rigor, viz. in the absence of ATP (29). It is, however, not fully clear to what extent cooperativity is applicable to the actin-myosin system under conditions corresponding to activation.

Conclusion

This brief survey has clearly not covered all problems in the area of contraction and its control and has certainly not covered any of them in detail. I hope, however, that it has pointed to some new findings and new problems, the resolution of which will eventually lead to a better understanding of the molecular mechanisms in normal muscle and will also provide new insights into the understanding of problems of cardiac muscle under pathological conditions.

References

1. Huxley, H. E.: The Mechanism of Muscle Contraction. Science **164,** 1356 (1969).
2. Huxley, A. F.: Review Lecture: Muscular Contraction. J. Physiol. **243,** 1 (1974).
3. Mendelson, R. A., M. F. Morales, J. Botts: Segmental Flexibility of the S-1 Moiety of Myosin. Biochemistry **12,** 2250 (1973).
4. Thomas, D. D., J. C. Seidel, J. S. Hyde, J. Gergely: Motion of Subfragment 1 in Myosin and Its Supramolecular Complex: Saturation Transfer Electron Paramagnetic Resonance. Proc. Nat. Acad. Sci. U.S. **72,** 1729 (1975).
5. Huxley, H. E., A. R. Faruqi, M. Kress, J. Bordas, M. H. J. Koch: Time-resolved X-Ray Diffraction Studies of the Myosin Layer-line Reflections During Muscle Contraction. J. Mol. Biol. **158,** 637 (1982).
6. Huxley, H. E., R. M. Simmons, A. R. Faruqi, M. Kress, J. Bordas, M. H. Koch: Millisecond Time Resolved Changes in X-Ray Reflections from Contracting Muscle During Rapid Mechanical Transients Recorded Using Synchroton Radiation. Proc. Nat. Acad. Sci. U.S. **78,** 2297 (1981).
7. Huxley, H. E., A. R. Faruqi, J. Bordas, M. H. Koch, J. R. Milch: The Use of Synchroton Radiation in Time Resolved X-Ray Diffraction Studies of Myosin Layer-line Reflections During Muscle Contraction. Nature **284,** 140 (1980).
8. Borejdo, J., S. Putnam, M. F. Morales: Fluctuation in Polarized Fluorescence:

Evidence that Muscle Crossbridges Rotate Repetitively during Contraction. Proc. Nat. Acad. Sci. U.S. **76,** 6346 (1979).
9. Mornet, D., R. Bertrand, P. Pantel, E. Audemard, R. Kassab: Structure of the Actin-Myosin Interface. Nature **292,** 301 (1981).
10. Amos, L. A., H. E. Huxley, K. C. Holmes, R. S. Goody, K. A. Taylor: Structural Evidence that Myosin Heads May Interact with Two Sites on F-Actin. Nature **299,** 467 (1982).
11. Engelhardt, V. A., M. N. Lyubimova: Myosin and Adenosinetriphosphatase. Nature **144,** 668 (1939).
12. Taylor, E. W.: Mechanism of Actomyosin ATPase and the Problem of Muscle Contraction. Crit. Rev. Biochem. **6,** 103 (1979).
13. Stein, L. A., P. B. Chock, E. Eisenberg: Mechanism of the Actomyosin ATPase: Effect of Actin on the ATP Hydrolysis Step. Proc. Nat. Acad. Sci. U.S. **78,** 1346 (1981).
14. Huxley, A. F., R. M. Simmons: Proposed Mechanism of Force Generation in Striated Muscle. Nature **233,** 533 (1971).
15. Tsong, T. Y., T. Karr, W. F. Harrington: Rapid Helix Coil Transitions in the S-2 Region of Myosin. Proc. Nat. Acad. Sci. U.S. **76,** 1109 (1979).
16. Ueno, H., W. F. Harrington: Conformational Transition in the Myosin Hinge Upon Activation of Muscle. Proc. Nat. Acad. Sci. U.S. **78,** 6101 (1981).
17. Cooke, R.: Stress Does Not Alter the Conformation of a Domain of the Myosin Crossbridge in Rigor Muscle Fibres. Nature **294,** 570 (1981).
18. Naylor, G. R. S., R. J. Podolsky: X-Ray Diffraction of Strained Muscle Fibers in Rigor. Proc. Nat. Acad. Sci. U.S. **78,** 5559 (1981).
19. Cooke, R., M. S. Crowder, D. D. Thomas: Orientation of Spin Labels Attached to Crossbridges in Contracting Muscle Fibres. Nature **300,** 776 (1982).
20. Ebashi, S.: Regulatory Mechanism of Muscle, in "Essays in Biochemistry" **10,** P. N. Campbell and F. Dickens, eds., p. 1 (1974).
21. Weber, A., J. M. Murray: Molecular Control Mechanisms in Muscle Contraction. Physiol. Rev. **53,** 612 (1973).
22. Gergely, J.: Ca^{2+} control of actin-myosin interaction. Basic Res. Cardiol. **75,** 17 (1980).
23. Trueblood, C. E., T. P. Walsh, A. Weber: Is the Steric Model of Tropomyosin Action Valid? In: "Basic Biology of Muscles: A Comparative Approach", B. M. Twarog, R. J. C. Levine and M. M. Dewey, eds., Raven Press, p. 223 (1982).
24. O'Brien, E. J., E. P. Morris, J. Seymour, J. Couch: Structure and Activity of the Thin Filament, in "Muscle Contraction: Its Regulatory Mechanisms". S. Ebashi et al., eds., p. 147. Springer-Verlag (Berlin 1980).
25. Taylor, K. A., L. A. Amos: A New Model for the Geometry of the Binding of Myosin Crossbridges to Muscle Thin Filaments. J. Molec. Biol. **147,** 297 (1981).
26. Chalovich, J. M., E. Eisenberg: Inhibition of Actomyosin ATPase Activity by Troponin-tropomyosin Without Blocking of the Binding of Myosin to Actin. J. Biol. Chem. **257,** 2432 (1982).
27. Lehrer, S. S., E. P. Morris: Dual Effects of Tropomyosin and Troponin-Tropomyosin on Actomyosin Subfragment 1 ATPase. J. Biol. Chem. **237,** 8073 (1982).
28. Brenner, B., M. Schoenberg, J. M. Chalovich, L. E. Greene, E. Eisenberg: Evidence for Cross-bridge Attachment in Relaxed Muscle at Low Ionic Strength. Proc. Nat. Acad. Sci. U.S. **79,** 7288 (1982).
29. Greene, L. E., E. Eisenberg: Cooperative Binding of Myosin Subfragment-1 to the Actin-Troponin-Tropomyosin Complex. Proc. Nat. Acad. Sci. U.S. **77,** 2616 (1980).

Author's address:

Dr. J. Gergely, Department of Muscle Research, Boston Biomed. Research, Institute, Boston, Massachusetts, U.S.A., 02114

Cardiac Adaptation to Hemodynamic Overload, Training and Stress
Dr. D. Steinkopff Verlag 33–38 (1983)

Effects of activity on some physiological properties of skeletal muscles

G. Vrbová

Department of Anatomy and Embryology and Centre for Neuroscience, University College London (UK)

Summary

The mechanism by which the motor nerve exerts its influence on some contractile and biochemical properties of skeletal muscle were discussed. Evidence to show that the contractile and biochemical characteristics of skeletal muscle are determined by the particular pattern of activity that is imposed upon the muscle by its motor nerve is presented. Each motoneurone can in this way induce in the muscle fibres it supplies the development of those properties that will match its particular activity pattern.

Key words: skeletal muscle, activity, contractile and biochemical properties

Introduction

In mammals, two distinct types of muscles with respect to the time course of their contraction and relaxation, as well as their biochemical properties, have been recognized: slow contracting muscles with high levels of oxidative and low levels of glycolytic anaerobic enzymes, and fast contracting muscles, with low levels of oxidative and high levels of glycolytic enzyme activities (Ranvier, 1874; Denny-Brown, 1929; Cooper and Eccles, 1930).

Although more recent findings suggest that such a clear distinction is arbitrary, and moreover many additional differences in the composition of muscle fibres have been reported, the distinction into slow and fast muscles is certainly valid for particular leg muscles of mammals. These characteristic properties of slow and fast muscles are well matched to the functional requirements imposed upon them by their respective motor nerves. Motor nerves to the slow soleus muscles of the cat and rabbit fire at low rates of about 8 to 15 Hz, more or less continually; whereas motor nerves to fast muscles fire only occasionally and at higher frequencies (Denny-Brown, 1929; Eccles, Eccles and Lundberg, 1957). Since for coordinated movement it is important for the contraction to be smooth, the slow contraction and relaxation of the soleus is well adjusted to the slow firing rate, and the fast contraction of the fast leg muscles to the fast firing rate. In addition, soleus develops maximal tetanic tension at lower rates of firing than fast muscles. The question as to how these contractile characteristics are determined is therefore of special interest.

The dependence of the muscle fibre on its neurone was most clearly demonstrated in experiments of Buller, Eccles and Eccles (1960). They sutured the motor nerve from the slow soleus muscle of the cat into the fast flexor digitorum longus and the nerve from this fast muscle into the soleus. Some time after this "cross-innervation", the characteristic contractile speeds of the two muscles were examined and compared to those of the contralateral, unoperated side. The fast muscles now supplied by the slow nerve became slow contracting, and the slow muscles supplied by a fast nerve became fast contracting. By this series of experiments it was clearly established that the contractile properties characteristic of a given muscle are not inherent but are determined by the motor nerve.

It was later found that many other properties characteristic of a slow muscle came to resemble those of a fast muscle when it had become innervated by a nerve from the fast muscle, and vice-versa. So, for example the enzyme pattern of the soleus muscle fibres changed from a homogeneously high oxidative, low anaerobic type to a heterogeneous population of muscle fibres resembling a fast muscle (Romanul and Van Der Meullen, 1967). The structure of contractile proteins is also different in slow and fast muscles. The myosin ATP-ase activity of soleus muscle is lower and that of fast muscle higher (Bárány, 1967), and this, too, changes after cross-innervation (Buller et al., 1969; Bárány and Close, 1971). Many other biochemical features are also altered by cross-innervation; for example, the ATP-ase activity of the sarcoplasmic reticulum also differs in slow and fast muscles and is transformed following cross-innervation. The myosin light chains are distinctly different in slow and fast muscles, and after cross-innervation the light chains of the fast muscle will become to resemble those of the slow muscle and those of the slow muscle will become similar to those in fast muscles (Weeds et al., 1974).

Not only does the structure of the thick filament and sarcoplasmic proteins change, but that of the thin filament is also influenced by the alien innervation. As expected, when the soleus muscle of a rabbit is reinnervated by the lateral popliteal nerve, which usually innervates fast muscle fibres, the contractile properties of the soleus muscle change, i.e., it becomes a fast contracting and relaxing muscle. This change of contractile properties is accompanied by a transformation of the structure of troponin I, which is one of the regulating proteins in skeletal muscles (Amphlett et al., 1976; Dhoot et a., 1981).

There are several possible explanations as to how the nerve exerts its influence over the muscle fibres it supplies. In their original paper, Buller et al. (1960) suggested that the nerve exerts a special "trophic" influence over the muscle fibres and that it is in this way that it determines what is to become of the muscle fibre. Another possible explanation of these results was put forward by A. F. Huxley and discussed by Buller et al. (1960). Huxley suggested to Buller et al. (1960) that the motor nerve maintains the slow time course of contraction of the soleus muscle fibres by imposing onto it a slow frequency activity, which may act as a "vibratory stress" (see Buller et al., 1960). Buller et al. did not favour this interpretation, and it was not until later that evidence was provided to show the crucial importance of the activity of the muscle in determining its characteristic properties.

It is known from the work of Sperry (1944) that the activity pattern of motor nerves remains unaltered when they are transposed into different muscles. Thus in the experimental situation of Buller et al. (1960) the nerve from a fast muscle, now supplying a slow muscle, would activate the slow muscle by the same activity pattern as the original fast muscle, and the nerve from the slow muscle would carry on activating the fast muscle by the type of activity of the original slow muscle. From this it is clear that after crossing the motor nerves from one type of muscle to another, the activity pattern of each muscle would be changed. The effects produced by crossing the motor nerves could be explained by the altered activity the muscle was made to perform, without having to involve a special trophic influence.

A simple situation was sought that would alter radically the activity pattern of skeletal muscle without interfering with its innervation. Soleus motoneurones have a low threshold to stretch but are inexcitable by flexor reflex afferens. It might therefore be expected that the stretch reflex would be of greater importance for the activity of soleus than for that of muscles involved in other types of movement. When EMG activity was recorded from the soleus muscles of conscious, unrestrained rabbits, it was found that continuous activity could be recorded from this muscle, no matter whether the rabbit was walking, standing or just sitting quietly in its cage. Other muscles like the tibialis anterior were activated during movement of the animal or on pinching its foot. After cutting the tendons of these muscles, and thus preventing them from being stretched, the continuous activity of the soleus muscle can no longer be seen, and only occasionally, activity of very small motor units can be detected. Tenotomy of the other calf muscles does not alter appreciably their phasic type of EMG activity (Vrbová, 1963a).

Thus tenotomy alters the activity pattern of soleus, but not that of tibialis anterior. When the contractile speeds of the tenotomized soleus muscle were examined some time after the operation, it was found that the tenotomized soleus muscle had become fast contracting. Thus in this experiment the innervation was unaltered and only the activity pattern of the soleus muscle was changed by tenotomy; nevertheless the contractile properties of the soleus muscle changed. The activity pattern of the tibialis anterior muscle was unaltered by tenotomy, and correspondingly the contractile speeds remained unaffected (Vrbová, 1963b).

In order to study the effects of activity at different frequencies on the contractile properties of muscle, it was thought desirable to work with muscles that had no, or extremely little reflex activity. As already mentioned, the tenotomized soleus, although quiescent, had some activity. If this residual activity was due to a supraspinal excitatory influence on soleus motoneurones, then cutting the spinal cord ought to abolish even this activity. Indeed, after section of the cord the tenotomized muscle is completely "silent", whereas reflex activity can readily be elicited from the tibialis anterior muscle. The tenotomized soleus of a spinal rabbit became fast contracting, suggesting that its normal activity maintains the slow contractile speed. Electrodes were implanted close to the motor nerve of the "silent" soleus muscle, and electrical activity was imposed upon the muscle via these electrodes. When the muscle was stimulated at 5 or 10 Hz for eight hours a day over a period of two to three weeks, the soleus muscle remained slow; when, however, higher frequencies of stimulation were used, 20 or 40 Hz, the soleus muscle became fast contracting. These results clearly show that the contractile speed of the rabbit soleus is determined by the particular activity pattern of the muscle (Vrbová, 1966).

Whether contractile properties of fast muscles can also be influenced by activity was the next question. Since it is practically impossible to prevent reflex activity from reaching these muscles, it was decided to superimpose a slow frequency activity onto the normal phasic activity of fast leg muscles. Electrodes were implanted so as to stimulate the motor nerves to tibialis anterior and extensor digitorum longus muscles of rabbits, and they were stimulated at 10 Hz. When the contractile characteristics of these stimulated muscles were examined two to four weeks after such stimulation, it was found that these fast muscles had become slower contracting. When stimulated for longer intervals such as two to three months, their contractile speeds were similar to those of the slow soleus muscle. Thus even though the slow frequency activity was superimposed onto the normal activity of the muscle, it had a dramatic, slowing effect (Salmons and Vrbová, 1969). From these results it is apparent that the nerve exerts its influence on the contractile properties by imposing a particular pattern of activity, and not by a special trophic influence.

Not only the contractile speeds but the enzyme composition of fast muscles is also altered after long-term electrical stimulation. The anaerobic muscles fibres of the tibialis anterior muscle and extensor digitorum longus muscles are transformed into predominantly aerobic ones, and this can be shown both by biochemical analysis of the muscles as well as by histochemical examinations (Pette et al., 1973). The heterogeneous appearance of the muscles disappears, and all the muscle fibres become of a similar size and similar staining intensity for the oxidative enzyme succinate dehydrogenase. This is not so for myosin ATP-ase, for with regard to this enzyme, the muscle fibres remain heterogeneous for a long time (Pette et al., 1976). This may be due to the fact that the normal activity of the muscle is still present. If different activity patterns are applied to completely "silent" muscles, like cat-tail muscles after they are deafferented and spinalized, the histochemical appearance of the muscles depended entirely on the activity pattern. Slow, tonic type of activity made muscle fibres with high oxidative enzymes and low anaerobic enzymes, fast phasic activity produced muscle fibres with low oxidative and high anaerobic enzymes and high activity of myosin ATP-ase (Riley and Allin, 1973). Changes of the sarcoplasmic reticulum and its ability to bind Ca^{++} are also altered by the long-term electrical stimulation (Ramirez and Pette, 1974) as are the myosin light chains of fast muscles (Sreter et al., 1973).

The mechanism by which the muscle fibre alters its biochemical composition and starts synthesizing a set of different proteins is poorly understood. Experiments where such changes are brought about by electrical stimulation seem to be a suitable model situation for studying this question. The time sequence of the development of particular changes may help to elucidate this problem, and an attempt was made to investigate the time sequence of the different changes induced by chronic electrical stimulation. The first apparent change in response to slow frequency activity is of course the well-recognized functional hyperaemia. This is followed by a growth of capillaries. It was found that such increase in capillary density can be brought about only by electrical activity at low frequencies, and not by stimulating the muscle at higher rates (Brown et al., 1976). The increase of capillary density is followed by an increase in the muscle oxidative enzyme capacity and a decrease of enzymes concerned with anaerobic metabolism. Activities of membrane-bound enzymes such as hexokinase and palmitoyl CoA synthetase that may be concerned with transport of "substrates" in and out of the muscle fibres are already increased four days after electrical stimulation of fast muscles had started, and the increase of oxidative enzymes followed ten days later. Another change that can be detected is the change of ATPase activity of the sarcoplasmic reticulum (Ramirez and Pette, 1974). Finally, after a long time of continuous electrical stimulation, the structure of the myosin light chains also changes (Sreter et al., 1973). It may be that the increased availability of oxygen produced by the denser capillary network may shorten the diffusion distance between the blood and working muscle cell, so that the muscle fibre will be working in an environment with a higher partial pressure of oxygen. It is possible that this induces the transformation from anaerobic to aerobic metabolism. How this is accomplished is unknown.

When muscles are stimulated continually for long periods of time, i.e., for 24 hours a day, the variation of changes in contractile speeds is small, and these muscles always become slower. Moreover, the myosin light chains are regularly transformed from the fast type to resemble those of the slow soleus muscle (Sreter et al., 1973). This complete transformation of a fast muscle activated for months, day and night, by slow frequency activity is probably only possible because the animal entirely stops the normal usuage of the stimulated muscles. That such a muscle is becoming very "abnormal" is apparent from the loss of weight and decrease of its tetanic tension, which does not take place in muscles stimulated for only eight hours a day (Pette et al., 1976).

Since activity is considered to be the major regulatory influence in determining the functional and biochemical properties of skeletal muscle fibres, it is not surprising that the effects of the muscle's "own" activity can be completely overridden only by the most strenuous regime. Normally the contractile and biochemical properties of skeletal muscles are determined by the activity pattern imposed upon the muscle by its motor nerve.

References

Amphlett, G. W., S. V. Perry, H. Syska, M. Brown, G. Vrbová: Cross innervation and the regulatory protein system of rabbit soleus muscle. Nature **257,** 602–604 (1975).

Bárány M.: ATP-ase activity of myosin correlated with speed of muscle shortening. J. Gen. Physiol. **50,** (suppl. part 2), 197–218 (1967).

Bárány, M., R. I. Close: The transformation of myosin in cross-innervated rat muscles. J. Physiol. **213,** 455–474 (1971).

Brown, M. D., M. A. Cotter, O. Hudlická, G. Vrbová: The effects of different patterns of muscle activity on capillary density, mechanical properties and structure of slow and fast rabbit muscles. Pflügers Arch. **361,** 241–250 (1976).

Buller, A. J., J. C. Eccles, R. M. Eccles: Interactions between motoneurones and muscles in respect of the characteristic speeds of their responses. J. Physiol. **150,** 417–439 (1960).

Buller, A. J., W. F. H. M. Mommaerts, K. Seraydarian: Enzymic properties of myosin in fast and slow twitch muscles of the cat following cross-innervation. J. Physiol. **205,** 581–597 (1969).

Cooper, S., J. C. Eccles: The isometric responses of mammalian muscles. J. Physiol. **69,** 377–385 (1930).

Denny-Brown, D.: The histological features of striped muscle in relation to its functional activity. Proc. R. Soc. **104,** 371–411 (1929).

Dhoot, G. K., S. V. Perry, G. Vrbová: Changes in distribution of the components of the troponin complex in muscle fibres after cross-innervation. Exp. Neurol. **72,** 513–530 (1981).

Eccles, J. C., R. M. Eccles, A. Lundberg: The action potentials of motoneurones supplying fast and slow muscles. J. Physiol. **142,** 272–291 (1958).

Pette, D., W. Müller, E. Leisner, G. Vrbová: Time dependent effects on contractile properties, fibre population, myosin light chains and enzymes of energy metabolism in intermittent and continuously stimulated fast twitch muscle of the rabbit. Pflügers. Arch. **364,** 103–112 (1976).

Pette, D., M. E. Smith, H. W. Staudte, G. Vrbová: Effects of long-term electrical stimulation on some contractile and metabolic characteristics of fast rabbit muscles. Pflügers Arch. **338,** 257–272 (1973).

Ramirez, B. U., D. Pette: Effects of long-term electrical stimulation on sarcoplasmic reticulum of fast rabbit muscle. Febs. Lett. **49,** 188–190 (1975).

Ranvier, L.: De quelques faits relatifs à l'histologie et à la physiologie des muscles striés. Archives of Physiological and Normal Pathology **6,** 1–5 (1974).

Riley, D. A., E. F. Allin: The effects of inactivity programmed stimulation, and denervation on the histochemistry of skeletal muscle fibre types. Experimental Neurology **40,** 391–413 (1973).

Romanul, F. C. A., J. P. van der Meulen: Slow and fast muscles after cross innervation. Enzymatic and physiological changes. Arch. Neurol. **17,** 387–402 (1967).

Salmons, S., G. Vrbová: The influence of activity on some contractile characteristics of mammalian fast and slow muscles. J. Physiol. **201,** 535–549 (1969).

Sperry, R. W.: The problem of central nervous reorganisation after regeneration and muscle transposition. Quart. Rev. Biol. **20,** 311–369 (1945).

Streter, F. A., J. Gergely, S. Salmons, F. Romanul: Synthesis by fast muscle of myosin light chains characteristic of slow muscle in response to long term stimulation. Nature New Biology, **214,** 17–19 (1973).

Vrbová, G.: Changes in motor reflexes produced by tenotomy. J. Physiol. **166,** 241–250 (1963a).

Vrbová, G.: The effect of motoneurone activity on the contraction speed of striated muscle. J. Physiol. **169,** 513–526 (1963b).

Vrbová, G.: Factors determining the speed of contraction of striated muscle. J. Physiol. **185,** 17–18P (1966).

Weeds, A. G., D. R. Trentham, C. J. C. Kean, A. J. Buller: Myosin from cross-innervated cat muscles. Nature. **247,** 135–139 (1974).

Author's address:

Dr. G. Vrbová, Dept. of Anatomy and Embryology and Centre for Neuroscience, Univ. College London, Gower Street, London WC1E 6BT, UK.

Cardiac Adaptation to Hemodynamic Overload, Training and Stress
Dr. D. Steinkopff Verlag 39–45 (1983)

Relationship between the synthesis rates and mRNA levels of the α and β cardiac myosin heavy chains in normal and thyrotoxic rabbits

A. W. Everett[1], A. M. Sinha[1], M. Rabinowitz[2], and R. Zak[1/3]

Departments of Medicine[1], Biochemistry[2], and Pharmacological and Physiological Sciences[3], The University of Chicago, Chicago, Illinois, 60637 (U.S.A.)

Summary

The role of transcription in the expression of cardiac myosin heavy chains (HC's) α and β has been investigated by comparing the relative synthesis rates and mRNA levels of these proteins in normal and thyrotoxic rabbits. The synthesis rates were determined in vivo from the incorporation of ^{3}H-leucine into each heavy chain after a continuous IV infusion of the labeled amino acid for 1 hour. We show that the synthesis rate of HCα increased 3-fold while that of HCβ was decreased at 1 and 2 days after administration of L-thyroxine. The relative amounts of mRNA were determined by S1 nuclease mapping using cloned cDNA sequences corresponding to the mRNAs of HCα and HCβ. The data show a close correlation between the relative amounts of the mRNAs and the relative synthesis rates for each heavy chain. This is consistent with pretranslational processes playing a major role in regulating the expression of myosin in the ventricles in both the euthyroid and thyrotoxic states.

Administration of D-thyroxine, like the naturally occurring isomer, also resulted in a relative accumulation of HCα in the ventricles.

Key words: heart, myosin heavy chains, transcriptional control, thyroxine, D-thyroxine, isomyosins, myosin synthesis

Introduction

A great deal of evidence indicates that the ventricles of a number of mammalian species contain at least two classes of myosin heavy chains; HCα and HCβ (1, 2), which assemble to form three isomyosins referred to as V1, V2 and V3. These two classes of heavy chain are most likely the products of different genes, based on analysis of the peptide maps (3, 4), immunochemical properties (4) and amino acid sequence of the proteins (5).

The expression of the heavy chains in the ventricles is controlled by a variety of means, since the ventricular content of these proteins changes continuously during the life of the animal (1, 6), and is also greatly influenced by a number of hormones (3, 7–10) and by change in the haemodynamic load (11, 12).

In rabbits, the V3 isomyosin, which is believed to consist of a homodimer of HCβ, is the predominant form of myosin during the late embryonic period. Soon after birth the V1 isomyosin (homodimer of HCα) begins to accumulate and may predominate by 2 weeks of age (6). After this time V1 is lost and is never normally re-expressed in significant amounts. Consequently, the ventricles of adult rabbits contain all or mostly the V3 isomyosin.

The transition in the isomyosin composition of the ventricles which occurs during normal life can be readily altered by thyroid hormone. Induction of the hyperthyroid state, both before and after birth, results in the accumulation of V1. Hypothyroidism, on the other hand, is associated with predominance of V3 when normally V1 is in the majority. As a first step therefore toward a more complete understanding of the control of myosin expression in the ventricles, we have compared the relative amounts of the mRNAs for HCα and HCβ with the relative synthesis rates of these proteins in euthyroid and thyrotoxic rabbits. Our preliminary results indicate that pretranslational events are of major importance in the regulation of myosin expression in the heart.

Methods

Myosin extraction

Myofibrils were isolated from ventricles by standard procedures and were washed with low salt buffer (40 mM NaCl, 1 mM $MgCl_2$, 0.1 mM DDT, 0.1 mM EGTA, 5 mM Na phosphate, pH 7.0). The myofibrils were extracted with 15 volumes of high salt buffer (as above with 0.6 M NaCl and 10 mM ATP). Myosin was then precipitated with ammonium sulfate between 39 and 50 % saturation followed by one cycle of dissolution and precipitation by dialysis against low salt buffer. Myosin was then dissolved in high salt buffer, centrifuged at 20,000 × g for 10 min and stored at −20 °C in 50 % glycerol for further analysis.

Separation of HCα and HCβ

V1 (HCα) and V3 (HCβ) were isolated by affinity chromatography using monoclonal antibodies RCM-37 (anti-V1) and CCM-52 (anti-V3) coupled to Sepharose-4B (6). Stored myosin was precipitated by dilution with water, dissolved in column buffer (0.5 M NaCl, 20 mM phosphate buffer, pH 7.5), and an aliquot (1–2 mg) was applied to each affinity column and recycled ten times. The unbound myosin fractions were collected and dialysed against 30 mM Na pyrophosphate, pH 7.0. The myosin was then boiled in the presence of 1 % each of SDS and 2-mercaptoethanol.

Determination of protein synthesis rate

Unrestrained rabbits (NZW) were infused via an ear vein with ^{3}H-leucine (70 Ci/mmol, Amersham Corp.) at a rate of 1.56 (1.5 mCi) ml/hr. Fractional synthesis rates were determined from the precursor (plasma) and protein specific radioactivities at the end of 1 hr infusion, as well as from the first order rate constant for the change in the precursor radioactivity during the infusion (6).

Determination of the leucine specific radioactivity

The heavy chains from the affinity purified isomyosins were separated from the light subunits by SDS-polyacrylamide gel electrophoresis. After staining the gels with Coomassie blue, the heavy chains were excised and hydrolyzed in 6 M HCl.

The specific radioactivity of leucine was then determined by the dansyl chloride procedure (13).

Quantitation of mRNA

The relative abundance of mRNA specific for each heavy chain was determined by S1 nuclease mapping using two cloned cDNA sequences corresponding to the mRNAs for HCα and HCβ (5).

Results

To study the relationship between the relative levels of mRNA and relative synthesis rates of both HC's in normal rabbits, we selected animals 4–6 weeks of age since only during neonatal development are both HC's expressed in similar amounts in the ventricles (6). After this time V1 (HCα) is lost, and only one isomyosin (V3, HCβ) predominates.

In 8 euthyroid rabbits, the mean fractional synthesis rates of both heavy chains were the same, averaging 0.14 day^{-1} (fig. 1). This means that in one day the heart synthesized an amount of each heavy chain equivalent to 14 % of the total heavy chain in the ventricles.

Daily administration of 200 μg thyroxine/kg body weight resulted in a rapid increase in the specific radioactivity of HCα and a concomitant decrease in that of HCβ (data not shown). At one day of hormone treatment the fractional synthesis rate of HCα was 3-fold that found in normal animals (fig. 1). No additional increase was noted on the second day. In

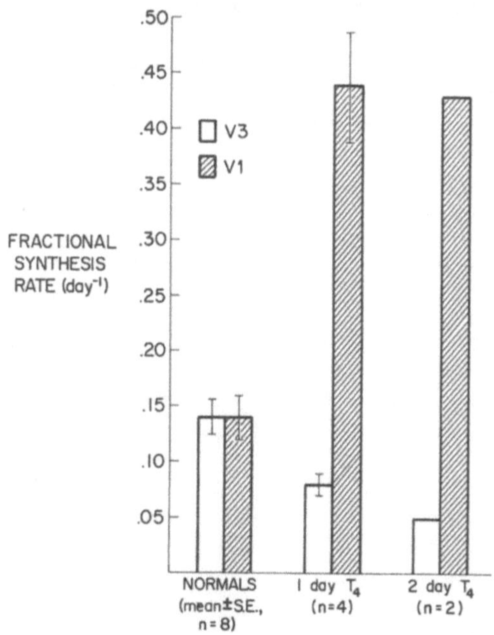

Fig. 1. Fractional synthesis rates of the V1 (HCα) and V3 (HCβ) cardiac myosin heavy chains in euthyroid and thyrotoxic rabbits. Rabbits (4–6 weeks old) were either untreated or given L-thyroxine (200 μg/kg/day) IM for 1 or 2 days.

contrast, the fractional synthesis rate of HCβ declined one day after injection of the hormone from 0.14 day^{-1} to 0.08 day^{-1}. The decline in HCβ synthesis continued reaching an average of 0.05 day^{-1} on the second day, well below the range found in normal animals.

The reciprocal changes in synthesis rates of HCα and HCβ were accompanied by a redistribution of the isomyosin profile in the ventricles to mostly V1. At one day this change is difficult to determine with accuracy, however, V1 accumulation is clearly indicated in these animals at 4-days treatment.

To gain some insight as to whether these changes in myosin synthesis resulted from direct and/or indirect actions of the hormone on the heart, we compared the affects of the D and L isomers of thyroxine. The D isomer at the dosage used here has no effect on whole body oxygen consumption (14) and did not result in a decrease in body weight. We still observed, however, a relative accumulation of V1 in the ventricles after administration of 250 μg D-thyroxine/kg/day to adult rabbits for 21 days (fig. 2). The conversion to V1 was not as complete as occurs with the L-isomer, which at a dose of 200 μg/kg/day leads to complete or almost complete conversion to V1 with an accompanying 30 % or more loss in body weight as well as some mortality (unpublished results).

These findings lend support to the hypothesis that at least some effect of the hormone on myosin synthesis occurs most likely through direct action(s) on the heart, and not necessarily by a change in haemodynamic load caused by the increased peripheral demand for oxygen.

The altered synthetic rates of ventricular myosin caused by administration of thyroxine could be a consequence of a change in either the rate of mRNA translation or rate of transcription (including RNA processing). In an attempt to distinguish between these two alternatives, we compared the synthesis rates of the two heavy chains with the relative amounts of

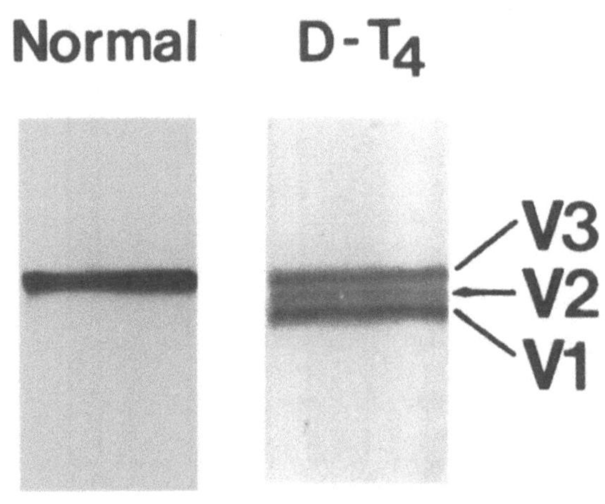

Fig. 2. Effect of D-thyroxine on cardiac myosin isozymes. Adult rabbits (>3 kg) were either untreated (normal) or given D-thyroxine (250 μg/kg/day) for 21 days. The cardiac isomyosin composition was determined by native gel electrophoresis (2).

their respective mRNAs. The relative amounts of mRNA for HCα and HCβ were determined by S1 nuclease mapping experiments with cDNA probes complimentory to the mRNAs for the heavy chains.

Total RNA extracted from each heart was analysed with both HCα and HCβ specific cDNA probes. Homology between the mRNA and its corresponding cDNA results in formation of a heteroduplex, which is resistent to the action of S1 nuclease. Consequently, the radiolabeled cDNA probe can be recovered in its original size after treatment with the nuclease. In contrast, when there is divergence in the nucleotide sequence between the cDNA probe and the mRNA, hybridization will not be complete and the S1 nuclease will split the probe at the point of nucleotide mismatch. The cDNA can then be recovered as a fragment of its original size.

When HCα and HCβ co-exist within the ventricle, the relative amount of mRNA for each heavy chain can be determined from the ratio of radioactivity associated with the full size and fragmented cDNA separated by electrophoresis. By this method we have determined that in normal and thyrotoxic rabbits, the relative amounts of mRNA specific for HCα and HCβ are in agreement with the relative synthetic rates for these two myosin heavy chains (fig. 3). The data support the thesis that the amount of myosin HCα and HCβ being synthesized/g tissue is most likely regulated by alteration in the mRNA levels in the cell. The possibility of thyroid hormone affecting the translation rate would only be evident in these experiments if a disparity existed between the relative mRNA levels

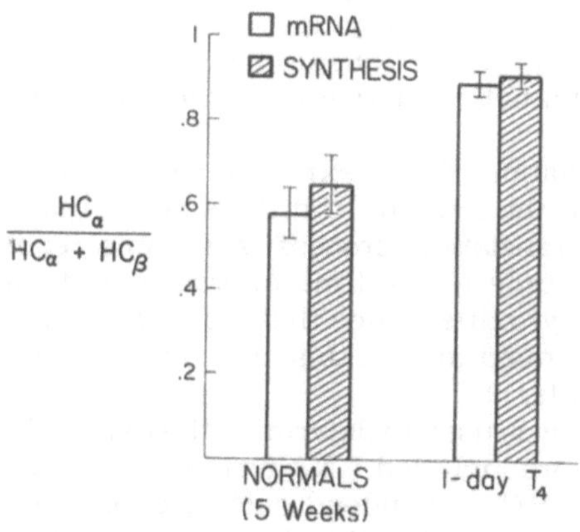

Fig. 3. Relationship between the relative synthesis rates and mRNA levels of the α and β cardiac myosin heavy chains in normal and thyrotoxic rabbits. The figure shows HCα synthesis rate and mRNA level expressed as a fraction of total heavy chain synthesis and total myosin mRNA in 4–6 week old rabbits. Bars represent the mean ± S.E. of 3 determinations. Synthesis rates are expressed in terms of mg HC synthesized/g tissue/day, and were calculated from the product of the fractional synthesis rate (day^{-1}) and the pool size of each heavy chain (mg/g tissue). The pool size of each HC was obtained by first measuring the total HC content of the myocardium (16), and then determining the relative contribution of each HC to this total from the ventricular content of V1 (HCα) and V3 (HCβ) as determined by native gel electrophoresis (2). The V2 isomyosin was ignored in this analysis.

and synthesis rates of the heavy chains. This did not appear to be the case, at least at 1 day thyroxine treatment.

Discussion

The thyrotoxic state in rabbits is associated with cardiac hypertrophy, and with a shift in the cardiac myosin composition toward the high ATPase V1 isomyosin. We show here that this results from an increase in the synthesis rate of myosin HCα (V1) and decrease in that of HCβ (V3). Furthermore, these changes in heavy chain synthesis were accompanied by similar changes in the relative amounts of the mRNAs for these proteins.

The alteration in myosin gene expression caused by thyroid hormone could result from direct and/or indirect actions on the heart. At least some direct effects might be anticipated based on the rapid and dramatic changes in the myosin synthesis rates and mRNA levels that were observed. This is further supported by our data obtained with D-thyroxine. This isomer resulted in the accumulation of V1 in the ventricles in the absence of significant change in peripheral metabolism that might indirectly effect the heart.

An additional component to the action of the hormone on myosin synthesis may be mediated via the sympathetic nervous system. Many of the cardiovascular changes seen in thyrotoxicosis are similar to those seen upon stimulation of sympathetic nerves. It is clear, however, that simple β-receptor blockade does not appear to affect myosin expression in the heart (6, 15) although chemical sympathectomy with 6-hydroxydopamine does (12, 15). Clearly, the relationship between thyroid hormone, myosin synthesis and sympathetic innervation of the heart deserves further attention.

As far as the regulation of gene expression by the hormone is concerned, our data imply that the amount of mRNA rather than the rate of mRNA utilization in the translation process is a prime regulatory event. This conclusion applies only to the time interval investigated, namely 1 day after injection of thyroxine. Since the effect of thyroid hormone on HCα synthesis is already maximum at this time, one has to direct future studies to even earlier events.

Total tissue RNA was used to determine the relative levels of the myosin mRNAs and therefore included RNA from the nucleus and cytoplasm, as well as any stored RNA, if indeed such a pool exists in the heart. At present we cannot say whether the change in the relative amounts of the mRNAs results from altered rates of transcription or from a change in the rate of HCα and/or HCβ mRNA processing. Additional experiments will be required to answer these questions.

Acknowledgements

This investigation was supported in part by United States Public Health Service Grants HL20592, HL16627, and HL09172 from the National Heart, Lung, and Blood Institute, and a grant from the Muscular Dystrophy Association of America.

A.W.E. is a Senior Research Fellow of the Chicago Heart Association.

References

1. Lompre, A. M., J. J. Mercadier, C. Wisnewsky, P. Bouveret, C. Pantaloni, A. d'Albis, K. Schwartz: Species and age-dependent changes in the relative amounts of cardiac myosin isoenzymes in mammals. Develop. Biol. **84,** 286–290 (1981).
2. Clark, W. A., R. A. Chizzonite, A. W. Everett, M. Rabinowitz, R. Zak: Species correlations between cardiac isomyosins: A comparison of electrophoretic and immunological properties. J. Biol. Chem. **257,** 5449–5454 (1982).
3. Flink, I. L., J. H. Rader, E. Morkin: Thyroid hormone stimulates synthesis of a cardiac myosin isoenzyme. J. Biol. Chem. **254,** 3105–3110 (1979).
4. Chizzonite, R. A., A. W. Everett, W. A. Clark, S. Jakovcic, M. Rabinowitz, R. Zak: Isolation and characterization of two molecular varients of myosin heavy chain from rabbit ventricle: Change in their content during normal growth and after treatment with thyroid hormone. J. Biol. Chem. **257,** 2056–2065 (1982).
5. Sinha, A. M., P. K. Umeda, C. J. Kavinsky, C. Rajamanickam, H.-J. Hsu, S. Jakovcic, M. Rabinowitz: Molecular cloning of mRNA sequences for cardiac α- and β-form myosin heavy chains: Expression in ventricles of normal, hypothyroid and thyrotoxic rabbits. Proc. Nat. Acad. Sci. U.S.A. **79,** 5847–5851 (1982).
6. Everett, A. W., W. A. Clark, R. A. Chizzonite, R. Zak: Change in synthesis rates of α- and β-myosin heavy chains in rabbit heart after treatment with thyroid hormone. J. Biol. Chem. 258 (1982), in press.
7. Hoh, J. F. Y., P. A. McGrath, P. T. Hale: Electrophoretic analysis of multiple forms of rat cardiac myosin: Effects of hypophysectomy and thyroxine replacement. J. Mol. Cell. Cardiol. **10,** 1053–1076 (1978).
8. Sartore, S., L. Gorza, S. Pierobon-Bormioli, L. Dalla Libera, S. Schiaffino: Myosin types and fiber types in Cardiac Muscle I. Ventricular Myocardium. J. Cell. Biol. **88,** 226–233 (1981).
9. Rupp, H.: Polymorphic myosin as the common determinant of myofibrillar ATPase in different haemodynamic and thyroid states. Basic Res. Cardiol. **77,** 34–46 (1982).
10. Dillman: Influence of thyroid hormone administration on myosin ATPase activity and myosin isoenzyme distribution in the heart of diabetic rats. Metabolism **31,** 199–204 (1982).
11. Mercadier, J. J., A. M. Lompre, C. Wisnewsky, J. L. Samuel, J. Bercovici, B. Swynghedauw, K. Schwartz: Myosin isoenzymes changes in several models of rat cardiac hypertrophy. Circulat. Res. **49,** 525–532 (1981).
12. Rupp, H., R. Jacob: Response of blood pressure and cardiac myosin polymorphism to swimming training in the spontaneously hypertensive rat. Can. J. Physiol. Pharmacol. **60,** 1098–1103 (1982).
13. Everett, A. W., G. Prior, R. Zak: Equilibration of leucine between the plasma compartment and leucyl-tRNA in the heart, and turnover of cardiac myosin heavy chain. Biochem. J. **194,** 365–368 (1981).
14. Gunning, J. F., C. E. Harrison, H. N. Coleman: Myocardial contractility and energetics following treatment with D-thyroxine. Amer. J. Physiol. **226,** 1166–1171 (1974).
15. Dowell, R. T.: Myofibrillar ATPase activity in rat heart after chronic propranolol administration. Amer. J. Physiol. **237,** C195–C199 (1979).
16. Everett, A. W., G. Prior, W. A. Clark, R. Zak: Quantitation of myosin in muscle. Anal. Biochem. (1983), in press.

Authors' address:

Prof. Radovan Zak, Department of Medicine Box 407, University of Chicago, 950 East 59 Street, Chicago, Illinois 60637, USA.

Cardiac Adaptation to Hemodynamic Overload, Training and Stress
Dr. D. Steinkopff Verlag 46–52 (1983)

Dissociation between factors resulting in hypertrophy and changes in myosin isoenzyme population of the pressure-loaded rat heart

H. Rupp, N. Popova, and R. Jacob

Physiologisches Institut II der Universität Tübingen (FRG)

Summary

The interrelationship between cardiac hypertrophy induced by increased pressure load and concomitant changes in the myocardial myosin isoenzyme population was studied. In order to induce severe load on predominantly one ventricle, 6-week-old Wistar rats were fed on seeds of the plant Crotalaria spectabilis for 4 weeks. The ensuing pulmonary hypertension resulted in significant hypertrophy of only the right ventricle (52 %). In contrast, the isoenzyme population of myosin was affected in both ventricles, more so, however, in the right ventricle, as shown by the proportion of ventricular myosin (VM)-3 given as a percentage of the 3 ventricular myosin isoenzymes (right ventricle 29.7 ± 4.8 % VM-3 vs. 20.6 ± 5.3 % VM-3 of left ventricle; VM-3 of left and right ventricles of control rats was 9.3 ± 1.8 %). Since thyroid hormones are major determinants of cardiac myosin isoenzymes and since Crotalaria spectabilis also affects other organs beside the lungs, serum thyroxine was determined. The thyroid hormone was significantly reduced, not, however, thyroxine binding index. The results suggest that reduced concentrations of circulating thyroid hormones contribute to the shift towards VM-3 in the myosin isoenzyme population. Since normal adult rats also exhibit an increased proportion of VM-3 in the predominantly loaded ventricle, it is concluded that beside the action of thyroid hormones, other mechanisms are responsible for the expression of the different myosin isoenzymes, such as those arising from altered adrenergic responsiveness and transmitter status of myocardium.

Key words: hypertrophy, myosin isoenzymes, Crotalaria spectabilis, pulmonary hypertension, thyroid hormones

Introduction

It is well documented that pressure load of the heart results in increased cardiac mass primarily due to hypertrophy of the myocytes. Generally, hypertrophy is induced only in the ventricle which is subjected to increased haemodynamic load. Beside the increase in muscle mass, the heart reacts to the altered haemodynamic load by a changed expression of genes coding for myosin isoenzymes. Increase in pressure load of the heart results in alteration of the ventricular myosin isoenzyme profile in favour of VM-3 (10, 11, 14, 17), which can be traced to altered myosin heavy chain structure (9, 10). Such a structural change results in reduced ATPase activity (5, 10–12, 15, 17, 18), velocity of shortening of muscle fibres (2, 21), and reduced oxygen consumption of the heart working under nearly isovolumetric conditions (8). In order to elucidate a possible relationship between mechanisms involved in the hypertrophy process and in the expression of different myosin isoenzymes, a model of hypertrophy was chosen which produced severe load predominantly on one ventricle and led to massive enlargement of the heart. For this purpose, rats were fed on seeds of the plant Crotalaria spectabilis, which led to pulmonary hypertension (3, 7). Myosin in the left and the right ventricle was analyzed using non-dissociating gel electrophoresis. Since thyroid hormone status represents a major determinant for the expression of myosin isoenzymes (2, 5, 10, 12, 15, 18, 20) and since Crotalaria spectabilis induces alterations in other organs (13) in addition to pulmonary hypertension, the concentration of thyroxine was determined in the serum.

Methods

Animals and materials

6-week-old Wistar (WU) rats were obtained from Ivanovas (Kisslegg, FRG). The control group was fed on a pellet diet (Ssniff, Soest, FRG) and the experimental group on the pellet diet C 1000 (Altromin, Lage, FRG) containing ground seeds of Crotalaria spectabilis (0.2 %, w/w). Water was ad libitum. Treatment extended over 4 weeks. In the first 3 weeks, there were no deaths, but in the 4th week, attrition amounted to 30 %. Blood was collected from the tail under ether anaesthesia; the heart was excised, trimmed and cut open to expose both ventricles, and blotted before weighing. The weights of the septum and left ventricle were combined and referred to as left ventricular weight. Reagents for electrophoresis were from Serva (Heidelberg, FRG). All other chemicals were of analytical grade whenever available. Seeds of the plant Crotalaria spectabilis were obtained from Beltsville Agricultural Research Center, Beltsville, Maryland 20705, U.S.A.

Thyroid hormones

Serum thyroxine concentrations were measured by a specific radioimmunoassay. Thyroxine binding index was determined using Enzymunassay TBI (Boehringer, Mannheim, FRG), which is based on an enzyme-linked immunosorbent assay. It can be used for indirect estimation of the protein-binding of thyroxine.

Pyrophosphate gel electrophoresis

Non-dissociating gel electrophoresis in the presence of pyrophosphate (5) was carried out as reported by Rupp and Jacob (19).

Results

Figure 1 shows the weight of left and right ventricles as a function of body weight of rats after Crotalaria spectabilis ingestion, and maturing control rats. The hypertrophy process induced by increased pulmonary resistance was restricted to the right ventricle. The mass of the right ventricle was increased by 52 %, whereas the left ventricle was not significantly affected when compared to control rats. When ventricular weight was related to body weight on the basis of the curve given in figure 1, then hypertrophy of the left ventricle was also small.

In figure 2, representative gels are shown containing myosins of left and right ventricles. The control rats exhibited predominantly VM-1 in the left

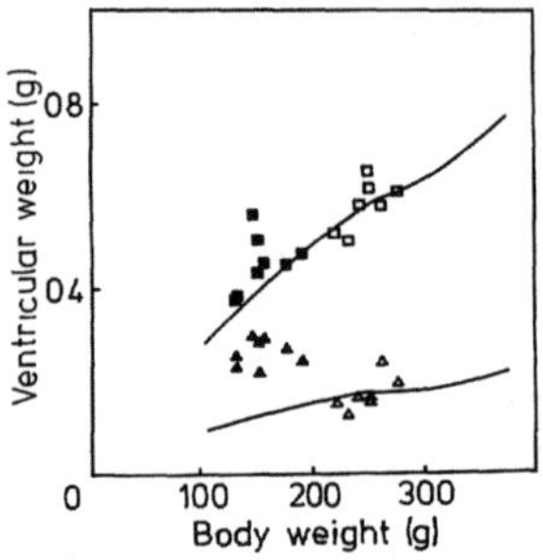

Fig. 1. Body weight was plotted versus weight of right (lower curve, triangles) and left ventricles (upper curve, squares) for (open symbols) control rats and (filled symbols) rats fed on seeds of the plant Crotalaria spectabilis. The curves were established in control rats (data points not shown) of the respective body weights using a least-squares procedure based on polynomials. Note, above approximately 300 g body weight, the ventricular weight vs. body weight relation can be described by a line-through-the-origin (for an example, see ref. 19).

and right ventricles. Following 4 weeks of pulmonary hypertension, the myosin population was changed in favour of VM-3 in left and right ventricles (figure 2). Electrophoretic mobilities of the three isoenzymes were identical in both groups of rats. Figure 3 shows the differences in the relative proportion of VM-3 given as a percentage for individual rats. There was no significant change in composition of left and right ventricular myosin in the 10-week-old control rats (also when taking into account a greater number of rats, not shown). The isoenzyme VM-3 was present only in a low amount (73.4 ± 1.8 % VM-1, 17.3 ± 1.4 % VM-2, 9.3 ± 1.8 % VM-3). In contrast, the proportion of VM-3 was markedly increased in rats with pulmonary hypertension. Right ventricle: 40.7 ± 5.7 % VM-1, 29.6 ± 3.3 % VM-2, 29.7 ± 4.8 % VM-3; left ventricle: 47.2 ± 7.7 % VM-1, 32.3 ± 2.9 %

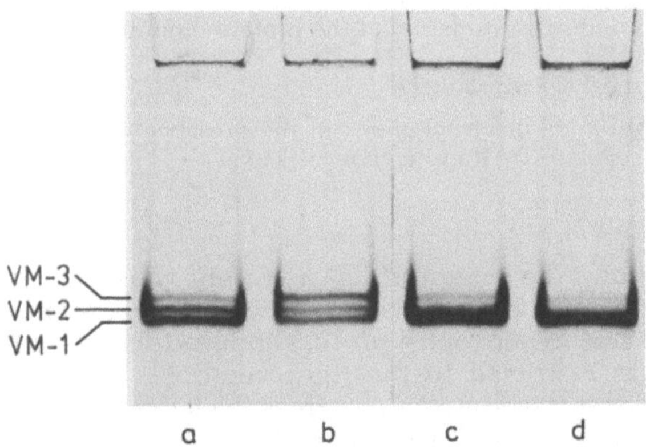

Fig. 2. Representative pyrophosphate gels of ventricular myosins isolated from a rat fed on seeds of Crotalaria spectabilis (a, left ventricle; b, right ventricle) and a corresponding control rat (c, left ventricle; d, right ventricle). Nomenclature as suggested by Zak (24).

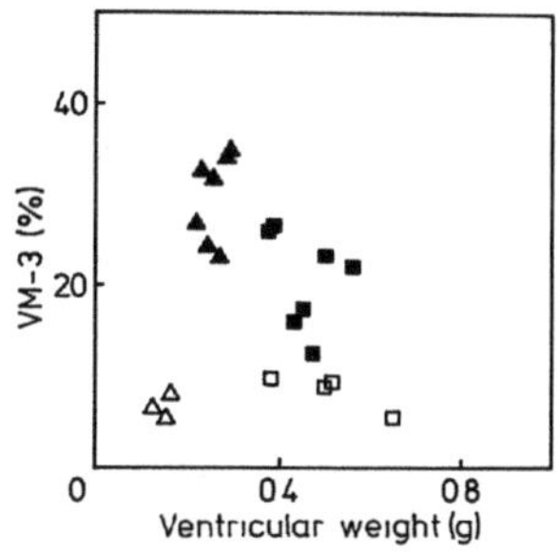

Fig. 3. Proportions of VM-3 of myosins isolated from individual ventricles were plotted versus ventricular weights for (open symbols) control rats and (filled symbols) rats fed on seeds of Crotalaria spectabilis. Myosins from right ventricles are represented by triangles, from left ventricles by squares.

VM-2, 20.6 ± 5.3 % VM-3. The differences between left and right ventricles were statistically significant ($P < 0.01$; Student's t-test) only for VM-3, not, however, for VM-1 or VM-2 ($P > 0.05$). Since thyroid hormone status is critical in determining the myosin isoenzyme population, the concentration of thyroxine and thyroxine binding index were determined in the serum (table 1). In rats fed on Crotalaria spectabilis seeds, the concentration of thyroxine was reduced significantly, whereas thyroxine binding index was not affected.

Discussion

Hypertrophy

Pulmonary hypertension induced by feeding of rats on Crotalaria spectabilis seeds resulted in massive hypertrophy of the right ventricle. Cardiac enlargement thus seems closely linked to work load. If hypertrophy in the present model was induced by factors arising from sites other than the heart, one would hardly expect to detect the selective regional response. One has to assume that a factor closely linked to haemodynamic load is responsible for the hypertrophy process. Among possible mechanisms (23), increased wall stress and a selective increase in sympathetic nerve activity in localized regions of the heart (16) should be considered.

Myosin isoenzyme population

In contrast to the mass increase of a selective region of the heart in the present model is the response of the myosin isoenzyme population:

Table 1. Serum thyroxine concentration and thyroxine binding index.

	Controls	Crotalaria spectabilis-treated
Thyroxine (µg/dl)	8.14 ± 0.44 (9)	5.48 ± 0.40 (5)^{x}
Thyroxine binding index	1.15 ± 0.05 (9)	1.14 ± 0.03 (6)^{NS}

Values are given as means ± SEM for (n) animals. The statistical significance was assessed with Student's t-test; ^{x} = $P < 0.001$ compared with control animals, ^{NS} = not significant ($P > 0.05$).

although mass of the left ventricle is not significantly changed, the myosin isoenzyme profile is altered in a manner characteristic for the pressure-loaded ventricle. A similar situation holds for 15–21 weeks spontaneously hypertensive rats (Rupp, unpublished).

As regards the determinants of myosin isoenzymes, thyroid hormone status should be considered (2, 5, 6, 15, 18, 20). Thyroid hormones are well documented to affect the myosin isoenzyme population following treatment of the rat with agents which induce hyperthyroidism or hypothyroidism (2, 5, 15, 18). Furthermore, there is good evidence that thyroid hormones play a major role in determining the myosin isoenzyme population during normal development of the rat. There exists a close correlation between thyroid hormone concentrations in the blood and the isoenzyme profile (6, 20): neonates exhibit very low thyroid hormone concentrations, which is reflected in the predominance of VM-3. 4–5 weeks rats exhibit the highest thyroid concentrations, due to the development of the hypothalamo-pituitary-thyroid axis in the neonatal rat (1). The high thyroid hormone concentration is associated with the exclusive presence of VM-1 in rat ventricles. During maturation, thyroid hormone concentrations decrease which is correlated with a redistribution towards VM-3. In the present study, the concentration of thyroxine was found to be decreased in the serum of rats treated with Crotalaria spectabilis. Since thyroid binding index was not altered significantly, the concentration of free thyroxine is expected to be reduced as well. The decreased thyroid hormone status is considered to be characteristic for the treatment with Crotalaria spectabilis and not for other forms of hypertension. The reduced concentrations of circulating thyroid hormones result most probably in an increased proportion of VM-3, whereby left and right ventricles are expected to be affected to the same extent. Since in rats treated with Crotalaria spectabilis (figure 3), in normal rats older than approximately 10 weeks and in spontaneously hypertensive rats (14; Rupp, unpublished), the ventricle exposed to the higher load exhibits more VM-3 than the other, one has to assume additional regulatory mechanisms. The observed isoenzymatic changes could thus be separated into changes arising from given concentrations of circulating thyroid hormones and additional factors linked with the haemodynamic load imposed on the heart. In this respect, it should be mentioned that catecholamines are probably also involved in the regulation of myosin isoenzymes (19; Sreter, personal communication). For example, transmitter depletion of myocardium resulting from treatment with 6-hydroxydopamine leads to a redistribution of the myosin isoenzyme population towards VM-3. Furthermore, isoproterenol in low doses results in an increased proportion of VM-1, whereas in high doses it induces a reduced proportion of VM-1 (unpublished data). Since transmitter depletion of pressure-loaded myocardium (22) and loss of adrenergic responsiveness (4) are also present in the ventricle not subjected to greatly increased load, but more pronounced in the loaded ventricle which responds with hypertrophy, mechanisms arising from altered sympathetic activity, adrenergic responsiveness, and transmitter depletion are good candidates for contributing to the different myosin isoenzyme profiles in left and right ventricles of normal and pressure-loaded hearts.

In sum, the results suggest a dissociation between the hypertrophy process and the expression of the myosin isoenzyme population. This differential regulation could arise from: (i) mechanisms which affect the myosin isoenzyme population, but do not alter cardiac mass; alternatively, stimuli may exist which are specific for the hypertrophy process. (ii) The responsiveness to a possible common trigger may be different as regards regulation of gene expression for myosin isoenzymes compared with regulation of the hypertrophy process. For example, a common stimulus could elicit an altered myosin isoenzyme population, but could be insufficient for inducing hypertrophy. The concept of a dissociation between hypertrophy and the expression of myosin isoenzymes seems noteworthy, since it suggests the principle possibility of changing the myosin isoenzyme population in the direction of VM-1 or VM-3 without necessarily affecting cardiac mass. Since a change in the myosin isoenzyme population is accompanied by changes in other cellular functions, one should be in a position to alter the functional state of heart at a given muscle mass which, in turn, would primarily depend on the haemodynamic load. Furthermore, it would thus be conceivable that depending on the model leading to pressure load, the functional state of heart could differ widely, although cardiac enlargement might be the same. Further work is required for defining the nature of the regulatory mechanisms involved in the induction of cardiac hypertrophy on the one hand, and the expression of genes coding for myosin isoenzymes on the other hand.

Acknowledgements

This study was supported by the Deutsche Forschungsgemeinschaft (Ja 172/13). Dr. N. Popova was supported by a fellowship of the Deutscher Akademischer Austauschdienst. The skilful technical assistance of L. Schwarz is gratefully acknowledged.

References

1. Dussault, J. H., P. Walker: The effect of iodine deficiency and propylthiouracil on the hypothalamo-pituitary-thyroid axis in the neonatal rat. Can. J. Physiol. Pharmacol. **56,** 950–955 (1978).
2. Ebrecht, G., H. Rupp, R. Jacob: Alterations of mechanical parameters in chemically skinned preparations of rat myocardium as a function of isoenzyme pattern of myosin. Basic Res. Cardiol. **77,** 220–234 (1982).
3. Gibson K., P. Harris: The distribution of microsomal (Na^+, K^+)-ATPase in the rat heart and the effects of induced right ventricular hypertrophy and feeding with digitalis, sodium, and potassium. Cardiovasc. Res. **4,** 6–13 (1970).
4. Hein, B., J. Janke: Restriction of β-adrenergic responsiveness in hypertrophied ventricular myocardium of rats. Basic Res. Cardiol. **72,** 279–285 (1977).
5. Hoh, J. F. Y., P. A. McGrath, P. T. Hale: Electrophoretic analysis of multiple forms of rat cardiac myosin: Effects of hypophysectomy and thyroxine replacement. J. Mol. Cell. Cardiol. **10,** 1053–1076 (1978).
6. Jacob, R., H. Rupp, G. Ebrecht, R. W. Gülch, G. Kissling: Chronic reaction of myocardium at the myofibrillar level. The functional significance of the isoenzyme pattern of myosin. In: Cardiac Structure and Metabolism, Nagano, M., I. Seki (eds.), pp. 1–28, Roppo Verlag (Tokyo 1981).
7. Kay, J. M., P. Harris, D. Heath: Pulmonary hypertension produced in rats by ingestion of Crotalaria spectabilis seeds. Thorax **22,** 176–179 (1967).

8. Kissling, G., H. Rupp, L. Malloy, R. Jacob: Alterations in cardiac oxygen consumption under chronic pressure overload. Significance of the isoenzyme pattern of myosin. Basic Res. Cardiol. **77,** 255–269 (1982).
9. Klotz, C., B. Swynghedauw, H. Mendes, F. Marotte, J. J. Leger: Evidence for new forms of cardiac myosin heavy chains in mechanical heart overloading and in ageing. Eur. J. Biochem. **115,** 415–421 (1981).
10. Litten, R. Z., III, B. J. Martin, R. B. Low, N. R. Alpert: Altered myosin isozyme pattern from pressure-overloaded and thyrotoxic hypertrophied rabbit hearts. Circulat. Res. **50,** 856–864 (1982).
11. Lompré, A.-M., K. Schwartz, A. d'Albis, G. Lacombe, N. Van Thiem, B. Swynghedauw: Myosin isoenzyme redistribution in chronic heart overload. Nature **282,** 105–107 (1979).
12. Martin, A. F., E. D. Pagani, R. J. Solaro: Thyroxine-induced redistribution of isoenzymes of rabbit ventricular myosin. Circulat. Res. **50,** 117–124 (1982).
13. McLean, E. K.: The toxic actions of pyrrolizidine (Senecio) alkaloids. Pharmacol. Rev. **22,** 429–483 (1970).
14. Mercadier, J.-J., A.-M. Lompré, C. Wisnewsky, J.-L. Samuel, J. Bercovici, B. Swynghedauw, K. Schwartz: Myosin isoenzymic changes in several models of rat cardiac hypertrophy. Circulat. Res. **49,** 525–532 (1981).
15. Pope, B., J. F. Y. Hoh, A. Weeds: The ATPase activities of rat cardiac myosin isoenzymes. FEBS Lett. **118,** 205–208 (1980).
16. Randall, W. C., M. Szentivanyi, J. B. Pace, J. S. Wechsler, M. P. Kaye: Pattern of sympathetic nerve projections onto the canine heart. Circulat. Res. **22,** 315–323 (1968).
17. Rupp, H.: The adaptive changes in the isoenzyme pattern of myosin from hypertrophied rat myocardium as a result of pressure overload and physical training. Basic Res. Cardiol. **76,** 79–88 (1981).
18. Rupp, H.: Polymorphic myosin as the common determinant of myofibrillar ATPase in different haemodynamic and thyroid states. Basic Res. Cardiol. **77,** 34–46 (1982).
19. Rupp, H., R. Jacob: Response of blood pressure and cardiac myosin polymorphism to swimming training in the spontaneously hypertensive rat. Can. J. Physiol. Pharmacol. **60,** 1098–1103 (1982).
20. Rupp, H., G. Kissling, R. Jacob: The hormonal and hemodynamic determinants of polymorphic myosin. In: Perspectives in Cardiovascular Research, Vol. 7, Myocardial Hypertrophy and Failure, Alpert, N. R. (ed.), 373–383 Raven Press (New York 1983).
21. Schwartz, K., Y. Lecarpentier, J. L. Martin, A. M. Lompré, J. J. Mercadier, B. Swynghedauw: Myosin isoenzymic distribution correlates with speed of myocardial contraction. J. Mol. Cell. Cardiol. **13,** 1071–1075 (1981).
22. Spann, J. F., Jr., R. A. Buccino, E. H. Sonnenblick, E. Braunwald: Contractile state of cardiac muscle obtained from cats with experimentally produced ventricular hypertrophy and heart failure. Circulat. Res. **21,** 341–354 (1967).
23. Zak, R., M. Rabinowitz: Molecular aspects of cardiac hypertrophy. Ann. Rev. Physiol. **41,** 539–552 (1979).
24. Zak, R.: Contractile function as a determinant of muscle growth. In: Cell and Muscle Motility, Vol. 1, Dowben, R. M., J. W. Shay (eds.) 1–33, Plenum Publishing Corporation (New York 1981).

Authors' address:

Physiologisches Institut II der Universität Tübingen, Gmelinstraße 5, 7400 Tübingen, FRG.

Cardiac Adaptation to Hemodynamic Overload, Training and Stress
Dr. D. Steinkopff Verlag 53–58 (1983)

Dissociation of hypertrophy and altered function in senescent rat myocardium

E. G. Lakatta

Gerontology Research Center, National Institute on Aging, National Institutes of Health, Baltimore, Maryland 21224 (U.S.A.)

Summary

In the rat aging model functional and biochemical alterations of senescence are accompanied by myocardial hypertrophy. The studies described herein indicate that this hypertrophy (1) does not involve a concomitant alteration in myofibrillar ATPase activity, (2) is not the cause of prolonged contraction times, i.e., time-to-peak force and relaxation time observed in the senescent heart.

Key words: adult aging, rat myocardium, isometric contraction, isolated cardiac muscle, myofibrillar ATPase, cardiac hypertrophy, chronic exercise

Introduction

Studies in several species, including man, have documented that myocardial hypertrophy occurs with adult aging, i.e., from adulthood to senescence (9). Structural, functional, and biochemical changes that accompany aging from maturation to senescence are similar to those induced by experimental hypertrophy produced in younger animals. These changes include an increase in collagen content, changes in passive viscoelastic properties, prolonged contraction duration, prolongation of the transmembrane action potential, a reduction in myocardial catecholamine levels, a diminished rate of Ca^{2+} sequestration in sarcoplasmic reticulum, diminished rate of hydrolysis of ATP by myofilaments, and a diminution in the rate of protein synthesis (6, 10, 19). Thus it might be postulated that myocardial aging over the adult range may be, in large part, explained by hypertrophy per se. Several recent studies in the rat aging model have addressed this issue and will be discussed in this presentation.

The effect of adult aging on relative heart mass has been quantitated in the Wistar rat (18). Figure 1 illustrates that left ventricular mass relative to body weight is fairly stable from young adulthood to late mid life, i.e., 6 mo through 16–18 mo; thereafter a progressive increase is observed through 24 mo, the magnitude of which is approximately 35–40 %. Left ventricular weight itself increases by about 15–20 % over this interval (18). While collagen content doubles during this period, it can only account for a 2–4 % increase in left ventricular weight (17). Histologic measurements estimate a 15–20 % increase in myocardial cell volume suggesting that most of the

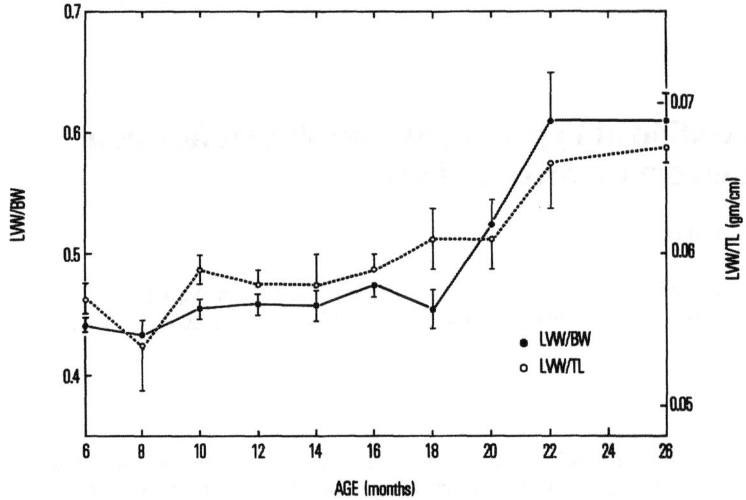

Fig. 1. The effect of adult age on the ratio of left ventricle + septal dry weight to body weight (LVW/WB) and to dry tibial length (LVW/TL) in the Wistar rat. From Yin et al. (18).

increase in cardiac mass is attributable to an increase in myocyte size (18). When tibial length, rather than body weight, is used as an estimate of body size, the extent of hypertrophy that occurs with senescence is 17 % (fig. 1) and agrees well with the measured increase in left ventricular weight and estimates of increased myocyte volume. Thus the estimate of the extent of left ventricular hypertrophy referencing left ventricular weight to body weight is falsely high, because beginning at about 18 mo, a decrease in body weight begins and progresses into senescence (18). It is interesting to note that right ventricular weight does not increase and the right ventricular to tibial length ratio is not significantly altered with age over this range (18).

It is often generalized that myofilament ATP hydrolysis declines with aging. However most of this age effect occurs over the maturational aging period (fig. 2A). Note that over the range in which myocardial hypertrophy occurs, i.e., between 18 and 24 mo (fig. 1), myofibrillar ATPase activity in the same (Wistar) rat strain is unaltered (2). Thus cardiac hypertrophy in the senescent rat occurs in the absence of a change in myofibrillar ATPase activity (closed symbol), indicating that hypertrophy, per se, need not produce an obligatory change in the rate of ATP hydrolysis by myofibrils. Note that ATPase activity in unregulated myofibrils, i.e., in an actomyosin preparation (open symbol) in the absence of troponin and tropomyosin, shows a similar pattern of age-related change but the magnitude of the age effect is substantially less (20 vs 50 %) than in purified myofibrils. A decline of similar magnitude over the maturational period has also been observed in the ATPase activity of actomyosin, myosin, and crude myofibrillar extracts in other studies (1, 5). The reduction in myosin ATPase activity occurring with maturation has been attributed to a change in the relative proportion of myosin isozymes (7, 11). However, the importance of

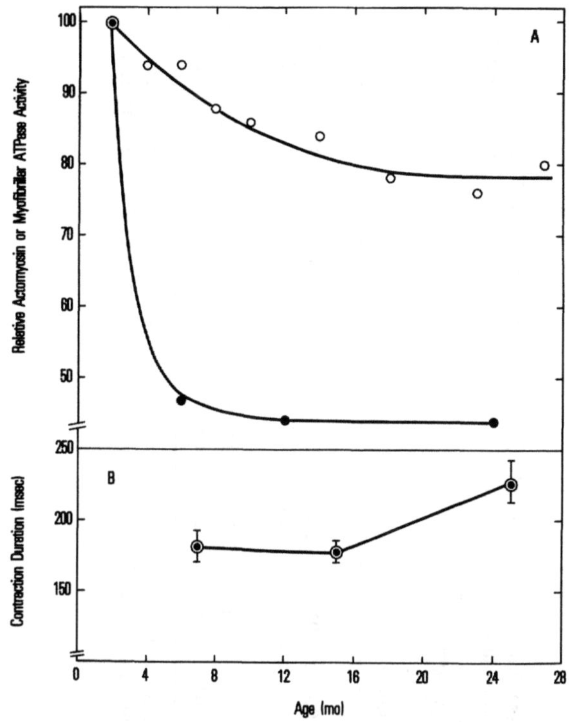

Fig. 2. A. The effect of age on actomyosin, ○, or myofibrillar ● ATPase activity in rat myocardium. The data have been normalized to that level measured at 2 mo of age. Actomyosin was prepared from hearts from Fischer 344 rats and ATPase activity was measured in fresh preparations by determining the amount of inorganic phosphate liberated from ATP after 3 minutes of incubation in [K^+] 60 mM, [ATP], 1.0 mM, pH 7.2; temperature 25 °C, and [Ca^{2+}] of 10 mM. At 2 mo of age ATPase activity was 260 nMol Pi min^{-1} mg $protein^{-1}$. Redrawn from Chesky and Rockstein (3). Myofibrils were prepared from the hearts of Wistar rats with slight modification of the procedure of Solaro et al. (13). ATPase activity was measured as the steady rate of Pi liberation at 25 °C in medium contain 100 mM KCl, 7 mM $MgCl_2$, 3 mM EGTA, 5 mM ATP, 25 mM imodizole, pH 7.0 and pCa 5.6. Myofibrillar ATPase activity at 2 mo of age was 0.17 μ moles Pi min^{-1} mg $protein^{-1}$. Redrawn from Bhatnagar et al. (1).
B. Contraction duration, measured as the time from stimulation to half relaxation of the isometric twitch as a function of age in left ventricular trabecular muscles from Wistar rats. From Yin et al. (19).

the present extent of phosphorylation of troponin on myofilament ATPase activity has also recently been emphasized (12). To establish to what extent functional changes in the myocardium that occur with maturation can be attributed to changes in myosin isoenzymes per se (7, 11), additional studies examining the effect of altered isoenzyme composition on *myofibrillar* ATPase are required.

The effect of adult aging on contraction duration of isolated isometric cardiac muscle (19) is illustrated in figure 2B. Note that contraction becomes prolonged over an age range in which myofibrillar ATPase is

Tab. 1. Effect of chronic exercise on left ventricular (LV) heart mass relative to tibial length (TL) and body weight (BW) and on time-to-peak force (TPF), half relaxation time (RT½), and their sum (CD) in isolated cardiac muscle from adult and senescent Wistar rats*).

	Age	LV WT (g)	$\frac{\text{LV WT}}{\text{BW}}$ (g/g × 10^3)	$\frac{\text{LV WT}}{\text{TL}}$ (g/cm)	TPT (m/sec)	RT½ (m/sec)	CD (m/sec)
Adult							
Control	7.9 ± 1.0	.254 ± .01	.421 ± .009	.056 ± .001	110.3 ± 3.9	77.4 ± 3.4	187.7 ± 6.7
Exercised	8.3 ± 0.9	.243 ± .01	.445 ± .013	.054 ± .001	110.9 ± 1.7	82.6 ± 3.5	193.5 ± 4.4
Senescent							
Control	23.5 ± 0.5	.280 ± .01	.565 ± .044	.060 ± .003	129.8 ± 6.3**)	102.9 ± 6.6***)	232.1 ± 12.3**)
Exercised	22.5 ± 0.9	.279 ± .01	.547 ± .037	.061 ± .037	112.9 ± 4.8***)	86.2 ± 2.0***)	191.1 ± 5.2***)

*) Experimental condition for contraction duration parameters were as in figure 2b. Resting and developed force, and maximum rate of force production were not age-related in control and were not altered by exercise in either age group. From Spurgeon et al. (15).

**) Significant age effect.

***) Significant exercise effect within age.

unchanged. Thus the prolonged contraction, i.e., time-to-peak force, relaxation time, or their sum in the senescent versus adult heart cannot readily be attributed to alterations in the rate of myofibrillar ATP hydrolysis. However, prolongation of contraction does occur over that age range in which hypertrophy occurs (fig. 1). Additional studies were undertaken to determine whether the two are related.

A chronic, low intensity, exercise protocol [running in motorized wheels driven at 0.7 Km/hr for 30 minutes, 5 days/week for 5 mo (15)], failed to alter heart weight, body weight, tibial length, heart mass relative to body weight, or tibial length in rats sacrified at 8 and 23 mo of age. Isometric contractions measured in left ventricular trabecular muscles from control, i.e., sedentary, aged matched, animals demonstrated the characteristic prolongation of-time-to-peak force and relaxation time with senescence. The mild exercise protocol did not alter the contraction in younger adult animals. Note, however, that in muscles from exercised senescent animals, both time-to-peak force and relaxation were markedly reduced to those levels in muscles from younger adults. Thus left ventricular hypertrophy persisted, but prolonged contraction was abolished by exercise in the senescent myocardium. This suggests that prolonged contraction in senescent myocardium is not the result of cardiac hypertrophy. A similar conclusion is also derived from other studies. In the absence of right ventricular hypertrophy, both the transmembrane action potential and contraction duration are prolonged in senescent versus younger adult papillary muscles isolated from right ventricles (16). Similarly, marked cardiac hypoplasia, i.e., a 50 % reduction in left ventricular weight relative to body weight or tibial length, in senescent animals produced by every other day feeding for 23 mo failed to alter contraction duration (14). This result is similar to that when atrophy of the senescent heart was caused by transplantation of the heart in a non-working mode into the abdominal cavity of another rat (8). In this regard, it is also noteworthy that the hyperthyroid state in senescent animals reduces contraction duration to those levels observed in the maturational period, without reducing heart mass or myofibrillar ATPase activity (4).

In conclusion, neither prolonged contraction duration, transmembrane action potential, or the level of myofibrillar ATPase activity can be directly linked to the concomitant myocardial hypertrophy in the senescent rat myocardium. Additional studies are required to determine whether other functional, structural, and biochemical alterations common to both hypertrophied myocardium produced experimentally and that naturally occurring in senescence (10) do in fact occur as a result of hypertrophy per se in the senescent heart.

References

1. Alpert, N. R., H. H. Gale, N. Taylor: The effect of age on contractile Protein ATPase activity and the velocity of shortening. In: Factors Influencing Myocardial Contractility, edited by R. D. Tanz, F. Kavaler, and J. Roberts, Academic Press, New York, pp. 127–133 (1967).
2. Bhatnagar, G. M., G. D. Walford, E. S. Beard, E. G. Lakatta: Dissociation of time to peak force (TPF) and myofibrillar ATPase activity (MF-ATPase) with aging of the myocardium (Abstract). Federation Proc. **41,** 1513 (1982).

3. Chesky, J. A., M. Rockstein: Reduced myocardial actomyosin adenosine triphosphatase activity in the ageing male Fischer rat. Cardiovasc. Res. **11,** 242–246 (1977).
4. Effron, M. B., G. Ruano-Arroyo, H. A. Spurgeon, G. M. Bhatnagar, E. G. Lakatta: Hyperthyroid state reverses prolonged contraction in rat cardiac muscle without altering myofibrillar ATPase activity (Abstract). Federation Proc. **42,** number 3, p. 465 (1983).
5. Heller, L. J., W. V. Whitehorn: Age-associated alteration in myocardial contractile properties. Amer. J. Physiol. **22,** 1613–1619 (1972).
6. Jacob, R., G. Ebrecht, A. Kammereit, I. Medugoras, M. F. Wendt-Gallitelli: Myocardial function in different models of cardiac hypertrophy. An attempt at correlating mechanical, biochemical, and morphological parameters. Basic Res. Cardiol. **72,** 160–167 (1977).
7. Klotz, C., B. Swynghedauw, H. Mendes, F. Marotte, J. J. Leger: Evidence for new forms of cardiac myosin heavy chains in mechanical heart overloading and in ageing. Eur. J. Biochem. **115,** 415–421 (1981).
8. Korecky, B.: The effects of load, internal environment and age on cardiac mechanics (Abstract). J. Mol. Cell. Cardiol. **11,** Suppl. 1, 33 (1979).
9. Lakatta, E. G.: Alterations in the cardiovascular system that occur in advanced age. Federation Proc. **38,** 163–167 (1979).
10. Lakatta, E. G., F. C. P. Yin: Myocardial aging: functional alterations and related cellular mechanisms. Amer. J. Physiol. **242** (Heart Circ. Physiol. 11), H927–941 (1982).
11. Mercadier, J.-J., A.-M. Lompre, C. Weisnewsky, J.-L. Samuel, J. Bercovici, B. Swynghedauw, K. Schwartz: Myosin isoenzymic changes in several models of rat cardiac hypertrophy. Circulat. Res. **49,** 525–532 (1981).
12. Resink, T. J., W. Gevers: Altered adenosine triphosphatase activities of natural actomyosin from rat hearts perfused with isoprenaline and ouabain. Cell Calcium **2,** 105–123 (1981).
13. Solaro, R. J., R. M. Wise, J. S. Shiner, F. N. Briggs: Calcium requirements of cardiac myofibrillar activation. Circulat. Res. **34,** 525–530 (1974).
14. Spurgeon, H. A., D. K. Ingram, E. G. Lakatta: Long-term food restriction causes cardiac atrophy but does not alter rat cardiac muscle performance (Abstract). Federation Proc. **42,** number 3, p. 466 (1983).
15. Spurgeon, H. A., M. F. Steinbach, E. G. Lakatta: Chronic exercise prevents characteristic age-related changes in rat cardiac contraction. Amer. J. Physiol. (in press) (1983).
16. Wei, J. Y., H. A. Spurgeon, E. G. Lakatta: Transmembrane action potential duration and contractile activation are lengthened in cardiac muscle of senescent rats (Abstract). Clin. Res. **28,** 619 (1980).
17. Weisfeldt, M. L., W. A. Loeven, N. W. Shock: Resting and active mechanical properties of trabeculae carneae from aged male rats. Amer. J. Physiol. **220,** 1921–1927 (1971).
18. Yin, F. C. P., H. A. Spurgeon, K. Rakusan, M. L. Weisfeldt, E. G. Lakatta: Use of tibial length to quantify cardiac hypertrophy: application in the aging rat. Amer. J. Physiol. **243** (Heart Circ. Physiol. 12), H941–947, 1982.
19. Yin, F. C. P., H. A. Spurgeon, M. L. Weisfeldt, E. G. Lakatta: Mechanical properties of myocardium from hypertrophied rat hearts. A comparison between hypertrophy induced by senescence and by aortic banding. Circulat. Res. **46,** 292–300 (1980).

Author's address:

Edward G. Lakatta, M.D., Cardiovascular Section, Gerontology Research Center, National Institute on Aging, Baltimore, Maryland 21224, USA.

Cardiac Adaptation to Hemodynamic Overload, Training and Stress
Dr. D. Steinkopff Verlag 59–64 (1983)

Differential effect of thyroid hormones on catecholamine enzymes and myosin isoenzymes in ventricles and atria of the rat heart

A. R. Bukhari and H. Rupp

Physiologisches Institut II der Universität Tübingen (FRG)

Summary

The effect of altered thyroid hormone status on myosin heterogeneity and catecholamine enzymes was investigated in ventricles and atria of the rat heart. Hypothyroidism (0.08 % propylthiouracil in drinking water for 6 weeks) and hyperthyroidism (daily 1 mg/kg thyroxine intraperitoneally for 2 weeks) resulted in homogeneous ventricular myosin (VM)-3 and VM-1, respectively, in rat ventricles. No such marked changes in the isoenzyme population were observed in atrial myosins using also as criterion the separation by non-dissociating pyrophosphate gel electrophoresis. Since the ventricular myosin isoenzyme population can additionally be altered by adrenergic agonists, the catecholamine enzymes phenylethanolamine-N-methyltransferase (PNMT), catechol-O-methyltransferase (COMT) and monoamine oxidase (MAO) were studied in ventricles versus atria of hypothyroid and hyperthyroid rats. As in the case of myosin isoenzymes, the response of PNMT, COMT and MAO to altered circulating thyroid hormones was different when determined in ventricles compared to atria. In ventricles, PNMT, COMT, and MAO activities were significantly reduced in hyperthyroid rats compared to hypothyroid rats, whereas an opposite change was found in atria: the enzyme activities were higher for the hyperthyroid relative to the hypothyroid state. The results suggest that ventricles and atria of rat heart differ in their response towards circulating thyroid hormones not only with respect to myosin heterogeneity, but also to catecholamine enzymes. The different action of altered thyroid status on catecholamine metabolism could thus be considered a factor contributing to the expression of the above myosin isoenzyme populations.

Key words: myosin, monoamine oxidase, catechol-O-methyltransferase, phenylethanolamine-N-methyltransferase, thyroid hormones

Introduction

Ventricular and atrial myosins of the rat are structurally different (3, 4, 6, 7, 10). Furthermore, ATPase activity of atrial myosin is higher compared to ventricular myosin (3, 6, 8, 10, 21). Maximal velocity of shortening of corresponding muscle fibres show a similar behaviour (8). These differences were detected in rats of normal thyroid status. A further difference seems to exist with respect to sensitivity towards thyroid hormones: Using separation by a non-denaturing gel system as a criterion, ventricular myosin isoenzymes proved to be very sensitive to changes in concentra-

Abbreviations: MAO = monoamine oxidase, COMT = catechol-O-methyltransferase, PNMT = phenylethanolamine-N-methyltransferase, VM = ventricular myosin.

tions of thyroid hormones (6, 16). Such behaviour has not been reported for atrial myosins. There is evidence that, beside thyroid hormones, catecholamines play a role in determining the myosin isoenzyme population (17; Sreter, personal communication). Furthermore, catecholamine metabolism (9) and adrenergic responsiveness (1, 20) are closely linked to thyroid hormone status. The question, therefore, arose as to whether enzymes involved in catecholamine metabolism also exhibit a differential response to thyroid hormones when studied in ventricles compared to atria. This approach should provide further evidence on possible links between mechanisms regulating myosin isoenzyme populations and catecholamine metabolism.

Methods

Animals and materials

12-week-old male Wistar (WU) rats were obtained from Ivanovas (Kissleg, FRG). Rats received a pellet diet (Ssniff, Soest, FRG) and tap water ad libitum. 6-n-propyl-2-thiouracil was from Sigma (München, FRG), l-thyroxine sodium salt from Serva (Heidelberg, FRG), S-adenosyl-L-[methyl-^{14}C] methionine from CEA (Saclay, France), and tryptamine bisuccinate, [side chain-2-^{14}C] from New England Nuclear (Boston, USA). All other chemicals were of analytical grade whenever available.

Experimental procedures

Hypothyroidism in 12-week-old rats was induced by adding 6-n-propyl-2-thiouracil to the drinking water (0.08 % in deionized water) for 6 weeks. Each rat received approximately 9–14 mg propylthiouracil per day. Hyperthyroidism was achieved by daily injections of l-thyroxine sodium salt in saline (1 mg/kg body weight, intraperitoneally) for 2 weeks. The rats were killed by decapitation approximately 17–20 h after the last thyroxine injection.

Assay of MAO, COMT, and PNMT

Left ventricles and left atria were homogenized in 0.9 % KCl, the homogenates were divided into two parts. The first part was diluted 1:10 (v/v) for determination of MAO activity, and protein determination according to Lowry et al. (11). The second part was centrifuged at 50,000 × g for 30 min at 1 °C. The supernatant was used for determination of COMT and PNMT activities. MAO was assayed using tryptamine[^{14}C] bisuccinate, and COMT, and PNMT were determined using S-adenosyl [methyl-^{14}C] methionine as described by Parvez and Parvez (14). The activities of MAO, COMT, and PNMT were expressed in cpm/mg protein. The extracted cpm was linearly proportional to the product formed.

Pyrophosphate gel electrophoresis

Gel electrophoresis in the presence of pyrophosphate was carried out as given elsewhere (17).

Results

Myosin isoenzyme population

Changes in concentrations of circulating thyroid hormones differentially affect ventricular and atrial myosin isoenzymes as judged from the electrophoretic mobility in pyrophosphate gels. In ventricles of hyperthyroid rats (daily 1 mg/kg thyroxine for 2 weeks), homogeneous VM-1 and in

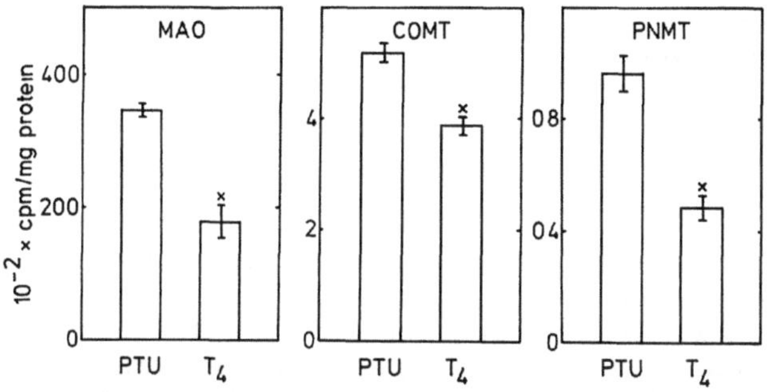

Fig. 1. Activities of MAO, COMT, and PNMT in left ventricles of rats made hypothyroid (n = 6) by treatment with propylthiouracil (PTU) and hyperthyroid (n = 6) by injections of thyroxine (T_4).
x = $P < 0.001$ (hyperthyroid vs. hypothyroid; Student's t-test)

hypothyroid rats (0.08 % propylthiouracil in drinking water for 5 weeks) homogeneous VM-3 were present. In contrast, atrial myosin, which was separated into 2 bands of higher electrophoretic mobility than VM-1, was not greatly affected. Irrespective of the treatment, 2 atrial myosin bands of nearly unchanged intensity were observed (not shown). Note, the nomenclature suggested by Zak (23) is used for ventricular myosins.

Catecholamine enzyme activities

The activities of the enzymes MAO, COMT, and PNMT of ventricular origin are given in figure 1. Rats were treated either with thyroxine or propylthiouracil. Hypothyroidism resulted in increased activities of the catecholamine degrading enzymes MAO, COMT, and of the adrenaline-synthesizing enzyme PNMT as compared to hyperthyroid rats. The enzyme activities in atria revealed an opposite phenomenon: in atria, hypothyroidism induced decreased enzyme activities relative to hyperthyroid rats (fig. 2). Thus there is a difference in the response of ventricular

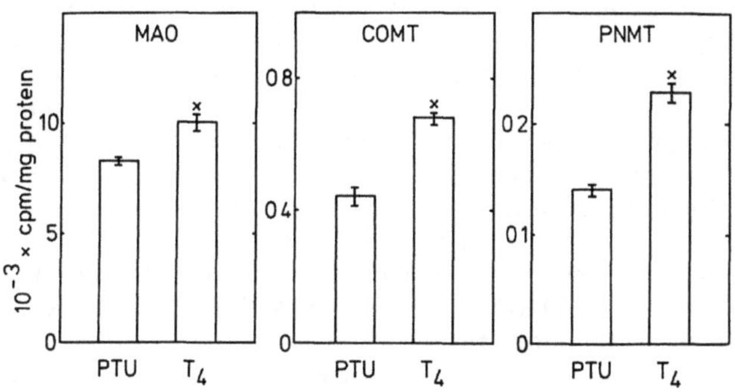

Fig. 2. Activities of MAO, COMT, and PNMT in left atria of rats made hypothyroid (n = 6) by treatment with propylthiouracil (PTU) and hyperthyroid (n = 6) by injections of thyroxine (T_4).
x = $P < 0.001$ (hyperthyroid vs. hypothyroid; Student's t-test)

and atrial catecholamine enzyme activities to changed concentrations of circulating thyroid hormones.

Discussion

Myosin isoenzyme population

According to Hoh (7), ventricular myosin isoenzymes in the rat heart differ in their heavy chain composition: VM-1 is considered to be a homodimer of $HC_\alpha HC_\alpha$ composition, VM-2 a heterodimer $HC_\alpha HC_\beta$ and VM-3 a homodimer of $HC_\beta HC_\beta$ composition. Since atrial myosin is structurally related to VM-1 (2), one might not expect a change in atrial myosin bands in pyrophosphate gels when rats become hyperthyroid. Intriguing is, however, the apparent lack of a change comparable to the shift towards VM-3 in ventricles subsequent to hypothyroidism. This could either be attributed to the failure of the pyrophosphate gel technique to detect an altered isoenzyme population or more probably to a different regulation of atrial myosin isoenzymes.

Catecholamine enzyme activities

Catecholamine enzymes in atria and ventricles were studied based on the observations of the different behaviour of ventricular and atrial myosins with respect to thyroid hormone status. Of the 3 enzymes studied in the present approach, only MAO is well characterized as regards the influence of thyroid hormones. In the young rat (up to approximately 200 g body weight), increased concentrations of circulating thyroid hormones induced an increase in MAO activity in the whole heart (12, 19). Hypothyroidism in young rats (up to approximately 175 g initial body weight) resulted in reduced MAO activity (12, 18). In contrast, hyperthyroidism in older rats slightly decreased MAO activity (5) or did not affect it (19) in agreement with the present data. The alterations in MAO activity were attributed to changes in the relative proportion of MAO-A (enhanced by hyperthyroidism) and MAO-B (enhanced by hypothyroidism) (13). In the present study, tryptamine was used as substrate for MAO which is predominantly deaminated by MAO-A (13, 22). Thus changes in overall MAO activity represent an altered proportion of MAO-A versus MAO-B (13) and/or an altered concentration of total enzyme molecules (15). The intriguing finding of the present study is that MAO in atria is influenced by thyroid hormones as would be expected for ventricles of young rats. Apparently, only ventricles undergo a change in their response with respect to thyroid hormones during maturation of the rat, not, however, atria. In this respect, it should be noted that COMT and PNMT, which are less well characterized with respect to thyroid hormone status, closely follow the pattern of MAO activities. COMT and PNMT activities were increased by 5 weeks of antithyroid treatment in rat ventricles. COMT and PNMT activities also followed the behaviour of MAO in atria: in hyperthyroid rats, both activities were increased relative to that of hypothyroid rats. In this respect it should be noted that the activities of MAO, COMT and PNMT in adrenal glands followed those in ventricles subsequent to altered thyroid hormone status.

We thus can conclude that the response of atria and ventricles to changed concentrations of thyroid hormones differs not only with respect to the myosin isoenzyme population, but also as regards catecholamine enzymes. The different action of altered thyroid hormone status on catecholamine metabolism could thus be considered a factor contributing to the expression of ventricular and atrial myosin isoenzyme populations. However, more work is required to determine the relative importance of the adrenergic system in different thyroid states as an additional determinant of myosin isoenzymes.

Acknowledgements

This study was supported by the Deutsche Forschungsgemeinschaft (Ja 172/13). We are indebted to Prof. Jacob for encouragement, support, and helpful discussions. The technical assistance of L. Schwarz is gratefully acknowledged.

References

1. Chang, H. Y., G. Kunos: Short term effects of triiodothyronine on rat heart adrenoceptors. Biochem. Biophys. Res. Commun. **100,** 313–320 (1981).
2. Clark, W. A., Jr., R. A. Chizzonite, A. W. Everett, M. Rabinowitz, R. Zak: Species correlations between cardiac isomyosins. A comparison of electrophoretic and immunological properties. J. Biol. Chem. **257,** 5449–5454 (1982).
3. Dalla Libera, L., S. Sartore, S. Schiaffino: Comparative analysis of chicken atrial and ventricular myosins. Biochim. Biophys. Acta **581,** 283–294 (1979).
4. Flink, I. L., J. H. Rader, S. K. Banerjee, E. Morkin: Atrial and ventricular cardiac myosins contain different heavy chain species. FEBS Lett. **94,** 125–130 (1978).
5. Ho-Van-Hap, A., L. M. Babineau, L. Berlinguet: Hormonal action on monoamine oxidase activity in rats. Can. J. Biochem. **45,** 355–362 (1967).
6. Hoh, J. F. Y., P. A. McGrath, P. T. Hale: Electrophoretic analysis of multiple forms of rat cardiac myosin: Effects of hypophysectomy and thyroxine replacement. J. Mol. Cell. Cardiol. **10,** 1053–1076 (1978).
7. Hoh, J. F. Y., G. P. S. Yeoh, M. A. W. Thomas, L. Higginbottom: Structural differences in the heavy chains of rat ventricular myosin isoenzymes. FEBS Lett. **97,** 330–334 (1979).
8. Korecky, B., L. Michael: Mechanical and biochemical relationship of atrial and ventricular contraction. Fed. Proc. Fed. Amer. Soc. Exp. Biol. **31,** 829 (1972).
9. Landsberg, L., J. Axelrod: Influence of pituitary, thyroid, and adrenal hormones on norepinephrine turnover and metabolism in the rat heart. Circ. Res. **22,** 559–571 (1968).
10. Long, L., F. Fabian, D. T. Mason, J. Wikman-Coffelt: A new cardiac myosin characterized from the canine atria. Biochem. Biophys. Res. Commun. **76,** 626–635 (1977).
11. Lowry, O. H., N. J. Rosebrough, A. L. Farr, R. J. Randall: Protein measurement with the folin phenol reagent. J. Biol. Chem. **193,** 265–275 (1951).
12. Lyles, G. A., B. A. Callingham: The effects of thyroid hormones on monoamine oxidase in the rat heart. J. Pharm. Pharmacol. **26,** 921–930 (1974).
13. Lyles, G. A., B. A. Callingham: Selective influences of age and thyroid hormones on type A monoamine oxidase of the rat heart. J. Pharm. Pharmacol. **31,** 755–760 (1979).
14. Parvez, H., S. Parvez: Microradioisotopic determination of enzymes COMT, PNMT and MAO in a single tissue homogenate. Clin. Chim. Acta **46,** 85–92 (1973).
15. Pletscher, A.: Regulation of catecholamine turnover by variations of enzyme levels. Pharmacol. Rev. **24,** 225–232 (1972).

16. Rupp, H.: Polymorphic myosin as the common determinant of myofibrillar ATPase in different haemodynamic and thyroid states. Basic Res. Cardiol. **77,** 34–46 (1982).
17. Rupp, H., R. Jacob: Response of blood pressure and cardiac myosin polymorphism to swimming training in the spontaneously hypertensive rat. Can. J. Physiol. Pharmacol. **60,** 1098–1103 (1982).
18. Skillen, R. G., C. H. Thienes, L. Strain: 5-hydroxytryptamine, 5-hydroxytryptophan decarboxylase and monoamine oxidase in hearts of normal, thyroid-fed and propylthiouracil-fed male and female rats. Endocrinology **70,** 743–746 (1962).
19. Tong, J. H., A. d'Iorio: Differential effects of L-thyroxine on cardiac and hepatic monoamine oxidase activity toward benzylamine and serotonin. Endocrinology **98,** 761–766 (1976).
20. Williams, L. T., R. J. Lefkowitz, A. M. Watanabe, D. R. Hathaway, H. R. Besch, Jr.: Thyroid hormone regulation of β-adrenergic receptor number. J. Biol. Chem. **252,** 2787–2789 (1977).
21. Yazaki, Y., S. Ueda, R. Nagai, K. Shimada: Cardiac atrial myosin adenosine triphosphatase of animals and humans. Distinctive enzymatic properties compared with cardiac ventricular myosin. Circ. Res. **45,** 522–527 (1979).
22. Youdim, M. B. H., M. Holzbauer: Physiological and pathological changes in tissue monoamine oxidase activity. J. Neural Transm. **38,** 193–229 (1976).
23. Zak, R.: Contractile function as a determinant of muscle growth. In: Cell and Muscle Motility, Vol. 1, Dowben, R. M., J. W. Shay (eds.) 1–33 Plenum Publishing Corporation (New York 1981).

Authors' address:

Physiologisches Institut II der Universität Tübingen, Gmelinstraße 5, 7400 Tübingen, FRG.

Cardiac Adaptation to Hemodynamic Overload, Training and Stress
Dr. D. Steinkopff Verlag 65–68 (1983)

The adrenals in experimental cardiac hypertrophy

F. Kölbel, V. Schreiber, J. Štěpán, T. Přibyl, and I. Gregorová

3rd Medical Department and the Laboratory for Endocrinology and Metabolism, Faculty of General Medicine, Charles University, Prague (CSSR)

Summary

1. The presence of the adrenals is essential for the development of experimental cardiac hypertrophy. In animals with experimental cardiac hypertrophy, the adrenal weight increases parallel to the heart weight. The increase of adrenal weight is not connected with increased plasma corticosterone or aldosterone levels.
2. The administration of digitoxin does not influence the extent of cardiac hypertrophy at the end of the third postoperative week following stenosis of the abdominal aorta in the rat. It does, however, block the increase of adrenal weight otherwise observed under these conditions.
3. In blood serum of animals with experimental cardiac hypertrophy, a factor was found reacting positively upon enzymoimmunoanalysis for digoxin. A positive correlation between the amount of this factor in the blood and the degree of cardiac and adrenal hypertrophy was found.
4. Several 14-OH derivatives of sex steroids, namely estradiol, display digoxin-like biological (inhibition of Na-K ATPase in situ) as well as immunological activity.

Key words: adrenal weight, experimental cardiac hypertrophy, heart weight, serum digoxin-like reactivity

Introduction

In this paper, we would like to focus the attention on three main topics:
1. the adrenal cortex and experimental cardiac hypertrophy,
2. digitoxin treatment in experimental cardiac hypertrophy,
3. endogenous digitalis-like activity in cardiac hypertrophy.

1 The adrenal cortex and experimental cardiac hypertrophy

Hypertrophy of the adrenals both in human (11) and in experimental cardiac hypertrophy (5) was described many years ago, but, for a long time, no special attention was paid to its significance. In 1964, Margaret Beznak has shown (1) that the adrenals are essential for the development of cardiac hypertrophy in rats with coarctation of the abdominal aorta. Several years later we have found that the adrenals are essential also for the development of isoproterenol cardiomegaly (7). In adrenalectomized rats, the administration of isoproterenol does not induce any significant increase of the heart weight. The reason for this phenomenon can be sought in decreased blood pressure accompanying adrenalectomy as well as in profound changes in the protein synthesizing system of all tissues of the adrenalectomized animal (8).

These old observations were followed only very recently by a more detailed analysis of the positive role of the adrenals in experimental cardiac hypertrophy. We found a positive correlation between the heart weight and the adrenal weight in rats with both the coarctation of the abdominal aorta and with experimental hyperthyroidism (16, 17). A similar observation in rats with cardiac hypertrophy induced by repeated exposures to cold stress was published by Tanaka and collab. (19).

The increased adrenal weight in rats with experimental cardiac hypertrophy was not connected with increased plasma levels of either corticosterone, the main rat adrenal glucocorticoid (9), or of aldosterone (13). On the contrary, in animals exposed to acute stress (swimming, hypoxia in a closed jar, laparotomy under ether anesthesia), the adrenal weight did not change, and the levels of corticosterone were increased (13).

2 Digitalis treatment in experimental cardiac hypertrophy

The effects of digitalis drugs in experimental cardiac hypertrophy have been investigated for almost 20 years. In 1973, Turto and Lindy (20) repeated the older experiments of Williams and Braunwald (21) and came to the conclusion that, at the end of the first postoperative week following stenosis of the abdominal aorta in the rat, the administration of digitoxin did not change significantly the extent of total heart RNA labelling, but it prevented a significant increase of the heart weight. This observation agrees with older observations of maximal yield of ribosomes from the cardiac muscle during the first postoperative week following coarctation of abdominal aorta and a significant increase of the heart weight between the 5th and 7th postoperative days (6). When, in repeated experiments, the observation period was prolonged to three weeks, the heart weight in animals with stenosis of abdominal aorta treated with digitoxin did not significantly differ from that in untreated rats. Surprisingly, the administration of digitoxin inhibited the increase of the adrenal weight, as if there existed a negative feedback between the exogenous digitoxin and adrenal reaction in animals with the coarctation of the abdominal aorta (17).

3 Endogenous digitalis-like activity in cardiac hypertrophy

The presence of specific digitalis receptors in the myocardium led us to the question why did these receptors develop, and to the search for hypothetical endogenous digitalis. The parallelity of the increase of adrenal and cardiac weights in cardiac hypertrophy discussed above and, further, the similarity of the basic chemical structure between digitalis aglycones and adrenal steroids led us to the idea this putative endogenous cardiotropic substance might be a steroid, and we started to call it endocardin (12). A little earlier, a similar question was raised by Gruber and collab. (3). He as well as some others (2, 4) came to the conclusion that the endogenous digoxin-like substance existed, and they postulated for it a peptidic structure.

For the proof of its presence we started to use at first commercial kits for enzymoimmunoassay of digoxin. In rats with coarctation of the abdominal aorta and with resulting cardiac and adrenal hypertrophy, we observed a well-pronounced correlation between the extent of cardiac hypertrophy and the spontaneous serum digoxin immunoreactivity (12, 13, 14). The same was true also for the serum of rats with experimental hyperthyroidism. Also in them the adrenal weight increased parallel to the heart weight, and the spontaneous serum digoxin immunoreactivity appeared, indicating the presence of a substance non-specifically cross-reacting with antidigoxin antibodies (14). Therefore we started a search among natural as well as among synthetic steroids for compounds possessing "digoxin" immunoreactivity. Upon thin layer chromatography of adrenal cortical extracts, a fraction was found different from aldosterone, corticosterone and deoxycorticosterone, reacting positively upon enzymoimmunoanalysis for digoxin (equivalent of 1 pg digoxin per 1 mg wet adrenal weight). At the same time, this fraction inhibited to the highest degree the ^{86}Rubidium uptake by red blood cells, which reflects its ability to inhibit the Na, K-activated ATPase (15).

Among pure steroids and their derivatives, the highest digoxin-like activity was found with 14-OH-estradiol and 14-OH-estrone (18).

The chemical structure of the putative endogenous digitalis-like factor(s) is unknown. Two categories of such substances may exist: one peptidic, possibly identical with the long-sought natriuretic hormone, and the other steroidal, probably from the adrenal cortex.

References

1. Beznak, M.: Hormonal influences in regulation of cardiac performance. Circulat. Res. **14–15**, Suppl. II. 141–162 (1964).
2. Godfraind, T., A. DePover, A. C. Hermandez, M. Fagoo: Cardiodigin: Endogenous Digitalis-like Material from Mammalian Heart. Arch. int. Pharmacodyn. **258**, 165–167 (1982).
3. Gruber, K. A., J. M. Whitaker, V. M. Buckalew, Jr.: Endogenous digitalis-like substance in plasma of volume-expanded dogs. Nature **287**, 743–745 (1980).
4. Haupert, G. T., Jr., J. M. Sancho: Sodium transport inhibitor from bovine hypothalamus. Proc. Nat. Acad. Sci. US **76**, 4658–4660 (1979).
5. Hort, W.: Morphologische und physiologische Untersuchungen an Ratten während eines Lauftrainings und nach dem Training. Virchows Arch. **320**, 197–237 (1951).
6. Kölbel, F.: Cardiac Hypertrophy – Clinical and Experimental Study, pp. 89–101 (Czech text). State Medical Publishing House (Prague 1969).
7. Kölbel, F., J. kapitola, O. Schreiberová, V. Kölbelová: Influence of adrenalectomy on the effects of Isoproterenol in the rat. Physiol. bohemosl. **19**, 281–285 (1970).
8. Kölbel, F., W. F. H. M. Mommaerts, V. Kölbelová, P. Vančura: Cardiac muscle and liver ribosomes of the rat: The influence of laparotomy and laparatomy combined with adrenalectomy. Experientia (Basel) **26**, 361–362 (1970).
9. Kölbel, F., V. Schreiber, T. Přibyl: Reflections on What Makes Heart Grow. In: Advances in Myocardiology, vol. 4. Eds. N. Dhalla, E. Chazov, Plenum Publ., New York, in press.
10. Kölbel, F., V. Schreiber, J. Štěpán, T. Přibyl: The endogenous digoxin-like substance – endocardin. In: Advances in studies on heart metabolism. Eds.: C. Caldarera, P. Harris. CLUEB Bologna 1982, pp. 527–530.

11. Liebegott, G.: Studien zur Orthogenie und Pathologie der Nebennieren. Beitr. pathol. Anat. **190,** 93–178 (1944).
12. Schreiber, V., F. Kölbel, J. Štěpán: Apparent (?) immunoreactivity of digoxin in the sera of rats with cardiac overload – on the problem of endogenous cardiotonic (Endocardin). Čas. lék. česk. **119,** 768–770 (1980).
13. Schreiber, V., J. Štěpán, I. Gregorová, F. Kölbel, T. Přibyl, J. Jahodová, V. Janovská: Digoxin-like Immunoreactivity in Serum of Hyperthyroid Rats with Hypertrophy of the Heart is not Caused by Aldosterone. Sborník lék. **82,** 305–308 (1980).
14. Schreiber, V., J. Štěpán, F. Kölbel, T. Přibyl, J. Jahodová, V. Kubová: Failure of the aldosterone antagonist spironolactone to inhibit myocardial hypertrophy produced by experimental hyperthyroidism and accompanied by "apparent" digoxin immunoreactivity in the blood. Physiol. bohemoslov. **29,** 577–579 (1980).
15. Schreiber, V., I. Gregorová, T. Přibyl, J. Štěpán: Digitalis-like Biological Activity and Immunoreactivity in Chromatographic Fractions of Rabbit Adrenal Extract. Endocr. Experiment. **15,** 229–235 (1981).
16. Schreiber, V., F. Kölbel, J. Štěpán, I. Gregorová, T. Přibyl: Digoxin-like immunoreactivity in the serum of rats with cardiac overload. J. Molec. cell. Cardiol. **13,** 107–110 (1981).
17. Schreiber, V., F. Kölbel, J. Štěpán, T. Přibyl, J. Jahodová, V. Kubová: Correlations between adrenal weight and heart weight in rats with a cardiac overload. Physiol. bohemoslov. **30,** 289–294 (1981).
18. Schreiber, V., J. Štěpán, T. Přibyl: Digitalis-like biological activity (inhibition of ^{86}Rb uptake by red blood cells in vitro) of certain steroids and other hormones. Biochem. Pharmacol. **30,** 3001–3002 (1981).
19. Tanaka, M., H. Yamada, T. Matsuura, K. Fukui, T. Kuribayashi, H. Katsume, A. Kizu, H. Ijichi, Y. Ibata: Morphological study on cardiac hypertrophy induced by cold stress in rats. J. Molec. cell. Cardiol. **13,** Suppl. 2, 42 (1981).
20. Turto, H., S. Lindy: Digitoxin treatment and experimental cardiac hypertrophy in the rat. Cardiovasc. Res. **7,** 482–489 (1973).
21. Williams, J. F., Jr., E. Braunwald: Studies on digitalis. 11. Effects of digitoxin on the development of cardiac hypertrophy in the rat subjected to aortic constriction. Amer. J. Cardiol. **16,** 534–539 (1965).

Authors' address:

Dr. František Kölbel, Third Medical Department, Charles University, U nemocnice 1, 128 21 Prague 2, Czechoslovakia.

Cardiac Adaptation to Hemodynamic Overload, Training and Stress
Dr. D. Steinkopff Verlag 69 (1983)

Myocardial nucleus in growing and hypertrophied heart

F. Cluzeaud, J. Perennec, E. de Amaral, M. Willemin, and P. Y. Hatt

I.N.S.E.R.M. U2, Hôpital Léon Bernard, 94450 Limeil-Brévannes (France)

Myocyte nucleus was studied at different ages in the normal rat and under acute and chronic types of heart overloading.

In normal young and adult rat. Nuclear chromatin was essentially dispersed. The condensed/dispersed chromatin ratio averaging 1/10. Nucleolus was spherical, the nucleolonema poorly designed and blurred.
In foetus the amount of condensed chromatin was greater than in adult. Condensed/dispersed chromatin ratio averaging 1/1.

The decrease in condensed chromatin from foetus to young rat is likely due to the loss of ability to mitosis after birth.

In recent isoproterenol overloading, evolution proceeded in 2 stages: a first stage of cell necrosis where condensed chromatin increased abruptly; a later one of cell overactivity where condensed chromatin contrariwise disappeared.

In heart hypertrophy of long duration (aorto-caval fistula, aortic constriction and insufficiency of 6 to 9 months duration) nucleus remained often "overactive". It was frequently grossly deformed. Some aspects could be interpreted either as nuclear fusion, or amitosis. In few cells, otherwise very damaged, karyolysis was present.

The number of nuclei per myocyte was evaluated in isolated cells. In adult rat, percentage of binucleated myocytes averaged 90 per cent. It decreased to 80 per cent in 21-day-long isoproterenol overloading and in heart hypertrophy of 6–9 months duration.

The nuclear size, measured with the aid of an image analyser, increased during growth. It increased relatively more in heart hypertrophy of long duration, as well as under isoproterenol overdosage.

The amount of nuclear DNA, as measured by cytophotometry, increased under isoproterenol overdosage as in hypertrophy of long duration in a proportion compatible with some polyploidy.

These "big" nuclei were predominant in mononuclear myocytes.

Key words: rat, cardiac growth, cardiac hypertrophy, isoproterenol, aorto-caval fistula, aortic constriction, myocardial nucleus, chromatin

References

1. Hatt, P. Y., K. Rakusan, F. Cluzeaud: Heart hypertrophy at the cell level. J. Mol. Cell. Cardiol. **11** (suppl. 2), 22 (abstract, 1979).
2. Hatt, P. Y., K. Rakusan, P. Gastineau, M. Laplace, F. Cluzeaud: Aorto-caval fistula in the rat. An experimental model of heart volume overloading. Basic Res. Cardiol. **75**, 105–108 (1980).
3. Hatt, P. Y., F. Cluzeaud, J. Perennec: Left ventricular hypertrophy experimental aspects. Eur. Heart J. **3** (suppl. A), 9–14 (1982).

Authors' address:

I.N.S.E.R.M. U2, Léon Bernard, 94450 Limeil-Brévannes, France

Cardiac Adaptation to Hemodynamic Overload, Training and Stress
Dr. D. Steinkopff Verlag 70–77 (1983)

A pathomorphological study on the diabetogenic drug-induced heart disease in the rat

S. Onishi, H. Nunotani, and Y. Tochino*

Department of Pathology, College of Biomedical Technology, Osaka University, Japan
* Department of Biological Science, Shionogi Central Laboratory, Osaka (Japan)

Summary

To clarify the mechanism of diabetic (DM) heart disease in man, a pathomorphological study on the heart of the DM rat was performed. 16 adult male Wistar rats were made DM by single injection of alloxan (ALX) or streptozotocin (STZ). ALX-DM animals were sacrificed 1.5 mos. later and STZ-DM rats after 4 and 6 mos., respectively. In all DM rats, serum glucose level was elevated. Blood pressure measured by tail cuff was also high up to the 23rd week. Histologically, DM heart showed a thickening of arteriolar wall and a tendency toward cardiac hypertrophy corresponding with hypertension. Ultrastructure revealed acute damage of various organelles in cardiomyocytes of the DM rat; subsequently cardiac cells were restored and normalized. The vascular smooth muscle cells (SMC) were modified and indicated activation and proliferation penetrating the inner elastic layer. Then marked thickening of arteriolar basal laminae was noted. Finally, degenerative change in the heart cells due to chronic cardiac failure was observed. The morphometrical results suggested a depressed myosin ATPase activity. Thus it is concluded that DM heart disease may be caused by DM microangiopathy associated with modulated SMC, thereafter it seems to develop into DM cardiomyopathy coexisting with hypertension.

Key words: diabetes mellitus, diabetogenic drug, myocardium, pathomorphology, morphometry, work overload, cardiac hypertrophy, cardiomyopathy, microangiopathy, smooth muscle cell

Introduction

Diabetes mellitus (DM) apparently affects the cardiovascular system, developing into congestive heart failure. Several clinical and experimental reports have suggested the concept of DM cardiomyopathy (4, 6, 16, 17) occurring independently of extramural coronary atherosclerosis, valvular disease, or systemic hypertension.

The research described here was designed to study the pathomorphology and the pathogenesis of the DM-genic drug-induced heart disease associated with DM cardiomyopathy.

Materials and methods

DM was induced in 16 adult male Wistar rats at 8 weeks of age by single intravenous administration of alloxan (ALX) (5 rats: 36 mg per kg body weight) or streptozotocin (STZ) (11 rats: 80 mg per kg body weight). ALX-injected DM animals were sacrificed 6 weeks later (DM-A) and STZ-DM rats after 17 (DM-B) and 23 weeks (DM-C), respectively. 18 littermates were used as controls. Serum glucose level was determined by the glucose oxidase method, and blood pressure was measured with an Electro-Sphygmomanometer PE-300. At the respective end of the experimental period, the animals were weighed, slightly anesthetized with pentobarbital and sacrificed. The hearts were immediately removed from the thoracic cavity. Following immersion in physiological saline, rings 1–2 mm in thickness were cut at the subvalvular level perpendicular to the long axis of the ventricle, and part of the myocardial tissue was fixed in 10 % formaldehyde solution for light microscopy; the rest was quickly fixed in Karnovsky's solution containing glutaraldehyde and then in OsO_4-solution for electron microscopy. Histologic sections were stained with hematoxylin-eosin for general observation, Mallory's method for connective tissue, elastica-van Gieson technique for elastic and connective tissue, and periodic acid Schiff (PAS) reaction with/without diastase step for glycogen and glycoprotein.

Measurement of heart size, i.e., semiquantitative macroscopy, was also performed. Each value on the histologic section of representative midventricular rings in both control and DM-B group were measured with slide-calipers on the line of perpendicular septum, as shown in figure 1.

For the ultrastructural study, the routine procedure was employed, and the sections were observed with JEM 100B electron microscope.

The morphometric analysis was done on the sections of six randomly selected rat hearts in DM-B group, cut at an angle of 32.4° to the longitudinal axis of the left ventricular posterior papillary muscle according to Mall's method (8). Mall et al. have recently demonstrated that this angle is optimal in the case of geometrically anisotropic surfaces. Various morphometric parameters in figures 2 and 3 were

Measurements of Hearts

Group (Number)		RW	RC	SW	LC	LW
Control (6)	mm*	0.90 (±0.06)	1.22 (±0.32)	2.05 (±0.27)	3.83 (±0.37)	2.07 (±0.15)
	%	8.9	12.1	20.4	38.0	20.6
Diabetic-B (6)	mm*	0.80 (±0.10)	0.28 (±0.04)	1.83 (±0.14)	2.22 (±0.27)	1.58 (±0.18)
	%	11.9	4.2	27.3	33.1	23.5

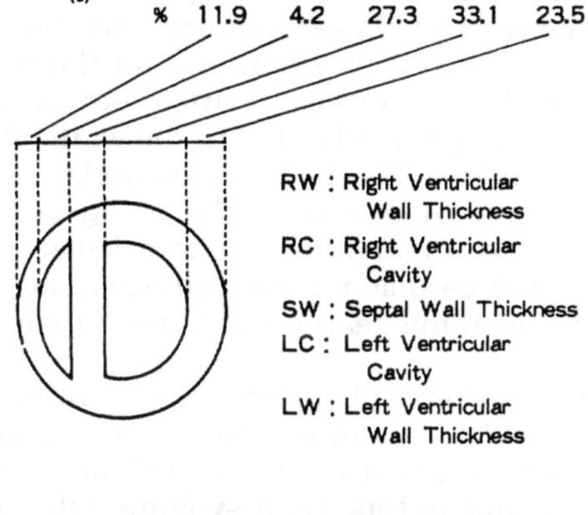

* Results are expressed as mean ± SD, respectively

Fig. 1.

evaluated in the group of the DM-B animals. These values were obtained by the well-known point-counting procedure, as described minutely in Mall's papers (9, 10).

Results and discussion

General characteristics of the groups given DM-genic drug showed overt DM, such as an evident increase of blood glucose (DM-B: 474.3 ± 68.7 mg/dl) compared with controls (227.2 ± 32.9 mg/dl). Furthermore, due to the DM-genic action of ALX or STZ, the heart increased in weight per gram body weight in each animal than in the controls (average percent increase in weight of heart relative to controls was 35.2 ± 0.28 %). Comparison with controls (always 130 to 145 mm Hg) revealed that blood pressure of DM-A animals rose acutely to 191 ± 6 mm Hg after 2 weeks and 232 ± 13 mm Hg after 5 weeks, and the STZ-induced DM rats showed 186 ± 2, 194 ± 5, 203 ± 6 and 154 ± 12 mm Hg after 4, 10, 14, and 23 weeks, respectively. It seemed that hypertension occurred until the 14th week, and then blood pressure was tending downward.

As shown in figure 1, macroscopic measurement revealed that the thickness of each wall of right ventricle, septum and left ventricle in the DM-B group was significantly greater than that of controls, while both right and left ventricular cavities in DM-B were relatively narrower than in controls. According to Laplace's law, this nearly symmetrical hypertrophy of DM heart seemed to be a cardiac transformation in conformity to pressure overload, i.e., hypertension.

Light microscopically, approximately 70 μm or smaller sized arterioles generally revealed a thicker wall than controls, with proliferating vascular smooth muscle cells (SMC) in the left ventricular myocardium of DM-A rats, that is, in early DM state. Increased PAS-positive materials were also observed in and around these arteriolar walls. Adjacent cardiac cells were degenerative, e.g., with vacuolar, cloudy swelling, sometimes eosinophilic with pyknosis of nucleus. In the hearts of animals with moderately severe DM, i.e., DM-B, marked thickening of walls of small vessels (ca. 70 μm in diameter or smaller) was noted. Generally speaking, the arteriolar lumen was hardly seen. A series of these vascular alterations may be called "microangiopathy" due to DM. Furthermore, in the severe DM-C state which was accompanied by hypertension up to 14th week, the myocardial cell hypertrophy occurred gradually, that is, the width of cardiomyocytes increased by approximately 20 % (17 μm in controls vs. 20 μm in DM on the average). At the same time, heart cells having two activated nuclei were frequently observed. In addition, left ventricular myocardium indicated a tendency toward cardiac muscle cell disorganization, one of the specific and sensitive anatomic features of hypertrophic cardiomyopathy (11).

Figure 2 shows the histomorphometric results in the left ventricular papillary muscle of the DM-B and control animals. Among the volume densities, the capillary volume/total tissue volume decreased, and the residual-interstitial-volume-to-total-tissue-volume ratio increased significantly in DM myocardium. Concerning the surface-to-volume ratio, the value of the myocardial-surface-area-to-cell-volume ratio in DM decreased

Histomorphometric Results in the Left Ventricle

Morphometric Parameters Component Parameter/ Reference Parameter	Control (6)* mean ± SD	Diabetic-B (6)* mean ± SD	p
Volume Densities (μ^3/μ^3)			
Myocardial Cell Volume/ Total Tissue Volume	0.788±0.013	0.805±0.019	N.S.
Capillary Volume/ Total Tissue Volume	0.195±0.015	0.173±0.018	#
Residual Interstitial Volume/ Total Tissue Volume	0.015±0.003	0.022±0.005	#
Surface to Volume Ratio (μ^2/μ^3)**			
Myocardial Surface Area/ Myocardial Cell Volume	0.252±0.013	0.213±0.022	##
Capillary Surface Area/ Capillary Volume	0.506±0.030	0.690±0.028	###

* In ( ) : Number of Animal.
** Based on Weibel (1969)'s formula ; $S_V = 4/d$ (d = diameter of cylinder)
The Student's t-test was used for statistical evaluation.
#p is smaller than 0.05, ## smaller than 0.01, ### smaller than 0.001.

Fig. 2.

significantly. These data suggest that the cardiac cell hypertrophy accompanies the increase of interstitial components in the DM animals.

Ultrastructurally, shortly after inducing the DM state the cardiomyocytes revealed acute damage of various cellular organelles such as great accumulation of beta-glycogen granules in cellular hyaloplasm, mitochondrial swelling with cristolysis, myofibrillar fragmentation, and some dissociation of intercalated discs. After that, the heart muscle cells tended gradually toward restoration and normalization adaptively. On the other side, also in the initial stage of DM, the endothelial cells were modulated, and the vascular SMC in the approximately 70 µm or smaller sized vessels were modified and revealed activation, with proliferation penetrating the electron clear inner elastic laminae into the subendothelial space in the arteriolar wall. In vascular lumen, several platelet-like particles also could be seen. In the interstitium, generally speaking, some thickening of electron-dense basal laminae was recognizable directly outside the approximately 70 µm or smaller sized arterioles. Besides them, the interstitial space was filled with collagen fibers and party with fragmented collagenous materials. Thereafter, hypertrophy of myocardial cells, being over 20 µm in width, was found in the advanced DM stage, accompanied by hypertension. Occasionally, a typical myofibrillar disarray was noticed in the heart muscle cells of DM animals. Finally, degenerative alteration of the various cellular organelles in the cardiomyocytes such as partial myofibrillolysis, irregularity of Z-band, and deterioration of mitochondria were observed prior to the cardiac failure.

Figure 3 shows the cytomorphometric results in the left ventricular papillary muscle of the DM and control rats. The statistically significant findings were a decreased mitochondrial mass, an increased myofibrillar

Cytomorphometric Results in the Left Ventricle

Morphometric Parameters Component Parameter/ Reference Parameter	Control (6)* mean ± SD	Diabetic-B (6)* mean ± SD	p
Volume Densities (μ^3/μ^3)			
Mitochondrial Volume/ Cytoplasmic Volume	0.338±0.013	0.298±0.024	##
Myofibrillar Volume/ Cytoplasmic Volume	0.525±0.010	0.555±0.019	##
Mitochondrial Volume/ Myofibrillar Volume	0.644±0.008	0.537±0.008	###
Surface to Volume Ratio (μ^2/μ^3)			
Outer Mitochondrial / Membrane Surface/ Mitochondrial Volume	8.80±0.33	7.39±0.21	###
Total Inner Mitochondrial/ Membrane Surface / Mitochondrial Volume	38.40±0.77	34.59±0.68	###

* In ( ) Number of Animal #,## & ### mean the same value as in Fig.2
The Student's test was used for statistical evaluation.

Fig. 3.

volume, i.e., a decreased mitochondrial volume per myofibrillar volume, and a decrease in both outer and inner mitochondrial membrane surfaces.

It is reported that mitochondrial volume density increases in the early stage of cardiac work overload (12, 13). On the contrary, a decreased mitochondrial volume density, as in this experiment, has been shown after chronic pressure overload (12, 14, 20), and in a cardiomyopathy of the Syrian golden hamster (2). On the other hand, the surface area of inner mitochondrial membrane is rather more important than the mitochondrial mass, with regard to the structure-function relationship. The ratio of surface area of inner mitochondrial membrane to myofibrillar volume reflects myosin ATPase activity (18). This data is in parallel with the findings that the myosin ATPase activity (7) and the mitochondrial volume density (1, 12, 20) decreased in cardiac hypertrophy. These findings suggest that the decreased mitochondrial volume density in this study, that is, the depressed myosin ATPase activity, is consistent with the results of a long-standing pressure overload, even though several weeks of STZ-DM alters myocardial function (15). Besides a decrease of total inner mitochondrial membrane surface, the index of outer mitochondrial membrane surface per mitochondrial volume was also depressed significantly. This result indicates that mitochondrial decrease and swelling associated with cristolysis occur due to acute and chronic myocardial cell damage (1), as well as injured biosynthesis of mitochondrial protein caused by a diminution in the myocardial protein synthesis and a reduction in the RNA-to-protein ratio in rats which were treated with STZ (19).

Thus the mechanism of experimental DM heart disease may be summarized as follows (fig. 4).

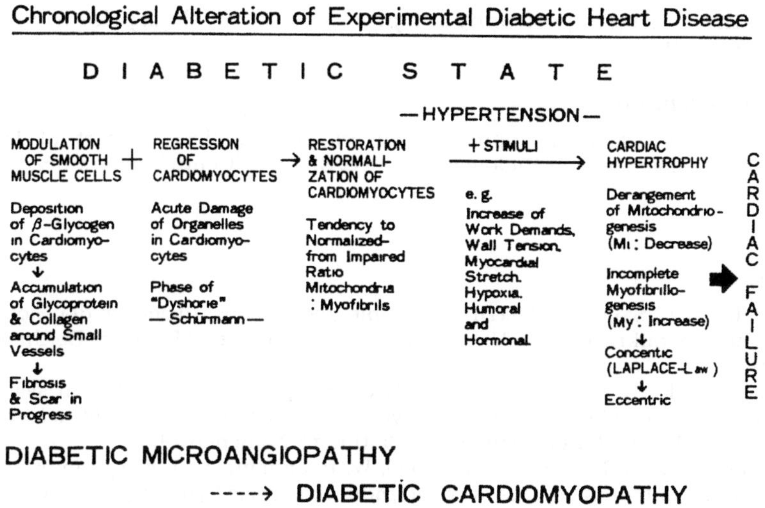

Fig. 4.

Shortly after the DM-genic drug administration, modulation and modification of the endothelial cells and SMC occurred prior to accumulation of glycoprotein and collagenous materials adjacent to small vessels. The SMC activity factor is obscure; however, it may occur in DM serum. As the result of the thickened wall and the narrowed lumen of the small vessels, so-called microangiopathy could produce not only hypoxia leading to myocardial fibrosis and scar, but also hypertension because of an increased peripheral vascular resistance. Furthermore, some disturbances in catecholamine secretion in the DM heart before the appearance of typical microangiopathic alterations may play an important role in a pathogenesis of hypertension (5).

On the other side, regressive alterations, i.e., acute damage of myocardial organelles, occurs in the DM state. After that, the heart muscle cells are restored and normalized gradually, and then the DM heart tends to be hypertrophic which may be attributed to the cardiomegalogenic factors, especially hypertension-induced work load and the volume overload caused by elevated mesenchymal components (3).

In the advanced DM stage, being accompanied by cardiac hypertrophy, a long-standing pressure and volume load were the cause of a decreased mitochondrial volume density, as well a decreased myosin ATPase activity, i.e., a depressed myofibrillar ATPase in spite of an increased myofibrillar volume density.

It is concluded that excessive hemodynamic loads produce myocardial hypertrophy, with functional derangement to cardiac failure, provided the excessive loads are maintained. The dynamic characteristics of DM are demonstrated by the finding that the diabetic, metabolic disorder-induced microangiopathy may lead to hypertension; thereafter, diabetic cardiomyopathy, having hypertrophy as a prerequisite, develops prior to congestive heart failure.

Acknowledgements

The authors gratefully appreciate the expert technical support of Dr. S. Funakawa, Department of Biological Science, Shionogi Central Laboratory, Osaka, Japan.

References

1. Büchner, F., S. Onishi: Herzhypertrophie und Herzinsuffizienz in der Sicht der Elektronenmikroskopie. Urban & Schwarzenberg (München–Berlin–Wien 1970).
2. Büchner, F., S. Onishi, A. Wada: Cardiomyopathy associated with systemic myopathy. Genetic defect of actomyosin influencing muscular structure and function. Urban & Schwarzenberg (Baltimore–München 1978).
3. Carey, R. A., G. Natarjan, A. A. Bove, W. P. Santamore, J. F. Spann: Elevated collagen content in volume overload induced cardiac hypertrophy. J. Mol. Cell. Cardiol. **12,** 929–936 (1980).
4. Factor, S. M., R. Bhan, T. Minase, H. Wolinsky, E. H. Sonnenblick: Hypertensive-diabetic cardiomyopathy in the rat. Amer. J. Pathol. **102,** 219–228 (1981).
5. Fushimi, H., T. Inoue, H. Namikawa, B. Kishino, M. Nishikawa, Y. Tochino, S. Funakawa: Increased norepinephrine content in diabetic rat heart: J. Biochem. **91,** 1805–1807 (1982).
6. Hamby, R. I., S. Zoneraich, L. Sherman: Diabetic cardiomyopathy. J. Amer. Med. Assoc. **229,** 1749–1754 (1974).
7. Jacob, R., G. Ebrecht, A. Kämmereit, I. Medugorac, M. F. Wendt-Gallitelli: Myocardial function in different models of cardiac hypertrophy. An attempt at correlating mechanical, biochemical, and morphological parameters. Basic Res. Cardiol. **72,** 160–167 (1977).
8. Mall, G., H. Reinhard, K. Kayser, J. A. Rossner: An effective morphometric method for electron microscopic studies on papillary muscles. Virchows Arch. A Path. Anat. Histol. **379,** 219–228 (1978).
9. Mall, G., H. Reinhard, D. Stopp, J. A. Rossner: Morphometric observations on the rat heart after high-dose treatment with cortisol. Virchows Arch. A Path. Anat. Histol. **385,** 169–180 (1980).
10. Mall, G., T. Mattfeldt, P. Rieger, B. Volk, V. A. Frolov: Morphometric analysis of the rabbit myocardium after chronic ethanol feeding – early capillary changes. Basic Res. Cardiol. **7,** 57–67 (1982).
11. Maron, B. J., W. C. Roberts: Distribution and significance of cardiac muscle cell disorganization in the left ventricle of patients with hypertrophic cardiomyopathy: Evidence of a diffuse cardiomyopathic process. In: Kaltenbach, M., S. E. Epstein (eds.). Hypertrophic Cardiomyopathy. The Therapeutic Role of Calcium Antagonists, pp. 38–57. Springer (Berlin–Heidelberg–New York 1982).
12. Meerson, F. Z., T. A. Zaletayeva, S. S. Lagutchev, M. G. Pshennikova: Structure and mass of mitochondria in the process of compensatory hyperfunction and hypertrophy of the heart. Exp. Cell Res. **36,** 568–578 (1964).
13. Onishi, S.: Die Feinstruktur des Herzmuskels nach Aderlaß bei der Ratte. Beitr. path. Anat. **136,** 96–132 (1967).
14. Onishi, S., F. Büchner, M. Thermann, R. Zittel: Das elektronenmikroskopische Bild des Herzmuskels bei experimenteller Hypertrophie in der Phase der Kompensation. Beitr. path. Anat. **140,** 38–53 (1969).
15. Penpargkul, S., T. Schaible, T. Yipintsoi, J. Scheuer: The effect of diabetes on performance and metabolism of rat hearts. Circulat. Res. **47,** 911–921 (1980).

16. Regan, T. J., P. O. Ettinger, M. I. Khan, M. U. Jesrani, M. M. Lyons, H. A. Oldewurtel, M. Weber: Altered myocardial function and metabolism in chronic diabetes mellitus without ischemia in dogs. Circulat. Res. **35,** 222–237 (1974).
17. Rubler, S., J. Dlugash, Y. Z. Yuceoglu, T. Kumral, A. W. Branwood, A. Grishman: New type of cardiomyopathy associated with diabetic glomerulosclerosis. Amer. J. Cardiol. **30,** 595–602 (1972).
18. Smith, H. E., E. Page: Morphometry of rat mitochondrial subcompartments and membranes: Application to myocardial cell atrophy after hypophysectomy. J. Ultrastruct. Res. **55,** 31–41 (1976).
19. Whitman, V., H. G. Schuler, J. R. Neely: Effect of alloxan-induced diabetes on the hypertrophic response of rat heart. J. Mol. Cell. Cardiol. **11,** 1275–1281 (1979).
20. Wollenberger, A., W. Schulze: Über das Volumenverhältnis von Mitochondrien im chronisch überlasteten, hypertrophierten Herzen. Naturwissenschaften **49,** 161–162 (1962).

Authors' address:

Shunzo Onishi, M.D., Department of Pathology, College of Biomedical Technology, Osaka University, 1-1 Machikaneyama-cho, Toyonaka-shi, Osaka, 560, Japan

Cardiac Adaptation to Hemodynamic Overload, Training and Stress
Dr. D. Steinkopff Verlag 78–82 (1983)

The role of cyclic nucleotides in the pathogenesis of myocardial hypertrophy

N. Popova, B. Bozhkov, R. Kolarova, and I. Petkova

Chair of Pathophysiology (Chairman: Prof. Z. Kemileva),
Medico-Biological Institute, Medical Academy, Sofia (Bulgaria)

Summary

The present study has been designed on renal hypertensive rats with myocardial hypertrophy. The hypertension was performed according to Selye's model and correlated with high plasma and cerebral renin activity, and low $PGF_{2\alpha}$-metabolite concentration in the serum.

The concentration of ATP, cAMP and cGMP, the synthetizing and hydrolyzing enzymes AC and FDE were estimated in the myocard during the different stages of myocardial hypertrophy (on the 3rd, 30th and 90th day of the study). The effect of β-adrenergic blockade on the same parameters was estimated as well.

The results showed a decrease of ATP and an increase of cAMP, which were maximal on the 30th day of hypertension, while during the whole 30-days period of examination a progressive decrease of cGMP was evident. During the initial stage there was no change in AC activity, which slowly increased later on, in agreement with an increased catecholamine's level in the myocard. PDE activity was increased.

Beta-blocker pretreatment of the experimental animals prevented the above-cited changes of ATP and cAMP without any significant effect on the enzymatic activity.

The results suggest a possible role of cyclic nucleotides on the metabolic changes in different stages of myocardial hypertrophy.

Key words: cyclic nucleotides, myocardial hypertrophy, beta-adrenergic blockade

Introduction

The participation of adrenergic receptor mechanisms in the metabolic and functional heart activity upon loading is a subject of clinical and experimental investigations. An increase in the number of myocardial beta-adrenergic receptors was found in patients with valvular aortic stenosis (4, 5) as well as in myocardial hypertrophy caused by thyreotoxicosis (13). The decrease of beta-adrenergic receptors was reported in spontaneous hypertensive rats (SHR) and in rats with renal hypertension (5, 14, 15). These data arouse the interest for the role of cyclic nucleotides (cAMP and cGMP) and their generating enzymes (adenylate and guanylate cyclase) in the pathogenesis of myocardial hypertrophy. A hypothesis was proposed for the triggering role of the cAMP in the metabolic processes of the separate stages of myocardial hypertrophy after relative hypoxy. In the same time there are a controversial data concerning the concentration of myocardial cyclic nucleotides under hypoxy. Some authors (5) established increased levels of cyclic AMP alongside with sharp decrease of cyclic GMP (11). Other authors reported unchanged level of cAMP and increased concentration of cGMP (7).

In our previous studies with hypertensive animals we have established increased serum (3) and brain renin activity (1) and decreased level of prostaglandin $F_{2\alpha}$ (9). The aim of the present paper was to study the changes of ATP concentration, cAMP and cGMP levels, and adenylate cyclase, and phosphodiesterase (PDE) activity in various stages of experimental myocardial hypertrophy, and the effect of the beta-adrenergic blockade on myocardial hypertrophy.

Material and methods

The experiments were carried out on male Wistar rats (mean weight 200 g). Experimental hypertension was produced on the first group of animals by the method of Selye (12) – ligating between the renal arteries. Thus the kidney below the ligature was transformed into an endocrine-like organ, increting pressor substances. The second group of animals were treated with the beta-adrenergic blocker Obsidan (1 mg/kg daily) prior to the operation. On the 3rd, 30th and 90th days after the operation the blood pressure, ATP concentration, cAMP, cGMP, and enzyme

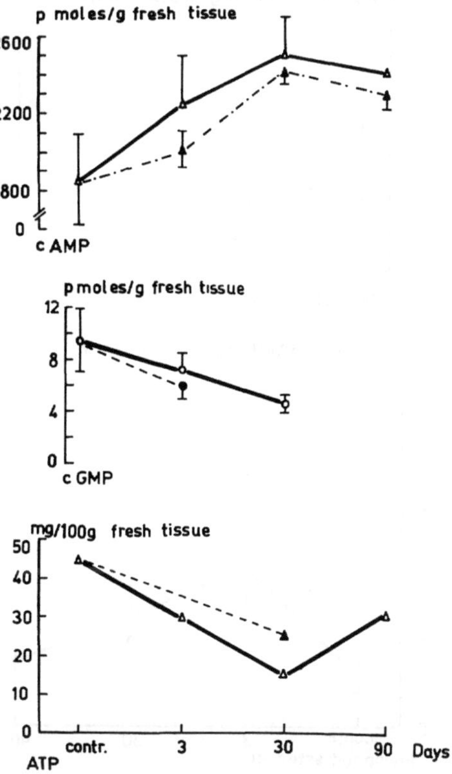

Fig. 1. The cyclic AMP and cGMP levels (in pmoles/g fresh tissue) and ATP concentrations (in mg = 100 g fresh tissue) in the myocards of hypertensive animals before the experiment and on the 3rd, 30th and 90th days of the experiment. The effects of the beta-adrenoreceptor blockade (Obsidan) are shown on the same figures with a dotted line.

activity of adenylate cyclase and PDE were determined. The same parameters were followed up in the 3rd (control) group of animals. Subsequently the animals were sacrificed by decapitation and myocardial tissue was taken from left ventricle of the heart by the Wollenberger's instrument in situ. The tissue was chopped under liquid nitrogen and homogenized in glass homogenizer. The ATP and cAMP concentrations were determined by Boehringer's kits, cGMP by the Amersham's RIA kits and the adenylate and PDE activity by the radioenzyme methods (Delaage et al., 1974).

Results

In the course of the study, the blood pressure of the test animals (1st group) was significantly elevated in comparison with the control animals (3rd group). In the animals treated with Obsidan (2nd group) the blood pressure was decreased.

There was a close correlation between the heart hypertrophy (confirmed by histomorphological methods) and the dynamics of the biochemical parameters followed. The ATP concentration was at its lowest on the 30th day after the beginning of the experiments, and showed a trend towards a slight increase by the 90th day of the study. At the same time, the cAMP concentration was increased in contrast to the decreased cGMP concentration (fig. 1). The adenylate cyclase activity after an initial decrease on

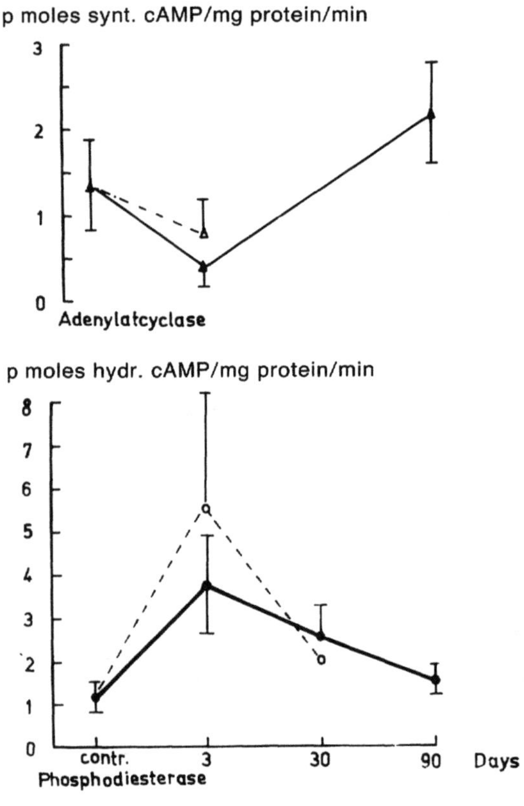

Fig. 2. Adenyl cyclase enzyme activity (in pmoles cAMP generated per minute) and phosphodiesterase activity (in pmoles cAMP hydrolysed per mg protein per min) in myocardial tissue of hypertensive rats, as well as the activity of the same enzymes after Obsidan pretreatment of the animals.

the 3rd day was found to be elevated in the late phase of myocardial hypertrophy. The PDE activity was elevated during the whole period of the investigation (fig. 2). The beta-adrenergic blockade by Obsidan reduced the ATP diminution as well as the increase of the cAMP concentration (fig. 1). At the same time, myocardial tissue of Obsidan-treated hypertensive animals showed increased adenylate cyclase and phosphodiesterase activity (fig. 2).

Discussion

The results obtained allow us to interpret the elevated cAMP concentration in myocardial tissue of hypertensive animals according to our previous results (10) about the changes of the myocardial oxidizing and glycolytic enzymes activity (MDH, isocitrat-DH, LDH, alpha HBD, pyruvat kinase, aldolase), glucose-6-P DH and creatin kinase activity. The participation of cAMP in some of these processes and the increased concentration of cAMP in myocardial hypertrophy is in some cases a valuable proof of the central role of beta-adrenergic mechanisms in this process. Our results obtained in experiments with blockade of beta-adrenergic receptors by Obsidan were in support of this view. Williams et al. (13) have shown under similar conditions that the increase in heart weight in thyreotoxic rats was accompanied with increase of the number of beta-adrenergic receptors. The cAMP elevation is probably a consequence of relative hypoxy due to hypertrophy caused by endogenous liberation of catecholamines and adenylate cyclase activation. The data showing decreased ATP concentrations and kreatin kinase activity (2) were also in support of this view.

The dynamics of ATP concentration, adenylate cyclase, kreatin kinase, and PDE activities have shown phase-dependent changes. The decrease of adenylate cyclase activity on the 3rd day after aortic constriction, found out by Krause et al. (4), might be interpreted as a protective mechanism against an increased catecholamine level. A similar protective mechanism was suggested by Limas (5) in rats with renal and deoxycorticosteron hypertension. The changes of adenylate cyclase and PDE-activity were also interpreted by Meerson (6) as an adaptive mechanism in myocardial hypertrophy. Another possibility for the explanation of these phenomena was the hypothesis proposed by Perkins (8), accepting a shift of the beta-adrenergic receptors from the outside to the inside of the cell membrane as a protective mechanism against catecholamine stress.

In summary, the observed phenomena related to cAMP metabolism might be associated with the complex neuro-humoral regulatory mechanisms for the maintaining of the homeostasis, which probably take place in the pathogenesis of myocardial hypertrophy.

References

1. Dimitrov, G. T., N. A. Popova, R. N. Kolarova, D. I. Kiprov: Kidney and brain renin concentration under experimental Selye hypertension in rats. Comptes rendus de l'Academie bulgare des Sciences **32**, 4, 537 (1979).
2. Kolarova, N. R.: Myocardial enzyme activity and influence of β-adrenergic blockade in experimental hypertension. Dissertation (Bulg.) (Sofia 1975).

3. Kolarova, N. R., I. Sirakova, N. Popova, L. Sirakov: Influence of β-adrenergic blockade on plasma renin activity and plasma renin concentration in experimental hypertension. Medico-Biological Problems **1,** 56, Sofia (1980).
4. Krause, F., H. Mest, C. Taube, W. Förster: Electrically induced tachyarrhythmia (TA) and the effect of propranolol (PROP) on the release of cyclic AMP and PG E by the canine left ventricle. Summary. J. Mol. Cell. Cardiol. **12,** Suppl. 1, 81 (1980).
5. Limas, J.: Effect of phospholipid methylation on β-adrenergic receptors in the normal and hypertrophied rat myocardium. Circulat. Res. **47,** 596 (1980).
6. Meerson, F.: Adaptation, stress and prophylaxis. Medicina (Moscow 1981).
7. Metsä-Ketelä, T., K. Laustiola, H. Vapaatalo: Regulation of the cardiac contractility and glycolysis by cyclic nucleotides during hypoxya. Summary. J. Mol. Cell. Cardiol. **12,** Suppl. 1, 106 (1980).
8. Perkins, J.: Catecholamine-induced modification of the functional state of β-adrenergic receptors. Trends Pharm. Sci. **12,** 326 (1981).
9. Petkov, O., L. Sirakov, Y. Belov, I. Sirakova, R. Kolarova, S. Torbova, N. Popova: Content of Prostaglandins E and $F_{2\alpha}$ in the blood plasma and kidneys in arterial hypertension (Clinical-experimental study). Acta physiologica et pharmacologica **7,** 4, 49 (1981).
10. Popova, N., R. Kolarova: Changes in the myocardial activity of some enzymes of the glycolytic and citric cycle in rats with experimental hypertension. Exper. Med. and Morph. **4,** 321 (1976).
11. Selivanova, P. L., L. M. Saburova: Cyclic nucleotides in acute myocardial ischemia. Summary. J. Mol. Cell. Cardiol. **12,** Suppl. 1, 147 (1980).
12. Selye, H.: Einführung in die Lehre vom Adaptationssyndrom, Georg Thieme, XI, **164,** 68 (Stuttgart 1953).
13. Williams, L. T., J. R. Lefkowitz, A. M. Watanabe, D. R. Hathaway, R. H. Besch: Thyroid hormone regulation of beta-adrenergic receptor number. J. Biol. Chem. **252,** 2787 (1977).
14. Will-Schahab, W. Warbanov, J. Kütner: Altered β-adrenergic reactivity of the hypertrophied heart. Summary. J. Mol. Cell. Cardiol. **12,** Suppl. 1, 179 (1980).
15. Woodcock, E. A., N. J. Funder, J. C. Johonston: Decreased cardiac β-adrenoreceptors in deoxycorticosterone-salt and renal hypertensive rats. Circulat. Res. **45,** 500 (1979).

Authors' address:

Dr. N. Popova, Chair of Pathophysiology, Medico-biological Institute, Medical Academy, Sofia, Bulgaria

Cardiac Adaptation to Hemodynamic Overload, Training and Stress
Dr. D. Steinkopff Verlag 83–93 (1983)

The role of cytoplasmic factors in RNA synthesis activation during hyperfunction of heart and liver

F. Z. Meerson and M. P. Yavich

Institute of General Pathology and Pathological Physiology,
U.S.S.R. Academy of Medical Sciences, Moscow 125315 (U.S.S.R.)

Summary

The effect of the cytoplasmic fraction (S-100) of the heart and liver on the rate of transcription in isolated nuclei was studied under normal conditions and during compensatory growth induced by hyperfunction. The cytoplasm of normal heart and liver contains factors which can accelerate RNA synthesis in the nuclei; the activity of RNA polymerase I is thereby increased to a greater degree than that of RNA polymerase II. In the heart in hyperfunction and in the saved liver lobe after partial hepatectomy the activity of the cytoplasmic factors accelerating the transcription is increased. It has been found that the cytoplasmic factors of the heart and liver which accelerate transcription have a protein nature and are not organ specific; their activity is correlated with the rate of cell RNA synthesis. It is assumed that the increase in the activity of protein cytoplasmic factors accelerating transcription is an essential mechanism of initiation of RNA synthesis acceleration in enhanced physiological function.

Key words: RNA polymerases, cytoplasmic factors, compensatory growth, heart, liver

Introduction

In the course of the heart adaptation to increased load caused by aortic stenosis, the rate of RNA synthesis in myocardium shows a drastic rise (1, 2). The acceleration of transcription results in enhanced production of polyribosomes in cardiac cells, activation of protein synthesis, and an increased organ mass (2, 3). Similar events are observed during compensatory growth of the liver after partial hepatectomy (4, 5) and the single kidney after unilateral nephrectomy (6). The molecular mechanisms which induce acceleration of transcription in physiological hyperfunction are still unclear.

It was demonstrated that the translation inhibitors p-fluorophenylalanine and puromycin, when injected in doses which do not change the rate of protein synthesis in intact organs, neither increase the rate of RNA synthesis in the heart and saved liver lobe in hyperfunction nor cause any compensatory growth of the organ (1, 4). This indicates that acceleration of transcription and, consequently, the development of hypertrophy require the presence of protein factors. The involvement of these factors of the cytoplasm in regulation of transcription has presently been shown for a number of animal cells (8–12).

Therefore it seemed promising to investigate the effects of cytosol from intact organs and from organs with hyperfunction on the rate of RNA synthesis. The aim of the present work was to check the effect of the cytoplasmic fraction of the heart and liver under normal conditions and during compensatory growth on the activity of RNA polymerases in isolated nuclei. The activities of RNA polymerase form I – transcribing ribosomal genes – and of RNA polymerase form II – transcribing structural genes – were determined in individual systems.

Materials and methods

The experiments were carried out on Wistar male rats weighing 180 to 200 g. The compensatory hyperfunction of the heart was induced by aortic coarctation as described previously (13). Partial hepatectomy was performed according to Higgins and Anderson by excising the lateral and medial lobes of the liver (14), amounting to 70 % removal of liver tissue.

Reagents

ATP, UTP and CTP were from "Serva" (West Germany). Creatine phosphate, creatine phosphokinase and actinomycin D were obtained from "Reanal" (Hungary). Dithiothreitol, EDTA, Tris-HCl, α-amanithine, pancreatic RNAase and DNAase, pronase and cycloheximide were purchased from "Sigma" (USA). Rifamycin AF/0.13 and [^{3}H]UTP with specific activity of 43.3 mCi/mM were from "Amersham" (England). Other reagents were of Soviet make and of the purest grades available.

Isolation of nuclei

The nuclei were isolated from the heart, liver and kidney tissues at +3 to +4 °C according to Pogo's method with some modifications (15). To remove blood, the tissues were washed with a solution containing 0.25 M sucrose, 0.010 M Tris-HCl, pH 7.5; and 0.003 M $MgCl_2$ and homogenized in the same buffer additionally containing Triton X-100 at a final concentration of 0.5 %, using a Downs homogenizer. The homogenate was centrifuged for 10 min at 1000 g. The pellet was resuspended in a 2.4 M sucrose solution containing 0.003 M $MgCl_2$ and was then layered on top of the same solution and centrifuged in a 'Spinco' SW-27.1 rotor for 60 min at 105,000 g, +3 °C. The 105,000 × g nuclear pellet was resuspended and washed with a solution containing 0.25 M sucrose, 0.050 M Tris-HCl, pH 7.9; 0.005 M $MgCl_2$; 0.025 M KCl; 0.1 mM EDTA; and 1 mM dithiothreitol. All the solutions used were prepared on clarified water. The isolated nuclear preparations were used immediately after isolation for an RNA polymerase assay. The DNA content in the nuclear suspensions was determined using diphenylamine (16).

Preparation of the cytosol fraction

The cytosol fraction was prepared according to Weil et al. (10) with some modifications. The tissues were homogenized in a solution (3:1) containing 0.25 M sucrose, 0.050 M Tris-HCl pH 7.6, 0.025 M KCl, 0.0025 M $MgCl_2$, 2 mM dithiothreitol and 0.10 mM EDTA, 3 °C. The 105,000 g supernatant (fraction S-100) was dialyzed (18 hrs, 3–4 °C) against a solution containing 0.25 M sucrose; 0.100 M KCl; 0.050 M Tris-HCl, pH 7.9; 0.5 mM dithiothreitol; and 0.2 mM EDTA. The dialyzate was decolorized by centrifugation at 2000–3000 g and was either used in a cell-free system of RNA synthesis immediately after centrifugation or was frozen in liquid nitrogen and stored at −25 to −30 °C for 2 or 3 days. Protein was determined by the Lowry method (17).

Determination of the RNA polymerase activity of nuclei

The activities of RNA polymerase forms I and II were determined separately and analyzed with α-amanithine. It is known that RNA polymerase I is insensitive to α-amanithine; the activity of RNA polymerase II is inhibited by small doses and that of RNA polymerase III by high doses of this compound (18–20). The assay mixture (0.5 ml) for RNA polymerase contained final concentrations of the following components (μmoles): a) for RNA polymerase I assay: Tris-HCl 50, pH 7.9; KCl 25; $MgCl_2$ 60; $(NH_4)_2SO_4$ 50; GTP and CTP 0.6; ATP 2.0; creatine phosphate 5.0; b) for RNA polymerase II assay: Tris-HCl 50, pH 7.9; KCl 25; $MgCl_2$ 2.0; $(NH_4)_2SO_4$ 120; UTP 0.06; creatine phosphate 5.0. Then creatine phosphokinase (one crystal) and 2 μCi of $[^3H]$UTP were added to both systems. The reaction was started by adding the nuclear suspension (50 μg DNA). Sometimes the cytoplasmic fraction S-100, α-amanithine (1 μg/ml), actinomycin D (100 μg/ml), rifamycin AF/0.13 (30 μg/ml), pancreatic ribonuclease (20 μg/ml) and DNAase (200 μg/ml) were added to the samples. RNAase was added to the nuclei after completion of RNA synthesis, and the samples were additionally incubated for 20 min. In some cases, fraction S-100 was treated with pronase (1 mg/ml) and pancreatic ribonuclease (100 μg/ml). Cytosol was incubated with the enzyme for 15 min at 37 °C. The nuclei-containing samples were incubated at 36 °C; after incubation, a cold solution of 10 % TCA containing 0.04 M sodium pyrophosphate was added to them. Then the pellets were washed on 'Aufs' millipore filters with a solution of 5 % TCA containing 0.02 M sodium pyrophosphate, alcohol and ester. The radioactivity was measured in a scintillation counter, in a toluene scintillator containing PPO and POPOP and was expressed as counts per min per sample.

Injection of cycloheximide

Cycloheximide was injected to the animals intraperitoneally in doses of 3 and 5 mg per 100 g body weight in order to inhibit protein synthesis in the liver and heart, respectively.

Results

The conditions for determination of the activities of RNA polymerase I and II in the heart and liver nuclei are shown in table 1. It can be seen that the incorporation of $[^3H]$UMP into the acid-insoluble nuclear fraction depends on the presence of DNA and the added triphosphates and is inhibited by 95 % by actinomycin D. The reaction product is split by 90 % by pancreatic ribonuclease. This suggests that the incorporation of $[^3H]$UMP into the nuclei reflects the RNA synthesis. It also appears that α-amanithine (1 μg/ml) inhibits the $[^3H]$UMP incorporation into the nuclei in system I by 15–20 %. The inhibited activity is that of RNA polymerase II (2). The bulk of radioactivity of the samples (80–85 %) reflects rRNA synthesis, since at low ionic strength the activity of RNA polymerase III is insignificant (10). In system II, α-amanithine represses the RNA polymerase activity by 80 %; consequently, this system is characterized by a predominant synthesis of DNA-like RNA. Upon increase in the ionic strength of the $(NH_4)_2SO_4$ reaction mixture up to 0.160–0.200 M, the α-amanithine-inhibited activity amounts to 90 %. However, there are some data indicating that high ionic strength causes structural damage of chromatin (21, 22). In further studies we therefore used $(NH_4)_2SO_4$ at concentrations not exceeding 0.120 M. The incorporation of $[^3H]$UMP into

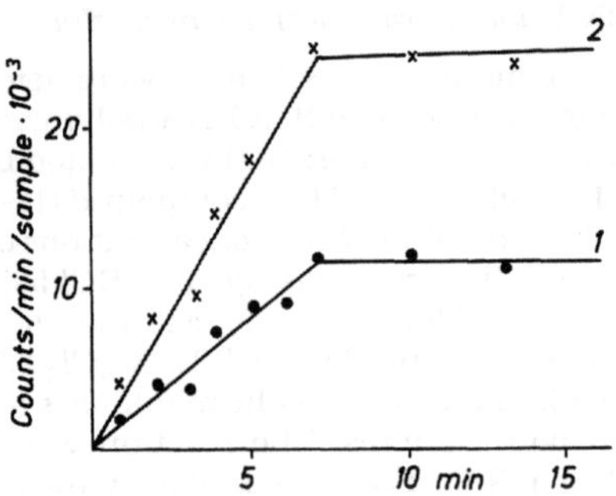

Fig. 1. Kinetics of [^{3}H]UTP incorporation into isolated liver nuclei. Abscissa – time (min); ordinate – counts per min·10^{-3} per sample. 1 – system I, 2 – system II.

the acid-insoluble nuclear fraction which was not inhibited by low doses of α-amanithine predominantly reflects the activity of RNA polymerase I, since the activity of RNA polymerase III is low in most tissues, i.e., 10 % of the total RNA polymerase activity (21, 22). Since system I is characterized by predominant synthesis of rRNA, and system II by predominant synthesis of DNA-like RNA, we will continue to refer to the activity of RNA polymerases I and II.

Figures 1 and 2 demonstrate the kinetics of [^{3}H]UMP incorporation into heart and liver nuclei (2a). It follows from the figures that RNA synthesis in both systems is linear only for the first 7 minutes, after which the plot has a plateau indicating the cessation of RNA synthesis. It is known that in most tissues the isolated nuclei can induce transcription only due to elongation of the polynucleotide chains initiated in vivo and that no reinitiation occurs under normal conditions (22).

The first step in our experiments was to study the effect of the cytoplasmic fraction (fraction S-100) from intact heart and liver on RNA synthesis

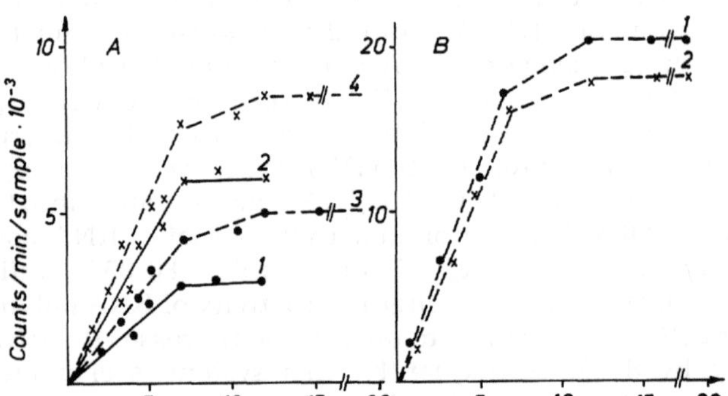

Fig. 2. Effect of the cytoplasmic fraction of heart and liver on the rate of [^{3}H]UMP incorporation into isolated liver nuclei. Abscissa – time (min); ordinate – counts per min · 10^{-3} per sample. A. 1 – system I, 2 – system II, 3 – system I + heart cytosol, 4 – system II + heart cytosol. B. 1 – system I + liver cytosol, 2 – system II + liver cytosol.

in isolated nuclei of these organs. The second step was to check the same effect in the cytoplasmic fractions of heart and liver during their compensatory hyperfunction. As can be seen from table 2, an addition of fraction S-100 from the heart to the incubation mixture of system I containing myocardial nuclei increases the rate of RNA synthesis by 70 % as compared to the effect of the cytosol-free buffer solution (the synthesis of DNA-like RNA in this mixture is inhibited by α-amanithine). An addition of liver cytosol to this system increases the RNA synthesis rate 7-fold as compared to the buffer system alone and more than 4-fold as compared to the cytoplasmic fraction of the heart. In system II, the rate of RNA synthesis in heart nuclei is increased by 50 % under the effect of a homologous fraction S-100 – and 2.5-fold as compared to the cytosol-free buffer solution after addition of liver cytosol. However, 15–20 % of the radioactivity in system II reflects the rRNA synthesis (table 1), which is sharply increased. Consequently, under our conditions the actual increase of the RNA polymerase II activity was considerably lower (by about 35 % in the case of heart cytosol and 75 % in the case of liver cytosol).

In liver nuclei, fraction S-100 also increases the rate of RNA synthesis. In system I, the rate of [^{3}H]UMP incorporation is increased by 190 %, while only by 26 % in system II. Incubation of liver nuclei with the cytoplasmic fraction of the heart enhances the rate of labelled triphosphate incorporation by 20 % in system I and only slightly in system II. In this way, the cytoplasmic fraction S-100 from heart and liver increases the activity of RNA polymerases I and II in homologous and heterologous nuclei, this being more pronounced for RNA polymerase I. In all cases studied, the effect of fraction S-100 from liver is stronger than that of the cytoplasmic fraction of the heart, which is probably correlated with the rate of RNA synthesis in these organs. Table 2 shows that the activity of RNA polymerase I in heart nuclei during incubation with liver cytosol exceeds that of liver RNA polymerase I in buffer solutions and is only 25 % lower than that of homologous cytosol. The protein concentration in the cytoplasmic

Table 1. Characteristics of a cell-free RNA-synthesizing system.

Conditions	Incorporation of [^{3}H] UMP into RNA (counts per min per sample)			
	liver nuclei		heart nuclei	
	system I	system II	system I	system II
Complete system	1200	2500	350	750
– ATP, CTP, GTP	12	20	5	10
+ RNAase*	120	200	35	70
+ DNAase**	150	150	30	50
+ actinomycin D	65	120	20	40
+ α-amanithine	960	200	290	160

* DNAase was initially added to the incubation mixture together with the nuclei.
** RNAase was added to the samples after completion of incubation and the reaction product was additionally incubated for 20 min.

fraction used in our studies was 8–10 mg/ml. Dilution of fraction S-100 to protein concentrations below 4 mg/ml decreases its activity (data not given).

Figure 2 shows the kinetics of RNA synthesis in heart nuclei incubated with cytosol from intact heart (A) and liver (B). These data suggest that the rate and mode of [^{3}H]UMP incorporation into the RNA in fraction S-100-containing systems differ from those in cytosol-free buffer systems. Firstly, the rate of the label incorporation into RNA is sharply increased during its linear synthesis, i.e., within the first 7 minutes; and, secondly, the time of the labelled triphosphate incorporation into the nuclei is increased to 12 min. This led us to the assumption that an addition of cytosol factors to the isolated nuclei results in partial reinitiation of the polynucleotide chains. To test this assumption we added rifamycin AF/013 to the incubation mixture of system I. This antibiotic is known to selectively inhibit the initiation of transcription (23). However, the level of the label incorporation into RNA (table 2) and the kinetics of its synthesis in the presence of rifamycin AF/013 remained unchanged (data not shown). Presumably the reinitiation of RNA synthesis in the presence of the cytoplasmic fraction does not take place either.

We made an attempt to elucidate the nature of cytoplasmic factors accelerating the transcription. For this purpose, fraction S-100 was preincubated with the proteolytic enzyme pronase and pancreatic ribonuclease. Table 2 shows that RNAase does not affect the activity of fraction S-100,

Table 2. Effect of cytosol on [^{3}H] UMP incorporation into RNA from isolated nuclei of heart and liver.

Conditions	Counts/min/sample	
	system I	system II
I – Heart nuclei		
without cytosol	220	560
+ heart cytosol	370	840
+ liver cytosol	1540	1500
Liver nuclei		
without cytosol	1120	2540
+ liver cytosol	2150	3200
+ heart cytosol	1300	2660
II – Heart nuclei		
without cytosol	300	620
+ heart cytosol	500	860
+ heart cytosol + pronase	290	610
+ heart cytosol + RNAase	500	850
+ heart cytosol (CHI-treated animals)	360	700
+ liver cytosol	2000	1700
+ liver cytosol + pronase	300	600
+ liver cytosol + RNAase	1900	1700
+ liver cytosol (CHI-treated animals)	810	1000

whereas the proteolytic enzyme causes its inactivation. This indicates that proteins or polypeptides are the active principle of the cytoplasmic fraction.

It also appears promising to investigate the problem as to whether the protein factors of the cytoplasm which accelerate transcription are long- or short-living components. For this purpose, we injected cycloheximide (CHI) to animals 2 hours prior to sacrifice. Our preliminary studies showed that CHI (2–5 mg per 100 g body weight) causes 97 % blocking of protein synthesis in the heart and liver 40 min after injection. The activity of fraction S-100 from heart and liver of CHI-treated animals is shown in table 2. It can be seen that the activity of the cytoplasmic fraction of the CHI-treated animals shows a 65–70 % fall. This is another proof of the protein nature of factors accelerating the transcription and of the unstability of these factors.

The next step in our studies was to investigate the effect of the cytoplasmic fraction from heart and liver isolated during the compensatory growth caused by increased load. The experimental results are presented in tables 3 and 4 and in figure 3. Fraction S-100 from the heart performing compensatory hyperfunction increases the RNA polymerase activity of the nuclei from normal myocardium as compared to the cytosol from a similar organ (table 3). Under the effect of the heart cytoplasmic fraction, the activity of RNA polymerase II is increased by 30 % 3 hours after the onset of hyperfunction (the activity of RNA polymerase I remains almost unaffected). Fraction S-100 from the heart 12 hours after the onset of hyperfunction enhances the activity of RNA polymerase I by 50 %, and that of RNA polymerase II by 35 %. The cytoplasmic fraction from the

Table 3. Effect of cytosol of the heart in hyperfunction on [^{3}H] UMP incorporation into RNA from isolated nuclei.

Conditions	Counts/min/sample	
	system I	system II
Heart nuclei		
+ cytosol from normal heart	400±25	900± 50
+ cytosol from heart at hyperfunction		
after 3 hrs of hyperfunction	450±20	1170± 60*
after 12 hrs of hyperfunction	600±30*	1280± 55*
after 24 hrs of hyperfunction	580±25*	1200± 70
after 48 hrs of hyperfunction	600±40*	1220± 70*
Kidney nuclei		
+ cytosol from normal heart	740±30	1420± 80
+ cytosol from heart 24 hrs after the onset of hyperfunction	1030±50*	1700± 100
Liver nuclei		
+ cytosol from normal heart	1000±50	2300±110
+ cytosol from heart 24 hrs after the onset of hyperfunction	1300±60*	2350±120

* $p < 0.05$

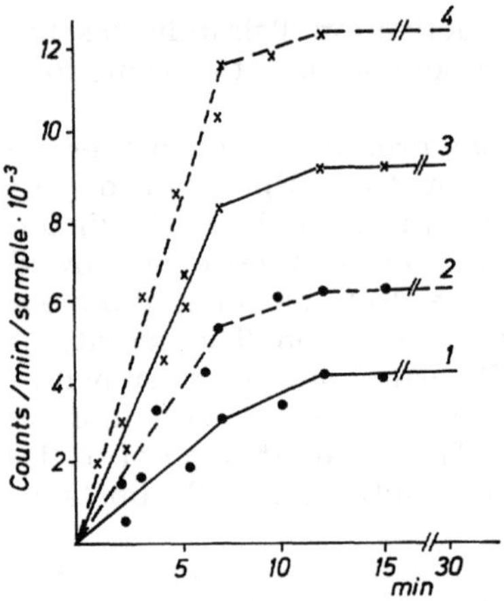

Fig. 3. Effect of the cytoplasmic fraction of the heart 48 hours after the onset of hyperfunction on the rate of [^{3}H]UMP incorporation into isolated heart nuclei. Abscissa – time (min); ordinate – counts per min · 10^3 per sample. 1 – system I + normal heart cytosol, 2 – system II + normal heart cytosol, 3 – system I + cytosol from heart at 48 hrs of hyperfunction, 4 – system II + cytosol from heart at 48 hrs of hyperfunction.

heart 24 and 48 hours after the onset of hyperfunction still increases the activity of RNA polymerase I by 45–50 %, and that of RNA polymerase II by 30–35 %. The cytoplasmic fraction from the heart 24 hours after the onset of hyperfunction was also tested in a system of liver and kidney nuclei. Table 3 shows that in this case the activity of RNA polymerase I in kidney nuclei is increased by 40 %, while that in liver nuclei by 30 % as compared to normal heart cytosol. The activity of RNA polymerase II in kidney nuclei under these conditions shows a 20 % increase; in liver nuclei no changes are observed thereby.

Figure 3 illustrates the kinetics of [^{3}H]UMP incorporation into myocardial nuclei after addition of fraction S-100 of the heart 24 hours after the onset of hyperfunction. It can be seen that the rate of RNA labelling during its linear synthesis is enhanced.

Table 4. Effect of cytosol from regenerating liver on [^{3}H] UMP incorporation into RNA of isolated nuclei.

Conditions	Counts/min/sample	
	system I	system II
Liver nuclei		
+ cytosol from normal liver	2000 ± 55	3000 ± 100
+ cytosol from regenerating liver		
3 hrs after hepatectomy	2900 ± 70	4000 ± 200
8 hrs after hepatectomy	3000 ± 200	3900 ± 150
	$p < 0.05$	$p < 0.05$
Heart nuclei		
+ cytosol from normal liver	1500 ± 100	1500 ± 50
+ cytosol from regenerating liver		
3 hrs after hepatectomy	1600 ± 120	1600 ± 70
8 hrs after hepatectomy	1650 ± 70	1550 ± 100

Table 4 sums up the results on the effects of fraction S-100 from the saved liver lobe on RNA synthesis in the nuclei of intact organs. The experimental results suggest that 3 hours after partial hepatectomy liver cytosol increases the rate of RNA synthesis in intact liver nuclei of system I by 45 % – and of system II by 35 %. 8 hours after surgery, fraction S-100 from the growing liver increases the rate of RNA synthesis in intact liver nuclei of systems I and II by 50 and 30 %, respectively. The changes in the RNA polymerase activity of heart nuclei induced by this fraction are hardly appreciable compared to a more pronounced effect of cytosol from normal liver.

The total activity of the cytoplasmic fraction of organs in hyperfunction is abolished during incubation with pronase (data not given).

Discussion

The experimental data suggest that heart and liver cytoplasm contain some factors which can accelerate RNA synthesis in isolated nuclei. Under the action of these factors the activity of RNA polymerase I – transcribing ribosomal genes – is increased to a larger degree than that of RNA polymerase II-transcribing structural genes. The stimulating effect of the cytoplasmic fraction (S-100) is exerted in systems of nuclei from homologous and heterologous organs. The activity of this fraction of the liver exceeds manifold that of the heart, irrespective of the type of nuclei. Consequently, the cytoplasmic factors of transcription are not organ-specific, and their activity is correlated with the rate of cell RNA synthesis. The activity of the cytoplasmic fraction is abolished after treatment with the proteolytic enzyme pronase and is sharply decreased after injection of CHI. This provides evidence for the protein nature of the cytoplasmic factors accelerating the transcription and for their unstability.

Earlier it was demonstrated that the extracts from Krebs ascites cells, Hela cells, and Chinese hamster oocytes can accelerate RNA synthesis in isolated nuclei of Krebs ascites cells (21). Lately it has been reported that heterologous cytoplasmic extracts (fraction S-100) from cell cultures of mammals and Xenopus oocytes in the presence of RNA polymerases of animal origin can control transcription of some structural genes and of genes coding 4S and 5S RNAs. These factors are of protein nature (8–12, 24), and some of them have been isolated (9, 12). Thus the organ nonspecificity is probably inherent to some cytoplasmic factors controlling the transcription.

It has later been established that during the hyperfunction-induced compensatory growth of the organs the activity of cytoplasmic factors accelerating RNA synthesis is enhanced. At first the activity of protein factors accelerating the synthesis of DNA-like RNA in the heart is increased followed by an increase in the activity of cytoplasmic factors accelerating rRNA synthesis. This correlates with the increased rate of rRNA and mRNA incorporation into the ribosomes and polyribosomes of the myocardium during its compensatory growth (13, 25). An enhanced activity of the cytoplasmic factors accelerating RNA synthesis was also observed in the saved liver lobe in hyperfunction. The increase of the RNA polymerase activity of normal liver nuclei and of Morris hepatoma nuclei under the action of the cytoplasmic fraction from the liver during compensatory growth was described earlier (26–28).

The cytoplasmic fraction isolated from heart and liver during their compensatory growth can accelerate RNA synthesis in different nuclei to a greater degree than the cytoplasmic fraction from intact organs. In this respect our experimental results are comparable to those obtained by Hammond et al. (7). These authors reported that when extracts from the myocardium or kidney after 24 hours of hyperfunction are added to a perfusate from isolated dog heart, the RNA obtained from this heart can accelerate protein synthesis in a reticulocyte system. Thus the literature data and our experimental findings suggest that the factors accelerating the transcription, which are additionally formed in the cytoplasm of organs at hyperfunction, are not organ-specific.

The total activity of fraction S-100 isolated from heart and liver during their compensatory growth is abolished under the action of a proteolytic enzyme. Hence this activity is also predetermined by protein factors. Our experimental results provide evidence for the phenomena described earlier by Fanburg et al. (1) and by Tsukado et al. (4), who demonstrated that an injection of small doses of the translation inhibitor, p-fluorophenylalanine, to the animals does not result in acceleration of RNA synthesis in the heart in hyperfunction, in the liver after partial hepatectomy, or during compensatory growth of these organs.

The mechanism of action of protein factors of the cytoplasm on transcription can be different. In our studies, rifamycin AF/013 did not cause any reinitiation of the polynucleotide chains in the systems used, but resulted in elongation of the polynucleotide complexes initiated in animal cells. At the same time, the rate of [^{3}H]UTP incorporation into RNA during its linear synthesis is increased, thus suggesting that the effect of protein factors on transcription consists in acceleration of the elongation process.

On the whole, the present data indicate that the animal cell cytoplasm contains organ-nonspecific protein factors which can accelerate transcription. In enhanced physiological function, the activity of these factors is increased – which is very essential for understanding the molecular mechanism initiating the accelerated synthesis of RNA.

References

1. Posner, B., B. Fanburg: Circulat. Res. **23,** 137–168 (1968).
2. Koide, F., M. Rabinowitz: Circulat. Res. **24,** 9–18 (1969).
3. Meerson, F. Z.: In: Hyperfunction, hypertrophy, cardiac insufficiency, 'Meditsina' Publishers (Moscow 1967).
4. Tsukada, K., I. Lieberman: J. Biol. Chem. **240,** 1731–1736 (1965).
5. Atzryzen, B., N. Fausto: Biochemistry **18,** 1281–1287 (1979).
6. Randen-Staron, I., W. Sendecki: Acta biochimica polonica **27,** 191–201 (1980).
7. Hammond, G., E. Wieben, C. Markert: Proc. Nat. Acad. Sci. USA **76,** 2455–2459 (1979).
8. Segal, J., T. Matsui, R. Roeder: J. Biol. Chem. **255,** 11986–11992 (1979).
9. Matsui, T., J. Segal, R. Weil, R. Roeder: J. Biol. Chem. **255,** 11992–11996 (1979).
10. Weil, A., D. Luse, J. Segal, R. Roeder: Cell **18,** 469–484 (1979).

11. Engelke, D., S. Wg, B. Shasy, R. Roeder: Cell **19,** 717–728 (1979).
12. Sakonju, S., D. Brown, D. Engelke, S.-Y. Na, B. Shastry, R. Roeder: Cell **23,** 665–669 (1981).
13. Yavich, M. P., M. I. Lerman, F. Z. Meerson: Biokhimiya (Russ.) **41,** 2110–2118 (1976).
14. Higgins, G. M., R. M. Anderson: Arch. Pathol. **12,** 186–200 (1931).
15. Pogo, A., V. Alfrey, A. Mirsky: Proc. Nat. Acad. Sci. USA **56,** 550–557 (1966).
16. Burton, K.: J. Biochem. **62,** 315–323 (1956).
17. Lowry, O. H., N. Rosebrough, A. Farr, R. Randall: J. Biol. Chem. **193,** 265–272 (1951).
18. Roeder, R., W. Rutter: Proc. Nat. Acad. Sci. USA **65,** 675–682 (1970).
19. Linder, T., F. Weinberg, P. Morris, R. Roeder, W. Rutter: Science **170,** 447–478 (1970).
20. Weinman, R., R. Roeder: Proc. Nat. Acad. Sci. USA **71,** 1790–1794 (1974).
21. Wu, G., G. Zabuy: Proc. Nat. Acad. Sci. USA **71,** 1803–1807 (1974).
22. Bitter, G., R. Roeder: Biochemistry **17,** 2198–2206 (1978).
23. Meilhac, M., Z. Tysper, P. Chambon: Eur. J. Biochem. **28,** 291–305 (1972).
24. Pelham, H., D. Brown: Proc. Nat. Acad. Sci. USA **77,** 4170–4174 (1980).
25. Meerson, F. Z., M. P. Yavich, G. G. Gorach: Voprosy meditsinskoi khimii (Russ.) **24,** 275–281 (1978).
26. Bastian, C.: Biochem. Biophys. Res. Commun. **83,** 893–900 (1978).
27. Bastian, C.: Biochem. Biophys. Res. Commun. **92,** 80–83 (1980).
28. Platonov, O. M., S. M. Zhelyabovskaya: Biokhimiya (Russ.) **45,** 1189–1195.

Authors' address:

Prof. Dr. F. Z. Meerson, Lab. of Heart, Pathophysiol. Institute, Physiol. of the USSR, Academy of Medical Sciences, Baltijskaya ul. 8, Moscow 125315, USSR

Cardiac Adaptation to Hemodynamic Overload, Training and Stress
Dr. D. Steinkopff Verlag 94–98 (1983)

New trends in biology of cardiac overload: plasma membranes, enzymes, cytoskeleton proteins and in vitro traduction of RNA

P. Mansier, K. Schwartz, L. Lelievre, J. M. Moalic, D. Charlemagne, J. L. Samuel, L. Rappaport, and B. Swynghedauw

I.N.S.E.R.M. Unité 127 – Hôpital Lariboisière – Paris (France)

Summary

It is now well established that chronic overload can induce, at least in the rat, an isoenzymic redistribution of myosin, which correlates with the diminution of the speed of shortening and which is reponsible for the improved myocardial efficiency. We are currently trying to extend this concept by exploring other systems. (i) Sarcolemma. A new preparative technique was developed in rat heart. Most of the vesicles were inside-out, and contained Na-K ATPase, as shown by blotting, with a high specific activity (110 μmole Pi $\cdot$ mg^{-1} $\cdot$ hour^{-1}). This preparation was as sensitive to ouabain as those from other species, providing the myocardium has been previously perfused with a relaxing solution. (ii) An immunofluorescence technique and an immunological assay were developed in order to show the tubulin network in isolated myocytes from overloaded tissue. (iii) A preparation of total RNA (1.3 mg/g f.t.), which contains 2.3 % of poly A + RNA, has been developed in adult rat heart. The population of mRNA (average nucleotide length 1,740) was characterized by *in-vitro* translation.

Key words: cardiac overload, tubulin, Na-K ATPase, sarcolemma, messenger RNA, immunofluorescence, digitalis, translation, rat heart

Introduction

Cardiac adaptation to chronic overload implies a modification of gene expression both quantitative and qualitative. A qualitative change in gene expression of myosin was found in rats (10, 12), which normally possess three isoenzymes V3, V2 and V1 in a relative ratio of 1:3:7. This pattern was reversed during chronic overload, and this inversion may account for both the change in the shortening speed (15) and the improvement in efficiency (1). It has been confirmed by several laboratories both in rat and in rabbit (7, 9).

We are currently trying to develop the concept according to which overload modifies not only the expression of myosin genes but also that of other genes and more specifically that of cytoskeleton and sarcolemma proteins.

This paper was essentially preliminary and presents three new approaches of the above-mentioned concept.

Methods

Sarcolemma. The heart was coronary perfused with a relaxing buffer made 0.025 M in KCl, 5 mM EDTA, and 0.039 M in Na-tetraborate, pH 6.8. The tissue was then homogenised into a hypotonic pyrophosphate solution in order to provoke a hypotonic lysis, and a highly enriched sarcolemma preparation was obtained by differential centrifugations. The Na-K ATPase was measured at 37 °C into 4 mM $MgCl_2$, 100 mM NaCl, 10 mM KCl, 40 mM imidazole. HCl pH 7.4 and 4 mM ATP. The maximal inhibition of this enzyme activity was obtained within 1 to 3 minutes after the exposure of the enzyme to ouabain. K^+-para-nitrophenylphosphatase (K^+-pNPPase), succinate dehydrogenase and myofibrillar ATPase were measured as described elsewhere (8). The isolation of inside-out vesicles was performed using ConA and methyl-αD-mannopyranoside as previously described (8).

Tubulin. Antibodies against rat brain microtubules were raised in rabbits and purified by affinity chromatography (14). Quantification ot tubulin was obtained by using the sandwich immunoassay (5) and a micro-ELISA reader Dynatechn. Pure myocytes were isolated from rat hearts by using the collagenase technique previously described (4). Indirect immunofluorescence was performed in a Ca^{2+}-free medium after treatment of the myocytes with Triton X-100, fixation with formaldehyde and incubation with purified sheep antitubulin immunoglobulins and fluorescein-labelled rabbit IgG (14).

mRNA. Total RNA was isolated from frozen adult rat heart by the guanidine-ethanol procedure (3) followed by a treatment with 3 M Na acetate, pH 5.2. Electrophoresis of glyoxalated RNA in agarose (16), in-vitro translation in a reticulocyte lysate system (13), fluorography, isolation of poly A + RNA on oligo-dT and estimation of the content in poly A + by using the ^{3}H-poly U assay (6) were performed as previously published.

Results

The rather high degree of purification of the sarcolemma was attested by a 35–130-fold enrichment in K^+-p NPPase and in 5' nucleotidase, and above all, by a very high activity in the ouabain-sensitive Na-K ATPase (110 μmole Pi · $hour^{-1}$ · mg^{-1}). Moreover, this preparation does not contain any significant amount of mitochondrial, myofibrillar and sarcoplasmic reticulum markers, which all were found in other fractions in the sucrose gradient.

This preparation was characterized by the predominance of inside-out vesicles, i.e., by vesicles which did not bind to a ConA affinity column. Other evidence for the internalization of the surface membrane was provided by the effect of low concentrations of SDS or of repetitive freezings and thawings. These experiments were based on the fact that the ATP binding site of the Na-K ATPase was internal, whilst the ouabain binding site was external. Therefore, when the vesicles were fragilized, they became permeable to ouabain, and consequently their ATPase became inhibited by G-strophanthidin. Simultaneously, the Na-K ATPase without ouabain was unaffected or slightly modified.

The most important characteristic of this preparation was its sensitivity to low amount of ouabain. The rat heart Na-K ATPase is generally considered to be insensitive to ouabain with an half-maximal inhibition at 6×10^{-5} M. This is in fact true when the sarcolemma was prepared from hearts either simply kept in ice and not perfused or perfused with 2 mM $CaCl_2$.

When the heart was perfused, as it is such in our technique, with EDTA, the sarcolemmal vesicles exhibited a two-step dose response curve to ouabain: 55 % of the Na-K ATPase was inhibited between 10^{-9} and 3×10^{-7} M ouabain and 45 % between 3×10^{-7} and 10^{-5}M. This was the same when membranes were prepared from isolated myocytes and was unaffected by opening the vesicles (8).

Tubulin. Tubulin content in adult rat heart myocytes was found to be approximetaly 10 µg per 100 mg of the total protein content which approximately represents $^{1}/_{1000}$ of that of the brain.

This low amount of tubulin was visualized by immunofluorescence both around the nuclei with usually a spreading at the poles and in the sarcoplasm as a tortuoùs network. The microtubular network disappears when disrupting reagents have been used, i.e., 2 hours after a colchicine injection, 3 hours after incubation of myocytes at 3 °C. Preincubation with taxol prevents the effects of cold and intensified the normal pattern (14). These treatments leave the cell shape unmodified.

Preliminary studies show that during ontogenesis the tubulin network appears to develop from the nucleus towards the periphery, and that it was intensified in the early stage of cardiac overload.

Messenger RNA. Our preparation of total RNA was deproteinized (260/280 = 1.70) without phenol treatment which usually gives scattered results for the estimation of mRNA. It was essentially free from DNA, the yield was 1.65 mg total RNA per g of fresh tissue and the content in Poly A + RNA, as estimated by hybridization with radioactive poly U, 2.30 %.

The average nucleotide length of the messenger RNAs was estimated after glyoxalation and elution from an agarose gel electrophoresis and hybridation with ^{3}H poly U. It was 1,640 for the heart and 1,740 for the liver. 15 to 20 % of the cardiac mRNA were heavier than the 28 S marker.

In vitro in presence of a reticulocyte lysate and in optimized conditions (2, 13) the messenger incorporates 40,000 to 60,000 dpm for 25 µl of assay. A plateau of incorporation was obtained for 400 ng of poly A + RNA, a larger amount having frequently an inhibitory effect (2). This was unaffected by using two different lysate systems which are commercially available.

During overload, both concentrations of total RNA and of poly A + RNA increase and peak by the 4th day, but the percentage of poly A + RNA apparently remains unchanged.

Discussion

Since a modification of the action potential has been clearly established by several people during cardiac overload, it is reasonable to think that, as for the sarcomere, a biochemical counter-part may exist in the sarcolemma. The literature, on this latter point, is rather confused, and it appears that the problem has to be considered on new basis.

We hope that our new preparation of sarcolemma will allow a careful examination of this problem. The preparation has several unique characteristics: (i) although we are dealing with rat heart, the preparation, made from a relaxed tissue (11), was sensitive to low concentrations of ouabain; (ii) the percentage of right-side-out and inside-out vesicles has been carefully estimated; (iii) this is, to date, the preparation with the highest specific activity in ouabain sensitive Na-K ATPase ever published.

To date there are no papers on the development of cytoskeleton proteins in hypertrophy. The main reason was very likely the difficulty in identifying these proteins, tubulin but also others such as vimentine, because of their low concentrations, of the dense structure of the heart, and of the predominancy of myofibrillar proteins.

To develop a good and reproducible preparation of total and poly A + RNA from adult rat heart was more difficult than expected. This is very likely due to the density of the tissue and the rather large amount of RNAase in adult heart. Several problems remain to be resolved before trying to know if the changes in gene expression are in this condition transcriptional or post-transcriptional.

References

1. Alpert, N. R., L. A. Mulieri: Increased myothermal economy of isometric force generation in compensated cardiac hypertrophy induced by pulmonary artery constriction in the rabbit. A characterization of heat liberation in normal and hypertrophied right ventricular papillary muscle. Circulat. Res. **50,** 491–500 (1982).
2. Benoff, S., B. Nadal-Ginard: Cell-free translation of mammalian myosin heavy-chain messenger ribonucleic acid from growing and fused-L6 E9 myoblasts. Biochemistry (Wash.) **18,** 494–500 (1979).
3. Chirgwin, J. M., A. E. Przybyla, R. J. MacDonald, W. J. Rutter: Isolation of biologically active ribonucleic acid from sources enriched in ribonuclease. Biochemistry (Wash.) **18,** 5294–5299 (1979).
4. Cutilletta, A. F., M. C. Aumont, A. C. Nag, R. Zak: Separation of muscle and non muscle cells from adult rat myocardium: an application to the study of RNA polymerases. J. Mol. Cell. Cardiol. **9,** 399–407 (1977).
5. Engvall, E.: Enzyme immunoassay ELISA and EMIT. Methods in Enzymology. A. H. van Vunakis, and J. J. Langone, ed. **70,** 419–439 (1980).
6. Gilles, D., S. Marshall, R. C. Gallo: RNA of RNA tumour viruses contains poly A. Nature New Biol. **236,** 227–231 (1972).
7. Gorza, L., P. Pauletto, A. C. Pessina, S. Sartore, S. Schiaffino: Isomyosin distribution in normal and pressure-overload rat ventricular myocardium. An immunohistochemical study. Circulat. Res. **49,** 1003–1009 (1981).
8. Lelievre, L. G., P. Mansier, M. Preteseille, G. Berson, B. Swynghedauw: Isolation of impermeable inside-out vesicles from an enriched sarcolemma fraction of rat heart. (To be published.)
9. Litten, R. Z., B. J. Martin III, R. B. Low, N. R. Alpert: Altered myosin isozyme patterns from pressure-overload and thyrotoxic hypertrophied rabbit hearts. Circulat. Res. **50,** 856–864 (1982).
10. Lompré, A. M., K. Schwartz, A. Albis, G. Lacombe, N. V. Thiem, B. Swynghedauw: Myosin isozymes redistribution in chronic heart overloading. Nature **282,** 105–107 (1979).
11. Mansier, P., L. Lelievre: Ca^{2+} free perfusion in rat heart reveals a (Na^{+}-K^{+})-ATPase form highly sensitive to ouabain. Nature **300,** 535–537 (1982).
12. Mercadier, J. J., A. M. Lompré, C. Wisnewsky, J. L. Samuel, J. Bercovici, B. Swynghedauw, K. Schwartz: Myosin isoenzymic changes in several models of rat cardiac hypertrophy. Circulat. Res. **49,** 525–532 (1981).
13. Pelham, H. R. B., R. J. Jackson: An efficient mRNA-dependent translation system from reticulocyte lysates. Europ. J. Biochem., **67,** 247–256 (1976).

14. Samuel, J. L., K. Schwartz, A. M. Lompré, C. Delcayre, F. Marotte, B. Swynghedauw, L. Rappaport: Immunological quantitation and localization of tubulin in adult rat heart isolated myocytes (Submitted.)
15. Schwartz, K., Y. Lecarpentier, J. L. Martin, A. M. Lompré, J. J. Mercadier, B. Swynghedauw: Myosin isoenzymic distribution correlates with speed of myocardial contraction. J. Mol. Cell. Cardiol. **13,** 1071–1075 (1981).
16. Thomas, P. S.: Hybridation of denatured RNA and small RNA fragments transferred to nitrocellulose. Proc. Nat. Acad. Sci. USA, **77,** 5201–5205 (1980).

Authors' address:

P. Mansier, I.N.S.E.R.M. Unité 127, Hôpital Lariboisière, 41 Bd de la Chapelle, 75010 Paris, France

Structural changes of contractile proteins

Cardiac Adaptation to Hemodynamic Overload, Training and Stress
Dr. D. Steinkopff Verlag 101–103 (1983)

Adaptive changes in cardiac isomyosins as visualized by immunofluorescence

S. Schiaffino, L. Gorza, S. Sartore, C. Valfré, and P. Pauletto

Istituto di Patologia Generale, Clinica Chirurgica, Centro per le cardiopatie operabili, Istituto di Medicina Clinica, Università di Padova (Italy)

Summary

Immunocytochemistry with specific antimyosin antibodies has been used to define the isomyosin composition of cardiac muscle cells in normal and stressed hearts. Heterogeneity of ventricular muscle cells and adaptive changes in cardiac isomyosins have also been observed in the human ventricular myocardium by the same procedures.

Key words: myosin, immunofluorescence, ventricular myocardium, human heart, cardiac hypertrophy

During the last few years there has been a growing interest in the study of myosin changes that accompany cardiac hypertrophy. This has been the result of the introduction of new methods for the analysis of the myosin composition of muscle cells (Hoh et al., 1978) and the demonstration that different myosin types are present in cardiac muscle. Several lines of evidence derived from the application of enzymatic, electrophoretic and immunochemical procedures have shown that the mammalian ventricular myocardium contains both high-ATPase, fast-type, and low-ATPase, slow-type isomyosins, whose relative concentration may vary during development and during hypertrophy. The finding that the proportion of fast and slow ventricular isomyosins is closely correlated with the velocity of shortening of cardiac muscle has strongly supported the notion that myosin is a major determinant of cardiac contractility (see Schwartz et al., 1981; Ebrecht et al., 1982; Alpert and Mulieri, 1982).

In this laboratory we have developed polyclonal antibodies specific for the fast-type (V1 using Hoh's nomenclature) and slow-type (V3) ventricular isomyosins. By immunofluorescence, these isomyosins appeared to be heterogeneously distributed among ventricular muscle cells in different mammalian hearts. In one study (Gorza et al., 1981), we found that immunoreactivity for V3 myosin is higher in the left compared to the right ventricle and in subendocardial compared to subepicardial layers in the normal rat heart. This heterogeneous pattern of reactivity was changed to

Work supported by CNR and Ministero della Pubblica Istruzione.

a homogeneous positive reaction in hypertrophied hearts of rats with renal hypertension. In another study (Sartore et al., 1981), we found that immunoreactivity for V1 myosins varies among ventricular muscle cells of the rabbit and bovine hearts, and that striking transformations to homogeneously positive or negative reactivity can be induced by hyper- or hypothyroidism, respectively. These findings are in agreement with the results of biochemical studies indicating that hemodynamic overload and thyroid hormone are major control factors of cardiac isomyosins.

We have now applied immunocytochemical methods to the study of isomyosin distribution in the human heart. Both autoptic and peroperatory specimens have been analyzed by immunofluorescence with an antibody that reacts specifically with the fast-type, V1 myosin. A number of labeled muscle cells were consistently found in samples obtained from patients without heart disease (fig. 1).

However, the proportion of labeled cells was seen to vary considerably from one heart to the other. In occasional specimens, the majority of muscle cells stained for V1 myosin, whereas in others only rare reactive fibers were encountered. Preliminary observations were also made on samples obtained from patients with cardiac hypertrophy or valvular heart disease. Almost no fiber stained for V1 myosin in hypertrophied hearts from hypertensive patients, as well as in papillary muscles from patients undergoing mitral valve replacement for mitral stenosis (fig. 2).

In the latter case, the papillary muscles were hypertrophied and stretched by the fibrotic transformation of the infravalvular apparatus.

These findings indicate that an antigenic form of ventricular myosin, analogous to the V1 isomyosin found in the rat and rabbit heart, is present in variable proportions in the normal human heart and disappears completely in cardiac muscle cells as a result of pressure overload or mechani-

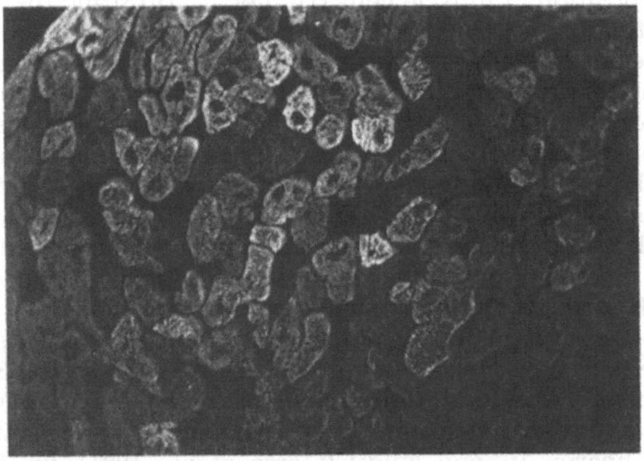

Fig. 1. Section of normal human ventricular myocardium processed for indirect immunofluorescence with anti-bAm, a policlonal antibody specifically reactive with the fast-type, V1 isomyosin (see Sartore et al., 1981). Several muscle cells stain with variable intensity for V1 myosin.

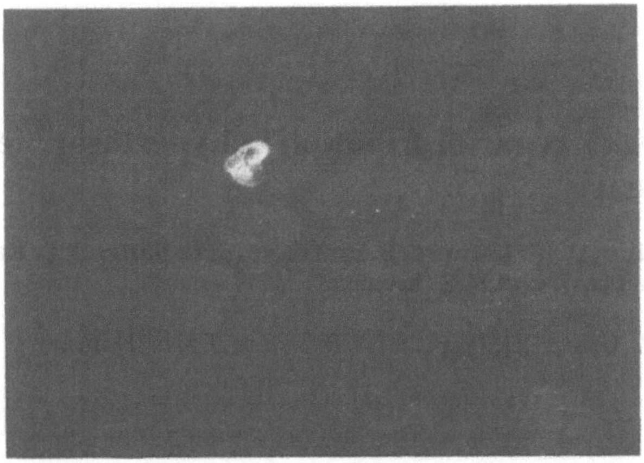

Fig. 2. Section of papillary muscle from a patient with mitral valve stenosis, stained with anti-bAm. Only one muscle cell stains for V1 myosin.

cal stretch. Further studies are necessary to quantify the amount of this V1-like myosin in the human heart in order to establish the physiological significance of isomyosin transitions in human heart disease.

References

Alpert, N. R., L. A. Mulieri: Heat, mechanics and myosin ATPase in normal and hypertrophied heart muscle. Fed. Proc. **41,** 192–198 (1982).

Ebrecht, G. H., R. Rupp, R. Jacob: Alterations of mechanical parameters in chemically skinned preparations of rat myocardium as a function of isoenzyme pattern of myosin. Basic Res. Cardiol. **77,** 220–234 (1982).

Gorza, L., P. Pauletto, A. L. Pessina, S. Sartore, S. Schiaffino: Isomyosin distribution in normal and pressure overloaded rat ventricular myocardium. An immunohistochemical study. Circulat. Res. **49,** 1003–1009 (1981).

Hoh, J. F., P. A. McGrath, P. T. Hale: Electrophoretic analysis of multiple forms of rat cardiac myosin: Effect of hypophysectomy and thyroxine replacement. J. Mol. Cell. Cardiol. **10,** 1053–1076 (1978).

Sartore, S., L. Gorza, S. Pierobon Bormioli, L. Dalla Libera, S. Schiaffino: Myosin types and fiber types in cardiac muscle. 1. Ventricular myocardium. J. Cell Biol. **88,** 226–233 (1981).

Schwartz, K., Y. Lecarpentier, J. L. Martin, A. M. Lompre, J. J. Mercadier, B. Swynghedauw: Myosin isoenzymic distribution correlates with speed of myocardial contraction. J. Mol. Cell. Cardiol. **13,** 1071–1075 (1981).

Authors' address:

Dr. S. Schiaffino, Istituto di Patologia Generale, Università di Padova, Via Loredan 16, 35100 Padova, Italia

Cardiac Adaptation to Hemodynamic Overload, Training and Stress
Dr. D. Steinkopff Verlag 104–112 (1983)

Myosin isoenzymic distribution in hyperthrophied rat and human hearts

J. J. Mercadier, A. M. Lompré, P. Bouveret, J. L. Samuel, L. Rappaport, B. Swynghedauw, and K. Schwartz

I.N.S.E.R.M. Unité 127, Hôpital Lariboisière, Paris (France)

Summary

Rat cardiac ventricular myosins were obtained from fetuses, from young, adult, and old normal animals, from hypophysectomised adults and from rats submitted to a chronic mechanical overload of the heart. The different proteins were compared by electrophoresis in non-denaturing conditions and by competitive enzyme-linked immunosorbent assay (ELISA). For the latter purpose, antibodies specific of the rat cardiac V_3 isomyosin were used. It was found that the V_3 isomyosin of fetuses is indistinguishable from that of adult hypertrophied heart. This result strongly suggests that adaptation to chronic increase in cardiac work is mediated through the synthesis of the fetal form of myosin. Double immunolabeling of isolated myocytes with antibodies specific of the rat V_1 or the rat V_3 isomyosins showed that this isoenzymic redistribution occurs throughout the whole length of the myocytes, without any preferential localization of the newly synthesized V_3 isoform. The existence of such a mechanism of adaptation was also searched for in human hearts. Competitive ELISA performed with antibodies against human cardiac heavy meromyosin indicated no differences in apparent affinities with the myosins of two "control" subjects and of three patients with noticeable cardiac hypertrophy.

Key words: pressure cardiac hypertrophy, rat and human ventricles, immunological and electrophoretical analyses, fetal and adult cardiac V_1 and V_3 isomyosins

Introduction

In the last 3 years, the existence of two basic types of cardiac ventricular myosins, V_1 and V_3, has been described in several mammalian species, and more especially in rats and rabbits (see ref. 27 for review). V_1 exhibits higher Ca^{++}-stimulated and actin-activated ATPase activities than V_3, and a faster electrophoretic mobility in non-denaturing conditions (5, 9, 12, 14, 19). The respective amounts of the two isomyosins is not constant, but varies during ontogenic development and ageing, and also in several pathological conditions such as chronic cardiac overloads. In all species so far tested, myosin is essentially V_3 during fetal life, and V_1 appears around the time of birth. Adult rats remain mostly V_1, while rabbits and pigs return to V_3 after several weeks of age (4, 9, 14). Hyperthyroidism (9, 12, 23) and physical training (20) favor apparition of V_1, whereas chronic mechanical overloads favor V_3 (8, 13, 16, 20). The close relationship between the velocity of shortening of cardiac fibers and myosin ATPase specific activities (see ref. 22 for review) can thus be now mostly explained in terms of isomyosin changes, and a correlation has indeed been found between V_1 or V_3 amounts and mechanical V_{max} (7, 25). These isomyosins' redistribution can be considered as true adaptative mechanisms as the tension-dependent heat per unit tension during an isometric contraction (2, 3) and oxygen consumption (10) are decreased when V_3 is increased.

The aim of the present study was to gather evidence in chronic mechanical overloads of the rat heart of the fetal nature of the adult V_3 and of its distribution within adult myocytes. We also tried to expand the isomyosin concept to the human heart.

Methods

Experiments were performed in 30 male Wistar rats. Abdominal aortic stenosis was performed at 2 months of age (i.e., 200 g b.w.) essentially as in (6), except that the partially occluded Weck hemoclip was positioned around the upper part of the abdominal aorta. The rats were killed at various times after surgery (1 to 3 weeks). Hypothyroidism was induced by hypophysectomy at 10 weeks of age, and the rats were killed at 7 weeks after the operation. The animals were housed in air-conditioned quarters with no more than six rats per cage. Fetal hearts were obtained from 18-day embryos. All animals were killed by a sharp blow on the neck and the hearts were rapidly excised. Both ventricles were dissected, blotted dry, and frozen in liquid nitrogen.

Pure myosins were obtained as in Lompre et al. (1979). Antibodies specific of rat V_1 isomyosin (a-rt V_1) were obtained by successive immunoaffinity chromatographies on columns of insolubilized rat V_3 and rat V_1 myosins (27). Antibodies specific of the rat V_3 isomyosin (a-rt V_3), in fact, antibodies directed against guinea-pig soleus myosin were prepared as in (18), and were a generous gift of S. Sartore and S. Schiaffino. Antibodies against human cardiac myosin were obtained by injecting sodium dodecyl sulfate-denatured human cardiac heavy-meromyosin to guinea pigs (26). Competitive enzyme-linked immunosorbent assays (ELISA) were performed as in (27) with human myosins either in their native state or denatured by sodium dodecyl sulfate after removal of excess sodium dodecyl sulfate by chromatography on Sephadex G-10 (26). Polyacrylamide gel electrophoresis in non-denaturing conditions was carried out as in (13) on 4 % polyacrylamide gels, using a Pharmacia GE-4II apparatus.

The procedures for isolation of pure cardiac myocytes and their double immunolabeling with a-rt V_1 or a-rt V_3 immunoglobulins are described in detail elsewhere (21).

The human myosins were prepared from autopsy samples of left ventricular myocardium of five adult subjects. Two patients (numbers 26 and 41) had no clinical evidence of heart disease. Their heart weights were inferior to 300 g, and they were considered as the control hearts. The three other patients (numbers 18, 36 and 37) had medical histories of chronic cardiac overload, and their heart weights, recorded from the autopsy report, were 300, 820 and 660 g, respectively. Patient 18 suffered from high blood pressure, patient 36 from mitral regurgitation and patient 37 from aortic incompetence. All specimens were frozen at the time of necropsy (8 h post mortem) and stored at −80 °C.

Results

Figure 1 summarizes the electrophoretic pattern of native myosins from several rat heart ventricles. Normal fetuses (F) and adult hypophysec-

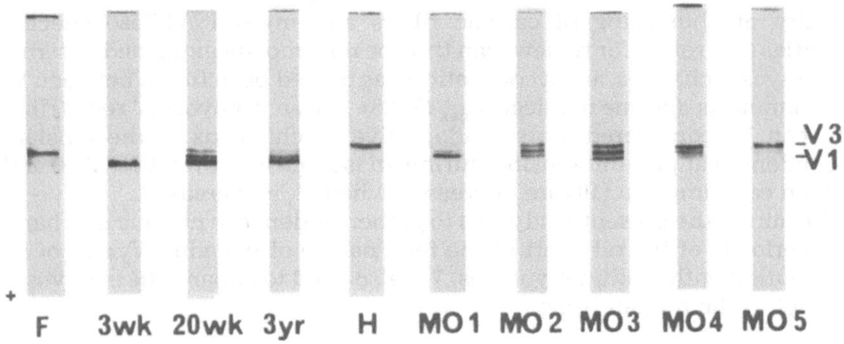

Fig. 1. Gel electrophoresis of native rat cardiac myosins under non-dissociating conditions. Ventricular myosins were purified from: F: fetuses (18 days *in utero*); 3wk: three-week-old controls; H: hypophysectomized animals; MO: hearts submitted to mechanical overload by abdominal aortic constriction. The degree of cardiac hypertrophy was calculated as in ref. 13 and was equal to 31 % for MO 1, 47 % for MO 2, 45 % for MO 3, 71 % for MO 4 and 94 % for MO 5. Myosin samples (1 to 3 μg) were run for 22 hours at 14 V cm^{-1} and 3 °C on cylindrical gels (5 by 60 mn) containing 3.88 % (w/v) acrylamide and 0.12 % (w/v) N-N' methylene-bisacrylamide in 20 mM sodium pyrophosphate buffer (pH 8.5), 1 mM EDTA, 0.01 % (v/v) 2-mercaptoethanol and 10 % (v/v) glycerol.

tomized animals (H) contained almost solely V_3. Myosins from hypertrophied hearts obtained after mechanical overloading (MO) were composed of a mixture of V_1, V_2 and V_3, the ratio of which varied with the degree of hypertrophy. Three-week-old animals (3 wk) contained only V_1. Myosin from hearts of very old animals (3 yr) was approximately 20–30 % V_3. All these patterns were in full agreement with previously published data (9, 14).

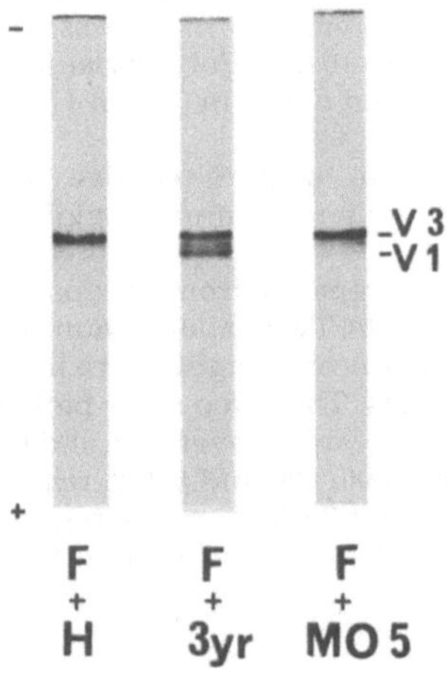

Fig. 2. Gel electrophoresis under non-dissociating conditions of mixtures of several native rat cardiac myosin. Abbreviations and experimental procedures as in figure 1.

To further characterize the electrophoretic mobilities of the different V_3 bands, comigrations were performed with myosins from the hearts of either fetuses or very old animals or hypophysectomized adults, or from a severely hypertrophied heart (fig. 2). All V_3 isomyosins appeared as single bands which strongly suggests that they are the same protein.

Myosins from fetal and hypophysectomized rats could precisely be compared as in the latter experimental model pure V_3 isoforms can be produced. As shown in (27), antibodies directed against guinea pig soleus myosin exhibit the same apparent affinity for both myosins, indicating that in this immune system and with this discriminant approach, fetal and adult hypophysectomized myosins appear very similar. Finally, monodimensional peptide maps were performed after partial proteolytic cleavage with *Staphylococcus aureus* protease in the presence of SDS (not shown). Although pure V_1 and V_3 isoforms differed by at least four peptides (27), careful analysis of myosins from 3-year-old and mechanically overloaded animals showed no additional peptides. This again was strongly suggestive of an identity between all V_3 forms, thus implying that

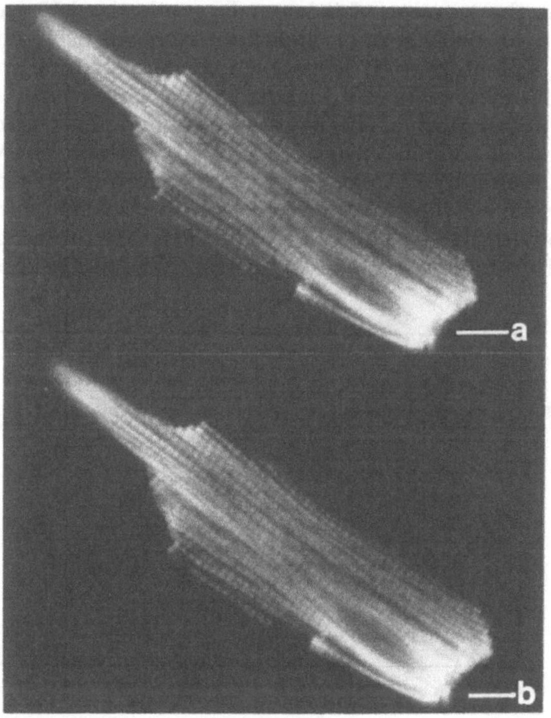

Fig. 3. Double indirect immunofluorescence micrographs (a and b) of a myocyte isolated from an hypertrophied rat heart. Hypertrophy was induced by constriction of the abdominal aorta, and the animal was sacrified 2 days after the operation. Incubations were performed with a-rat V_1 myosin immunoglobulins revealed with rhodamine-labeled goat a-guinea pig IgG (a) and a-rat V_3 myosin immunoglobulins revealed with fluorescein-labeled goat a-rabbit IgG (b) (Bar = 10 μm).

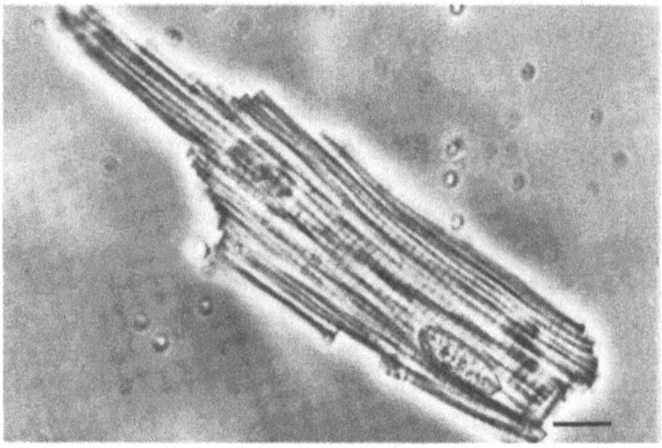

Fig. 4. Phase contrast image of myocyte from figure 3.

in adults the fetal form of the heavy chain is synthetized in some pathological conditions.

To determine the location of this newly synthetized V_3 isoform within the myocytes, a double immunological approach was used with antibodies specific of the V_1 isoform (a-rt V_1) labeled with rhodamine and antibodies specific of the V_3 isoform (a-rt V_3) labeled with fluorescein. After 2 days of stenosis, the population of myocytes contained 3 types of cells: one labeled only with a-rt V_1 (20 %), one labeled only with the a-rt V_3 (20 %), and the third one labeled by both antibodies. An example of a double-labeled myocyte is shown on figure 3 together with the phase-contrast image of the same myocyte (fig. 4). The selectivity of the immunological staining towards myosin is evidenced by comparison of the images obtained either

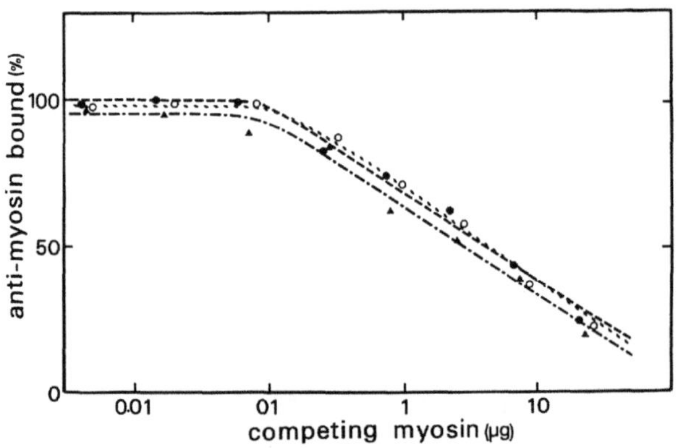

Fig 5. Competitive ELISA assays with native human cardiac myosins. Microtiter polystyrene plates were coated with myosin from the control heart n° 36, and the antibodies to normal cardiac human heavy meromyosin were reacted in the presence of increasing amounts of competing myosin. Results are expressed as a percentage of the amount of antibody bound in the absence of competing myosin. Competing human myosins: ●– – – –● control heart n° 36, ▲– · – · –▲ hypertrophied heart n° 37, ○– – – –○ hypertrophied heart n° 41.

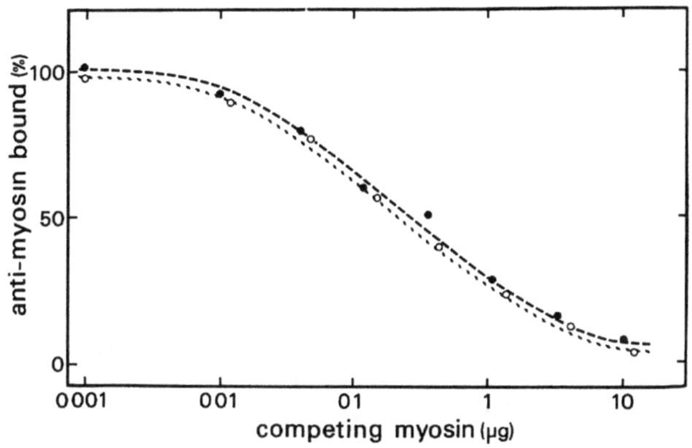

Fig. 6. Competitive ELISA assays with SDS-denatured human cardiac myosin. Experimental procedures as in figure 4. Competing myosins: ● - - - - ● control heart n° 18, ○ - - - - ○ hypertrophied heart n° 26.

in phase-contrast or after the double immunological labeling. Both types of antibodies stained all the sarcomeres, and there was no specific localization of one or the other isoform. Such an identical repartition of both isomyosins was in very good agreement with observations previously made in normal adult rats (21).

According to pyrophosphate gel analysis, adult human myosin is composed of a unique band, which appears to be very close to the rat V_3 isoform (24, Mercadier et al., in preparation). Using antibodies prepared against normal human ventricular myosin, we have tried to detect some structural differences between myosins from normal and hypertrophied hearts. For this, competitive ELISA were performed with native (fig. 5) and sodium dodecyl sulfate-denatured (fig. 6) myosins and antibodies directed against human heavy meromyosin. In both cases, the curves obtained with the myosins from normal hearts were superimposable to those from hypertrophied hearts, indicating that both myosin types shared the same antigenic determinants in these immune systems.

Discussion

Cardiac isomyosin redistributions have been well characterized in rats and rabbits, under several physiological and pathological situations (see 27 for review). The results presented here show that adaptation to chronic mechanical overload of the adult rat heart is probably also mediated through synthesis of the fetal myosin form and that this synthesis occurs harmoniously throughout the myocyte. Some data also indicate that human myosin from hypertrophied heart is closely related to that of normal hearts.

Precise comparisons of two myosin isoforms require very discriminant techniques and pure isoforms. This could easily be done with V_3 isoforms from fetal and hypophysectomized adults (27), because the latter experimental model yields pure V_3. In contrast, mechanical overloads induce mixed isoenzymic pattern with various degrees of V_3 amount (fig. 1). In these conditions, isolation of V_3 requires immunoaffinity columns, and indeed this procedure has been used by Chizzonite et al. (4) when these authors compared the structures of V_1 and V_3 in the rabbit heart. We have used pyrophosphate gel, which enables comparisons of individual isoforms in a mixture (fig. 2), and found no differences between V_3 from old animals, hypophysectomized adults and fetuses. Moreover, on the basis of monodimensional peptide maps, we saw no evidence of new peptides suggestive of an additional unknown isoenzyme. It is, of course, possible that the same band contains two isomyosins as mono-dimensional analysis is not extremely resolutive, especially when the comparisons are performed with mixtures and not with pure isomyosins. It remains, nevertheless, that in rats, rabbits, and pigs pyrophosphate gel plus peptide maps analysis enabled to differentiate V_1 and V_3 isoforms (5, 9, 12, 27). Only methods yielding amino-acid sequence will give the definitive answer, but it seems reasonable to assume at the present time that in rats an equilibrium exists between only two heavy chains, and that in adults, as a response to one or several triggers, the synthesis of the fetal form is derepressed. Identical conclusions were recently drawn concerning the balance of rabbit cardiac isozymes (4).

We found no difference in the distribution of the two myosin forms within one myocyte during the transformation process from V_1 to V_3 in chronic overload (fig. 3). During normal growth, or the differentiation of cardiac cells in culture, the two isoforms also appear identically distributed (21). It is thus interesting to note that the basic mechanisms which underly the replacement of one sarcomeric protein by the other is probably the same during normal growth and in response to increase in work. Since the two isomyosins hydrolyze ATP at different rates, one might postulate that the rate of cycling of the cross-bridges is different, and the question is, how in the same myocyte and probably in the same sarcomere these two proteins can function. Winegrad et al. (28) have recently proposed that the utilization of one isoform is under adrenergic control, and indeed this would be an attractive explanation of the mean by which one myocyte could select V_1 or V_3.

In humans, the experiments reported here are not in favor of the existence of significant isomyosin changes in response to chronic cardiac overload. Neither native nor SDS-denatured myosins from hypertrophied hearts exhibited different antigenic epitopes from the control hearts (fig. 5–6). It should however been pointed out that the antibodies used here were raised against whole myosin from control hearts and thus, if several isozymes exist, our antibodies will not allow to discriminate them. It might thus be postulated that, in these experimental conditions, small structural differences (for example 5 %) could hardly be detected, although this method is very sensitive if antibodies specific of one isomyosin form are used. Preliminary experiments performed with specific anti-rat V_1 myosin antibodies indicated that small amounts of V_1 indeed existed in the human ventricle. No differences, on the other hand, were found between myosins from cardiomyopathic and normal subjects (15, 24), and Ca^{++}-stimulated ATPase activities were not significantly lower in autopsy material from hypertrophied hearts as compared to controls

(Mercadier et al., in preparation). Significant decreases in myofibrillar ATPase activities nevertheless have been described on severely hypertrophied hearts with congestive failure (1, 11, 17). If this is confirmed, it implies that other mechanisms exist at the sarcomeric level to regulate human myofibrillar ATPase.

Acknowledgements

We wish to thank F. Marotte for performing the abdominal aorta constrictions, C. Wisnewsky for preparing the antiserum to human cardiac heavy meromyosin, S. Sartore and S. Schiaffino for the gift of the a-guinea pig soleus myosin antibodies, and P. Cagnac for the secretarial work. This work was supported in part by Institut National de la Santé et de la Recherche Médicale, grant n° 80 5034.

References

1. Alpert, N. R., M. S. Gordon: Myofibrillar adenosine triphosphatase activity in congestive heart failure. Amer. J. Physiol. **202,** 940–946 (1982).
2. Alpert, N. R., L. A. Mulieri: Heat mechanics and myosin ATPase in normal and hypertrophied heart muscle. Fed. Proc. **41,** 192–198 (1981).
3. Alpert, N. R., L. A. Mulieri: Increased myothermal economy of isometric force generation in compensated cardiac hypertrophy induced by pulmonary artery constriction in the rabbit. Circulat. Res. **50,** 491–500 (1982).
4. Chizzonite, R. A., A. W. Everett, W. A. Clark, S. Jakovcic, M. Rabinowitz, R. Zak: Isolation and characterization of two molecular variants of myosin heavy-chain from rabbit ventricle. Change in their content during normal growth and after treatment with thyroid hormone. J. Biol. Chem. **257,** 2056–2065 (1982).
5. Clark, W. A., R. A. Chizzonite, A. W. Everett, M. Rabinowitz, R. Zak: Species correlations between cardiac isomyosins. J. Biol. Chem. **257,** 5449–5454 (1982).
6. Cutilletta, A. F., M. Rudnik, R. Zak: Muscle and non-muscle cell RNA polymerase activity during the development of myocardial hypertrophy. J. Mol. Cell. Cardiol. **10,** 677–687 (1978).
7. Ebrecht, G. H., R. Rupp, R. Jacob: Alterations of mechanical parameters in chemically skinned preparations of rat myocardium as a function of isoenzyme pattern of myosin. Basic Res. Cardiol. **77,** 220–234 (1982).
8. Gorza, L., P. Pauletto, A. L. Pessina, S. Sartore, S. Schiaffino: Isomyosin distribution in normal and pressure-overloaded rat ventricular myocardium. An immunohistochemical study. Circulat. Res. **49,** 1003–1009 (1981).
9. Hoh, J. F. Y., P. A. McGrath, P. T. Hale: Electrophoretic analysis of multiple forms of rat cardiac myosin: Effect of hypophysectomy and thyroxine replacement. J. Mol. Cell. Cardiol. **10,** 1053–1076 (1978).
10. Kissling, G., H. Rupp, L. Mallay, R. Jacob: Alterations in cardiac oxygen consumption under chronic pressure overload. Significance of the isoenzyme pattern of myosin. Basic Res. Cardiol. **77,** 255–269 (1982).
11. Leclercq, J. F., B. Swynghedauw: Myofibrillar ATPase, DNA and hydroxyproline content of human hypertrophied heart. Europ. J. Clin. Invest. **6,** 27–33 (1976).
12. Litten, R. Z., B. J. Martin, R. B. Low, N. R. Alpert: Altered myosin isozyme patterns from pressure-overloaded and thyrotoxic hypertrophied rabbit hearts. Circulat. Res. **50,** 856–864 (1982).
13. Lompré, A. M., K. Schwartz, A. d'Albis, G. Lacombe, N. V. Thiem, B. Swynghedauw: Myosin isoenzyme redistribution in chronic heart overload. Nature **282,** 105–107 (1979).
14. Lompré, A. M., J. J. Mercadier, C. Wisnewsky, P. Bouveret, C. Pantaloni, A. d'Albis, K. Schwartz: Species and age-dependent changes in the relative amounts of cardiac isoenzymes in mammals. Develop. Biol. **84,** 286–290 (1981).

15. Maron, B. J., V. J. Ferrans, R. S. Adelstein: Isolation and characterization of myosin from subjects with asymmetric septal hypertrophy. Circulat. Res. **40,** 468–473 (1977).
16. Mercadier, J. J., A. M. Lompré, C. Wisnewsky, J. L. Samuel, J. Bercovici, B. Swynghedauw, K. Schwartz: Myosin isoenzymic changes in several models of rat cardiac hypertrophy. Circulat. Res. **49,** 525–532 (1981).
17. Peters, T. J., G. Wells, C. M. Oakley, A. B. Brooksby, B. S. Jenkins, M. M. Webb-Peploe, D. J. Coltart: Enzymic analysis of endomyocardial biopsy specimen from patients with cardiomyopathies. Brit. Heart J. **39,** 1333–1339 (1977).
18. Pierobon-Bormioli, S., S. Sartore, M. Vitadello, S. Schiaffino: Slow myosins in vertebrate skeletal muscle. An immunofluorescence study. J. Cell. Biol. **85,** 672–681 (1980).
19. Pope, B., J. F. Y. Hoh, A. Weeds: The ATPase activity of rat cardiac myosin isoenzymes. FEBS Lett. **118,** 205–208 (1980).
20. Rupp, H.: The adaptive changes in the isoenzyme pattern of myosin from hypertrophied rat myocardium as a result of pressure overload and physical training. Basic Res. Cardiol. **76,** 79–88 (1981).
21. Samuel, J. L., L. Rappaport, J. J. Mercadier, A. M. Lompré, S. Sartore, C. Triban, S. Schiaffino, K. Schwartz: Distribution of myosin isozymes within single cardiac cells. An immunohistochemical study. Circulat. Res. (in press).
22. Scheuer, J., A. K. Bhan: Cardiac contractile proteins. Adenosine triphosphatase activity and physiological function. Circulat. Res. **45,** 1–12 (1979).
23. Schiaffino, S., L. Gorza, S. Pierobon-Bormioli, S. Sartore: Myosin polymorphism, cellular heterogeneity and plasticity of cardiac muscle. In: Plasticity of the muscle, edited by D. Pette, pp. 559–568. Walter de Gruyter (Berlin–New York 1980).
24. Schier, J. J., R. S. Adelstein: Structural and enzymatic comparison of human cardiac muscle myosins isolated from infants, adults and patients with hypertrophic cardiomyopathy. J. Clin. Invest. **69,** 816–825 (1982).
25. Schwartz, K., Y. Lecarpentier, J. L. Martin, A. M. Lompré, J. J. Mercadier, B. Swynghedauw: Myosin isoenzymic distribution correlates with speed of myocardial contraction. J. Mol. Cell. Cardiol. **13,** 1071–1075 (1981).
26. Schwartz, K., A. M. Lompré, P. Bouveret, C. Wisnewsky, B. Swynghedauw: Use of antibodies to sodium dodecyl sulfate-denatured heavy-meromyosins to probe structural differences between muscular myosin isoenzymes. Eur. J. Biochem. **104,** 341–346 (1980).
27. Schwartz, K., A. M. Lompré, P. Bouveret, C. Wisnewsky, R. G. Whalen: Comparison of rat cardiac myosins at fetal stages, in young animals and in hypothyroid adults. J. Biol. Chem. **257,** 14412–14418 (1982).
28. Winegrad, S., G. McClellan, R. Horowitz, M. Tucker, L. E. Lin, A. Weisberg: Regulation of cardiac contractile proteins by phosphorylation. Fed. Proc. **42,** 33–38 (1983).

Authors' address:

Dr. J. J. Mercadier, I.N.S.E.R.M. Unité 127, Hôpital Lariboisière, 41, Boulevard de la Chapelle, 75010 Paris, France

Cardiac Adaptation to Hemodynamic Overload, Training and Stress
Dr. D. Steinkopff Verlag 113–122 (1983)

Thyroxine-induced molecular alteration of heavy and 27,000-dalton light chains of rabbit ventricular myosin. Reconstitution of heavy and light chain molecules of subfragment-1 isozymes of cardiac myosin

S. Ueda and Y. Yazaki

The Third Department of Internal Medicine, Faculty of Medicine, University of Tokyo, Hongo, Tokyo (Japan)

Summary

Thyroxine-induced molecular alteration of heavy and light chains of ventricular myosin was studied by reconstitution of myosin subfragment-1 (S-1) molecules. Crosswise reconstitutions were performed with a S-1 heavy chain (89,000 daltons) from euthyroid and hyperthyroid rabbit hearts with an excess of appropriate light chain 1 (27,000 daltons) from euthyroid or hyperthyroid hearts (NLC-1, TLC-1). The elevation of Ca^{2+}-activated and actin-activated ATPase activities of TS-1 was mainly due to molecular alteration of the heavy chain molecule. By reconstitution, TLC-1 increased the actin-activated Mg^{2+}-ATPase activity of NS-1 more than did NLC-1. These results suggest that thyroid hormone induces the molecular alteration of both heavy chain and light chain 1 of ventricular myosin.

Key words: thyroxine, cardiac myosin isozyme, reconstitution, heavy chain, light chain, subfragment-1

Introduction

Since the first observation by Thyrum et al. (1970), it has been established that cardiac ventricular myosin from hyperthyroid animals exhibits elevated Ca^{2+}-activated and actin-activated ATPase activities (Hjalmarson et al., 1970; Kuczynski et al., 1973; Yazaki and Raven, 1975; Katagiri et al., 1975). Flink et al. (1979) have recently reported through two-dimensional maps of CNBr peptides of myosin that the primary structure of the heavy chain of cardiac ventricular myosin from hyperthyroid rabbits differs from that of euthyroid animals. The isozymic pattern of rabbit cardiac ventricular myosin has recently been shown on sodium pyrophosphate gel electrophoresis (Martin et al., 1982), like rat cardiac ventricular myosin (Hoh et al., 1977). These findings suggest that cardiac ventricular myosin from hyperthyroid animals is a new isozyme universally found in animal hearts. However, it has not yet been determined whether the structural and functional alterations of two light chain subunits (light chain 1, 27,000

Abbreviations: NLC-1 = light chain 1 from euthyroid rabbit heart. *TLC-1* = light chain 1 from hyperthyroid rabbit heart. *NS-1* = subfragment-1 from euthyroid rabbit heart. *TS-1* = subfragment-1 from hyperthyroid rabbit heart.

daltons; light chain 2, 20,000 daltons) are involved in isozymic change in ventricular myosin. It is also unknown whether these structural alterations of the heavy chain are responsible for the elevated myosin ATPase activity. To further examine the relationship in the hyperthyroid state between molecular alteration and ATPase activity of ventricular myosin isozymes, we have modified the reconstitution technique originally described by Wagner and Weeds (1977) and applied it to subunits of this new cardiac myosin isozyme.

Methods

Myosin preparation

Young male white rabbits weighing 2.5 to 2.8 kg were given daily injection of l-thyroxine (300 μg/kg) for 14 days as described previously (Yazaki and Raven, 1975). Myosin was prepared from the ventricles of normal control and hyperthyroid rabbit hearts according to a dilution technique. Actin was extracted from the aceton powder from rabbit back muscles according to the method described by Spudich and Watt (1971).

Subfragment-1 (S-1) preparation

S-1 was prepared by chymotryptic digestion of cardiac myosin by a modification of the method described by Wagner and Weeds (1977). Myosin (10 mg/ml) was digested for 10 min at 25 °C in 0.12 M NaCl, 20 mM sodium phosphate (pH 7.0), 1 mM dithiothreitol and 1 mM EDTA (ethylenediaminetetra acetic acid) with chymotrypsin at 0.1 mg/ml. Undigested myosin and precipitated myosin rods were removed by centrifugation at 45,000 *g* for 45 min. The supernatant was applied to a DEAE-cellurose column equilibrated with 50 mM Tris-HCl (pH 8.0) and 20 mM NaCl and eluted with a linear NaCl gradient (0.02 to 0.3 M).

Preparation of light chain 1 (27,000 daltons)

Cardiac light chains (light chain 1 and 2) were dissociated from purified myosin by incubating for 4 hours at 4 °C in 5 M guanidine-HCl, 10 mM EDTA, 5 mM dithiothreitol and 0.1 M Tris-HCl (pH 8.0), then dialyzed against an excess of 20 mM NaCl and 5 mM sodium phosphate, and finally centrifuged at 30,000 *g* to remove the precipitated heavy chain. The supernatant was then dialyzed against 50 mM potassium phosphate (pH 6.0). The protein was applied to a DEAE 52-cellurose column and eluted with a linear potassium phosphate gradient (0.05 to 0.3 M). The early fractions of the single peak eluted with the gradient were pooled and lyophilized as light chain 1. Labeled light chain 1 was obtained by the incubation with [^{14}C]-N-ethylmaleimide. The protein was separated from unincorporated reagents on a Sephadex G-25 column.

Reconstitution of S-1 with purified light chain 1

S-1 (20 μM) and purified light chain 1 (200 μM) were mixed together in 0.1 M imidazole-HCl (pH 7.0), 2 mM EDTA and 2 mM dithiothreitol, and NH_4Cl was added to a final concentration of 4.7 M. After being stirred for 10 min at 4 °C, the mixture was dialyzed against 50 mM imidazole-HCl (pH 7.0) and 0.1 mM dithiothreitol. Reconstituted S-1 and free light chain were separated on a Sephadex S-200 column equilibrated in the same buffer. Eluted fractions of S-1 were concentrated by pressure filtration through an Amicon PM-30 membrane, followed by dialysis against 3 mM imidazole-HCl (pH 7.0), 6 mM KCl and 0.1 mM dithiothreitol, prior to enzyme assays.

ATPase assays

Ca^{2+}-activated ATPase activity was assayed in 10 mM $CaCl_2$, 5 mM ATP, 0.05 M Tris-HCl (pH 7.5), and K^+EDTA-activated ATPase activity in 0.6 M KCl, 1 mM EDTA, 5 mM ATP and 0.05 M Tris-HCl (pH 7.5). Mg^{2+}-activated ATPase activity was determined in 30 mM KCl, 1 mM ATP, 0.05 M Tris-HCl (pH 7.5) and 1.5 mM $MgCl_2$. Actin-activated Mg^{2+}ATPase activity was similarly assayed. The concentration of S-1 was determined in 0.5 mg/ml and that of actin between 0.1 and 1.5 mg/ml. All assays were run at pH 7.5 and 25 °C for 5 min and stopped by adding 10 % trichloroacetic acid. Precipitated protein was removed by centrifugation and inorganic phosphate in the reaction was measured according to the method of Fiske and Subbarow (1925).

Protein concentration

Concentration of myosin, S-1, light chain 1 and actin were determined by absorption at 280 nm (molar ratio extinction coefficients: $E^{280}_{1\%}$ of 5.6, 7.5, 2.0 and 10.9, respectively) and by the method of Lowry et al. (1951).

Results

Cardiac S-1 subunit structure

After chymotryptic digestion of cardiac myosin, polyacrylamide gel electrophoresis of cardiac S-1 in the presence of sodium dodecyl sulfate (SDS) showed three prominent molecular weight bands. Comparison of the mobilities with proteins of known molecular weights gave values of 89,000, 70,000 and 22,000 daltons, respectively. The two larger bands represented hydrolytic heavy chains and the smaller bands a slightly degraded light chain 1. Cardiac light chain 2 completely disappeared from S-1 after chymotryptic digestion. Cardiac S-1's prepared from the hearts of euthyroid and hyperthyroid rabbits had similar banding patterns.

Preparation of cardiac light chain 1

Cardiac light chain 1 was purified on a DEAE-cellurose column as described in Methods. The early fractions of the one peak gave a single band of light chain 1 of 27,000 daltons on SDS-polyacrylamide gel electrophoresis (fig. 1). There was no difference in SDS-7.5 % polyacrylamide gel electrophoresis between euthyroid (NLC-1) and hyperthyroid light chain 1 (TLC-1).

ATPase activities of cardiac S-1

Ca^{2+}-activated ATPase activities of TS-1 and NS-1 were 1.33 ± 0.05 μmoles Pi/mg/min and 0.51 ± 0.04 μmoles Pi/mg/min, respectively ($p < 0.01$), and K^+EDTA-activated ATPase activities of TS-1 and NS-1 0.44 ± 0.04 μmoles Pi/mg/min and 0.50 ± 0.03 μmoles Pi/mg/min, respectively (not significant). In the pH range of 5.0 to 10.0, Ca^{2+}-activated ATPase activity of TS-1 was increased to about 2.6 times that of NS-1. However, there was no difference in K^+EDTA-activated ATPase activity. Both the high level of Ca^{2+}-activated ATPase activity and the pH dependence of TS-1 were similar to those of myosin from hyperthyroid heart. Ca^{2+}-activated

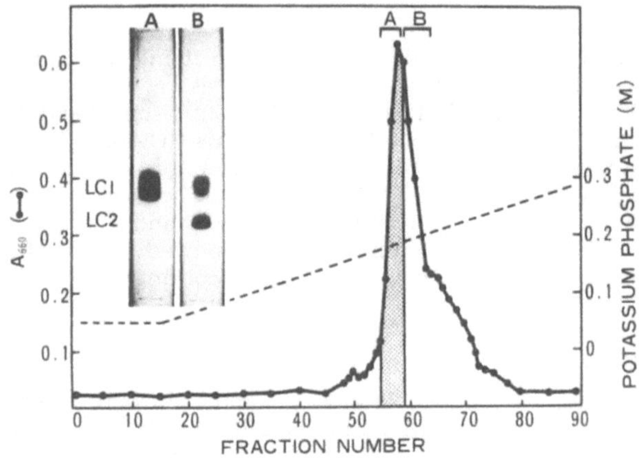

Fig. 1. DEAE elution profiles of light chain 1 (A) and light chain 2 (B). (A) was eluted as 0.15 to 0.18 M potassium phosphate, and (B) at 0.18 to 0.2 M potassium phosphate. Inserts: SDS-7.5 % polyacrylamide gel electrophoresis of light chain 1 (A), and light chain 1 and light chain 2 (B). Loading level, approximately 45 µg, respectively.

ATPase activity of NS-1 was increased from 0.11 ± 0.02 to 0.30 ± 0.02 µmoles Pi/mg/min by titration with N-ethylmaleimide (NEM) from 0 to 5 times the molar ratio. In contrast, Ca^{2+}-activated ATPase activity of TS-1 was not activated by NEM (0.59 ± 0.02 to 0.54 ± 0.04 µmoles Pi/mg/min) in this concentration range and inhibited at a higher concentration of NEM. Mg^{2+}-activated ATPase activity of TS-1 (0.070 ± 0.003 µmoles Pi/mg/min) was increased to 2.3 times that of NS-1 (0.030 ± 0.002 µmoles Pi/mg/min).

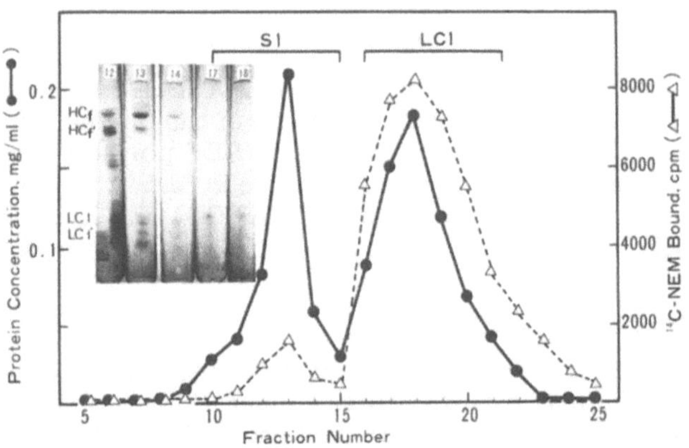

Fig. 2. Separation of reconstituted S-1 and excess [^{14}C]-N-ethylmaleimide-labeled light chain 1 on Sephadex S-200 column, which was equilibrated with 50 mM imidazole-HCl (pH 7.0) and 0.1 mM dithiothreitol. Reconstitution of S-1 and excess radio-labeled light chain 1 was done as described in "Methods". Inserts: SDS-7.5 % polyacrylamide gel electrophoresis of aliquots containing 50 µg of fractions 12, 13, 14, 17 and 18.

V_{max} of actin-activated ATPase of TS-1 (0.533 ± 0.050 μmoles Pi/mg/min) was 3.5 times that of NS-1 (0.153 ± 0.039 μmoles Pi/mg/min) ($p < 0.01$). The Kapp of TS-1 was twice that of NS-1 (table 1). These results reveal that S-1 completely retains the same enzymatic properties of its parent myosin, whether from euthyroid or hyperthyroid rabbits.

Determination of reconstitution of S-1

To determine the percentage of reconstituted NS-1 in the presence of excess NLC-1, NS-1 was reconstituted with excess NLC-1 labeled with [^{14}C]-N-ethylmaleimide, and both reconstituted and non-dissociated native S-1's were separated from free NLC-1 on Sephadex S-200. Radioactivity was associated with both NS-1 (reconstituted) and radiolabeled NLC-1 (fig. 2). About 6 % of the radiolabeled NLC-1 was reconstituted with dissociated NS-1. Light chain 1 and the heavy chain of native NS-1 could be completely separated on a column of a Sephadex S-200 run with 4 M LiCl, after dialysis against the same buffer for 36 hours. By this method, the degraded light chain 1 of NS-1 was found to be about 22 % of the weight of NS-1. As 6 % of the added light chain 1 bound to NS-1, about 54 % of degraded light chain 1 of native S-1 was exchanged with labeled NLC-1. When NS-1 was reacted with NH_4Cl in the absence of excess light chain 1, NS-1 lost 55 % of its own light chain 1. TS-1 similarly lost 55 % of its own light chain 1 in the absence of excess light chain 1 by NH_4Cl treatment. TLC-1 had the same affinity for [^{14}C]-N-ethylmaleimide as had NLC-1. The amounts of reconstituted S-1 were equal among the four crosswise reconstitutions (NS-1 with NLC-1 55 %, NS-1 with TLC-1 53 %, TS-1 with NLC-1 55 %, and TS-1 with TLC-1 52 %). Therefore, quantitative estimation of reconstituted S-1 component enabled the assay of their ATPase. The relative ATPase activities of non-dissociated or reconstituted S-1 after NH_4Cl treatment showed 97 % to 99 % of the values of native control S-1 ATPase activity.

ATPase activities of reconstituted S-1

The NH_4Cl-treated NS-1 showed 52 % and 48 % of the native control NS-1 in the Ca^{2+}-activated and K^+EDTA-activated ATPase activities in the absence of added light chain 1, respectively (table 1). The enzymatic activities of NH_4Cl-treated TS-1 similarly showed 52 % and 54 % of those of the native control TS-1, respectively. Ca^{2+}-activated and K^+EDTA-activated ATPase activities of NH_4Cl-treated NS-1 were recovered after reconstitution with NLC-1 (94 % and 93 %, respectively) or TLC-1 (92 % and 95 %, respectively) similarly. Similar recovery rate of ATPase activity was observed in NH_4Cl-treated TS-1 after reconstitution with NLC-1 or TLC-1. However, there was a difference in reconstituted S-1 ATPase activity between TS-1 and NS-1. The reconstitution with the mixture of NLC-1 and TLC-1, at various ratios of 3:1 or 1:1 or 1:3, also resulted in the same recovery in S-1 Ca^{2+}-activated ATPase as did that with only NLC-1 or TLC-1. These results indicate that S-1 ATPase activity (Ca^{2+}-activated and K^+EDTA-activated) is determined by the source of heavy chain molecule, but not affected by that of light chain 1 molecule. In the presence of actin, V_{max} for actin-activated Mg^{2+}ATPase of NH_4Cl-treated NS-1 was recovered

Table 1. ATPase activities of reconstituted S-1.

	Ca^{2+}	K^+EDTA	Actin-activated	
			V_{max}	Kapp
	µmoles Pi/mg/min (%)	µmoles Pi/mg/min (%)	µmoles Pi/mg/min (%)	mg/ml
NS-1	0.51 ± 0.04 (100)	0.50 ± 0.04 (100)	0.153 ± 0.031 (100)	0.63
NH_4Cl-treated NS-1	0.26 ± 0.04 (52)	0.24 ± 0.03 (48)	0.077 ± 0.010 (50)	0.50
+ NLC-1	0.48 ± 0.04 (94)	0.47 ± 0.03 (93)	0.141 ± 0.015 (93)	0.60
+ TLC-1	0.47 ± 0.03 (92) N.S.	0.48 ± 0.03 (95) N.S.	0.218 ± 0.020 (150) *	1.02
+ NLC-1 + TLC-1				
(75 %) (25 %)	0.45 ± 0.05 (88)	0.45 ± 0.04 (90)	0.080 ± 0.020 (52)	0.53
(50 %) (50 %)	0.49 ± 0.04 (96)	0.47 ± 0.03 (94)	0.170 ± 0.040 (111)	0.75
(25 %) (75 %)	0.47 ± 0.04 (92)	0.48 ± 0.03 (96)	0.200 ± 0.025 (131)	1.00
TS-1	1.33 ± 0.05 (100)	0.44 ± 0.04 (100)	0.533 ± 0.050 (100)	1.43
NH_4Cl-treated TS-1	0.71 ± 0.04 (52)	0.24 ± 0.03 (54)	0.263 ± 0.018 (49)	1.00
+ NLC-1	1.26 ± 0.04 (96)	0.37 ± 0.03 (85)	0.352 ± 0.040 (66)	1.01
+ TLC-1	1.25 ± 0.04 (95) N.S.	0.38 ± 0.04 (85) N.S.	0.502 ± 0.037 (95) *	1.40
+ NLC-1 + TLC-1				
(75 %) (25 %)	1.23 ± 0.04 (92)	0.36 ± 0.04 (82)	0.380 ± 0.020 (71)	1.10
(50 %) (50 %)	1.27 ± 0.05 (95)	0.39 ± 0.04 (88)	0.400 ± 0.030 (75)	1.20
(25 %) (75 %)	1.24 ± 0.04 (93)	0.37 ± 0.03 (84)	0.490 ± 0.035 (92)	1.40

Assays were performed as described in Methods. Ca^{2+}-activated, K^+EDTA-activated and actin-activated Mg^{2+}ATPase activities of S-1 after reconstitution reveal the summation of nondissociated (native) and reconstituted S-1 ATPase activities, as certified by using radio-labeled light chain 1. The increase in S-1 ATPase activity after reconstitution is due to the reconstituted component of S-1 molecules. Number of experiments is three to four in each group.
Values are means ± S.E.
* $P < 0.02$

Table 2. Ca^{2+}-activated and actin-activated Mg^{2+}ATPase activities of S-1 reconstituted with NEM-treated light chain 1.

	Ca^{2+}	Actin-activated	
		V_{max}	Kapp
	µmoles Pi/mg/min	µmoles Pi/mg/min	mg/ml
NS-1 +			
NLC-1	0.48	0.141	0.50
NEM · NLC-1	0.44	0.150	0.50
TLC-1	0.50	0.200	0.98
NEM · TLC-1	0.49	0.173	1.20
TS-1 +			
NLC-1	1.26	0.250	0.90
NEM · NLC-1	1.23	0.263	1.01
TLC-1	1.15	0.502	1.25
NEM · TLC-1	1.20	0.480	1.40

Purified light chain 1 (NLC-1 and TLC-1) was treated with [^{14}C]-NEM or cold NEM for 60 min, as described in Methods, and then reconstituted with NS-1 or TLC-1. The assay of S-1 reconstituted with NEM-treated light chain 1 was the same as that used in table 1.

again (93 % of native control NS-1) after reconstitution with NLC-1, and further elevated (150 % of native control NS-1) after reconstitution with TLC-1. NH_4Cl-treated TS-1 after reconstitution with TLC-1 was recovered from 49 % of native control TS-1 to 95 % in V_{max} of actin-activated Mg^{2+}ATPase. By reconstitution, NLC-1 increased V_{max} (66 % of native control TS-1) for NH_4Cl-treated TS-1 less than did TLC-1 (95 % of native control TS-1). Furthermore, the mixture of NLC-1 and TLC-1, at various ratios as shown in table 1, also showed a gradual effect on S-1 ATPase in the presence of actin. These results indicate that TLC-1 functionally differs from NLC-1 in terms of actin activation of S-1 ATPase.

Reconstitution with [^{14}C]-N-ethylmaleimide-labeled light chain 1

In the absence of cold N-ethylmaleimide, [^{14}C]-N-ethylmaleimide bound was saturable for 60 min both in 1.3 cysteine/mol of NLC-1 and in 1.2 cysteine/mol of TLC-1. In the presence of cold N-ethylmaleimide, no bound of [^{14}C]-N-ethylmaleimide occurred in both light chains. Saturable cysteinyl modification of NLC-1 or TLC-1 led to no loss of the recovery of S-1 ATPase after reconstitution (table 2).

Discussion

The present study has shown that both TS-1 heavy chain and TLC-1 are related to the elevation of TS-1 ATPase activity in the presence of actin, and that the isozymic alteration of cardiac myosin involves not only the functional alteration of the heavy chain molecule but also that of the light chain 1 molecule. However, the major effect on the enzymatic activity of S-1 was due to the source of the heavy chain molecule like other types of myosin.

TS-1 completely retained the specific enzymatic properties of parent myosin. There was no difference in the SDS-gel electrophoretic pattern of heavy chain and degraded light chain 1 between TS-1 and NS-1. Purified TLC-1 also did not differ from purified NLC-1 in SDS-gel electrophoresis. The NH_4Cl-mediated dissociation of degraded light chain 1 from S-1 heavy chain was identical in TS-1 and NS-1. The association of purified light chain 1 to S-1 heavy chain, estimated by using [^{14}C]-N-ethylmaleimide(NEM)-labeling, was also identical in TLC-1 and NLC-1, and the reconstituted molecules were equally stable at lower ionic strength. Cardiac light chain 2 (20,000 daltons) was completely lost during chymotryptic digestion. This indicates that the specific properties of hyperthyroid cardiac myosin, such as high ATPase activity and NEM-nonenhancement of ATPase, are limited to the single-headed S-1 molecule consisting of a heavy chain (about 89,000 daltons) and light chain 1 (about 22,000 daltons). The high level of ATPase activity of hyperthyroid cardiac myosin, therefore, is not related to the role of light chain 2, nor to its phosphorylation.

Reconstitution experiments showed that Ca^{2+}-activated ATPase of NS-1 and TS-1, in the absence of actin, was affected by the heavy chain source, but not by the light chain 1 source. K^+ EDTA-activated ATPase of NH_4Cl-treated TS-1 was recovered to a lesser degree (about 85 % of native NS-1). Although NH_4Cl treatment of S-1 at 4 °C for 10 min gave a higher level of reconstitution and enzymatic recovery, K^+EDTA-activated ATPase of TS-1 was more susceptible to inactivation of NH_4Cl than was that of NS-1. In the presence of actin, V_{max} for actin-activated Mg^{2+}ATPase of S-1 reconstituted between NS-1 heavy chain and TLC-1 increased to 150 % of the control NS-1 ATPase activity, whereas the level of ATPase activity of NS-1 was 93 %. The Kapp values in reconstituted S-1 were almost unaltered. In the presence of actin, although the heavy chain mainly determined S-1 ATPase activity, TLC-1 had some influence on reconstituted NS-1 ATPase activity, as did NLC-1. These experiments in the presence of actin were done at higher ionic strength (30 mM KCl). In contrast to the previous study (Wagner et al., 1979), higher ionic strength did not reduce the difference in ATPase activity between TS-1 and NS-1.

It has recently been reported that the heavy chain derived from fast skeletal myosin S-1 with alkali 2 light chain shows full ATPase activity (Wagner and Giniger, 1981; Sivaramakrishnan and Burke, 1982), like the heavy chain of non-muscle cell myosin of Acanthamoeba Ib (Maruta et al., 1978). The decline and recovery of the ATPase activity of S-1, as shown in the present study, indicates that the ATPase of S-1 was labile to NH_4Cl treatment after loss of the light chain 1 molecule. When the S-1 heavy chain was denaturated by 60-min treatment with NH_4Cl, the heavy chain reconstituted with native light chain 1 did not regain its ATPase activity. These observations suggest that the decline in the ATPase activity of dissociated S-1 after 10-min treatment with NH_4Cl is not due to the denaturation of the heavy chain molecule, but to the loss of light chain 1. The addition of light chain 1 from canine ventricular myosin also resulted in about 60 % to 70 % recovery of the ATPase activity of dissociated NS-1 and TS-1, while the addition of light chain 2 (20,000 daltons) from rabbit ventricular myosin, containing 3 % to 5 % light chain 1, did not increase the ATPase activity of dissociated NS-1 and TS-1 (unpublished data). Thus the association of light chain 1 stabilizes the heavy chain molecule, the active site of which conformationally may be changed by NH_4Cl treatment.

As shown by Wagner and Weeds (1977) and Burke and Sivaramakrishnan (1981), the ATPase activities of fast skeletal myosin S-1 (A1), containing alkali 1 light chain of 20,000 daltons, and S-1 (A2), containing alkali 2 light chain of 16,500 daltons, are identical in the absence of actin, whereas their actin-activated Mg^{2+}ATPase activities differ in V_{max} and Kapp for steady-state kinetics. Our results also reveal that the heavy chain is the major determinant of the actin-activated Mg^{2+}ATPase activity of myosin, and that the light chain is the minor determinant. The results obtained from the present study using uncommon type myosin TS-1 is consistent with these results. It is not known why light chain 1 influences the actin-activated Mg^{2+}ATPase of myosin and S-1. There is a possibility that the light chain 1 regulates the rate of release of ADP and phosphate from S-1 · ADP · Pi complex, as reported previously (Wagner and Weeds, 1977).

It has been found that chemical modification of a "homologous" or "essential" cysteine in the alkali light chain of canine fast skeletal myosin inhibits myosin ATPase activity and actin binding (Wagner and Yount, 1975). Our reconstitution experiment showed that thiol modification with [^{14}C]-NEM and cold NEM of purified light chain 1 molecules from euthyroid or hyperthyroid cardiac ventricular myosin did not inactivate either ATPase activity or actin-activated Mg^{2+}ATPase activity of reconstituted S-1. These findings indicate that the various active sites (Sekine and Kielley, 1964; Morkin et al., 1979) of the heavy chain molecule are susceptible to chemical modification and have a major role in ATPase activity, although light chain 1 is related, in part at least, to actin-activated Mg^{2+}ATPase.

Furthermore, different effects on actin-activated S-1 ATPase of light chain 1 molecules, which are not due to the cysteinyl modification, suggest their structural alteration. We found the heterogeneity of light chain 1 of rabbit ventricular myosin on sodium pyrophosphate gel electrophoresis (Ueda and Yazaki, 1981). Therefore, it is possible that thyroid hormone induces the new production of a light chain 1 molecule, which differs from that in the euthyroid state, in addition to that of the heavy chain molecule.

In conclusion, the present reconstitution study shows that thyroid hormone induces the molecular alteration of heavy chain and light chain 1 of ventricular myosin.

References

Burke, M., M. Sivaramakrishnan: Subunit interactions of skeletal muscle myosin and myosin subfragment-1. Formation and properties of thermal hybrids. Biochemistry **20,** 5908–5913 (1981).

Fiske, C. H., Y. Subbarow: Colorimetric determination of phosphorus. J. Biol. Chem. **66,** 375–400 (1925).

Flink, I. L., J. H. Rader, E. Morkin: Thyroid hormone stimulates synthesis of a cardiac myosin isozyme. Comparison of the two-dimensional electrophoretic patterns of the cyanogen bromide peptides of cardiac myosin heavy chains from euthyroid and thyrotoxic rabbits. J. Biol. Chem. **254,** 3105–3110 (1979).

Hjalmarson, A. C., C. H. Whitfield, H. E. Morgan: Hormonal control of heart function and myosin ATPase activity. Biochem. Biophys. Res. Commun. **41,** 1548–1589 (1970).

Hoh, J. F. Y., P. A. McGrath, P. T. Hale: Electrophoretic analysis of multiple forms of rat cardiac myosin: Effects of hypophysectomy and thyroxine replacement. J. Mol. Cell. Cardiol., 1053–1076 (1977).

Katagiri, T., A. S. Freedberg, E. Morkin: Effects of N-ethylmaleimide on the ATPase activities of cardiac myosin from thyrotoxic rabbits. Life Sci. **16,** 1079–1087 (1975).

Kuczynski, S. H., M. A. Inchiosa: ATPase activity of cardiac actomyosin and myosin in thyroxine-induced myocardial hypertrophy (abstr). 164th National Meeting, American Chemical Society (Biology Abstracts 128) (1973).

Lowry, O. M., N. J. Rosebrough, A. L. Farr, R. J. Randall: Protein measurement with the Folin phenol reagent. J. Biol. Chem. **193,** 265–275 (1951).

Martin, A. F., E. D. Pagani, R. J. Solaro: Thyroxine-induced redistribution of isozymes of rabbit ventricular myosin. Circulat. Res. **50,** 117–124 (1982).

Maruta, H., H. Gadasi, J. H. Collin, E. D. Korn: The isolated heavy chain of an Acanthamoeba myosin contains full enzymatic activity. J. Biol. Chem. **243,** 6297–6300 (1978).

Morkin, E., I. L. Flink, S. Banerjee: Phenylglycoxal modification of cardiac myosin S-1. Evidence for essential arginine residues at the active site. J. Biol. Chem. **254,** 12647–12652 (1979).

Sekine, T., W. W. Kielley: Enzymatic properties of N-ethylmaleimide modified myosin. Biochim. Biophys. Acta **81,** 336–345 (1964).

Sivaramakrishnan, M., M. Burke: The free heavy chain of vertebrate skeletal myosin subfragment-1 shows full enzymatic activity. J. Biol. Chem. **257,** 1102–1105 (1982).

Spudich, J. A., S. Watt: The regulation of rabbit skeletal muscle contraction. I Biochemical studies of the interaction of the tropomyosin-troponin complex with actin and proteolytic fragments of myosin. J. Biol. Chem. **246,** 4866–4871 (1971).

Thyrum, P. T., E. M. Kritcher, R. J. Luchi: Effect of l-thyroxine on the primary structure of cardiac myosin. Biochim. Biophys. Acta **197,** 335–336 (1970).

Ueda, S., Y. Yazaki: Heterogeneity of 27,000 dalton-light chain of cardiac ventricular myosin. J. Biochem. (Tokyo) **90,** 555–558 (1981).

Wagner, P. D., E. Giniger: Hydrolysis of ATP and reversible binding to F-actin by myosin heavy chains free of all light chains. Nature **292,** 558–562 (1981).

Wagner, P. D., C. S. Slater, B. Pope, A. G. Weeds: Studies on the actin activation of subfragment-1 isozymes and the role of myosin light chains. Eur. J. Biochem. **99,** 385–394 (1979).

Wagner, P. D., A. G. Weeds: Studies on the role of myosin alkali light chains. Recombination and hybridization of light chains and heavy chains in subfragment-1 preparations. J. Mol. Biol. **109,** 455–473 (1977).

Wagner, P. D., R. G. Yount: Subunit location of sulfhydryl groups of myosin labeled with a purine disulfide analog of adenosine triphosphate. Biochemistry **14,** 1908–1914 (1975).

Yazaki, Y., M. S. Raben: Effect of the thyroid state on the enzymatic characteristics of rat and rabbit cardiac myosin. Circulat. Res. **36,** 208–215 (1975).

Authors' address:

Seigo Ueda, M.D., The Third Department of Internal Medicine, Faculty of Medicine, University of Tokyo, 7-3-1 Hongo, Bunkyo-ku, Tokyo, Japan 113

Cardiac Adaptation to Hemodynamic Overload, Training and Stress
Dr. D. Steinkopff Verlag 123–128 (1983)

Structural variants of heavy and light chains of atrial and ventricular myosins in hypertrophied human hearts

C. R. Tuchschmid, T. Srihari, H. O. Hirzel, and M. C. Schaub

Institute for Pharmacology, University of Zürich, and Dept. of Cardiology, University Hospital, Zürich (Switzerland)

Summary

In human cardiac hypertrophy the myosin light chain complement varies in its relative composition as well as in its tissue-specific composition in both atrium and ventricle. In support of recent results (P. Cummins [1982] Biochem. J., **205**, 195–204), we also found ventricular VLC-2 and to a lesser extent VLC-1 to occur in hypertrophied atrium in addition to its own light chain complement. Our new findings concern the additional occurrence of atrial ALC-1 in hypertrophied ventricle. We further observed a large predominance of light chain of type-1 over that of type-2 in both ventricle and atrium of adult hypertrophied hearts. On the other hand, no differences were observed in the peptide patterns containing a total of around 180 distinguishable peptides produced by two different proteinases from the isolated myosin heavy chains, between normal and hypertrophied ventricular or atrial tissues. However, a number of differences in the peptide patterns from normal atrium and ventricle indicates different primary structures of the myosin heavy chains in these two heart tissues.

Key words: human heart, cardiac hypertrophy, myosin subunits, myosin isoenzymes

Introduction

Transitions in myosin isoenzymes in response to different types of stimuli and functional requirements have been investigated in different muscles of various species. They involve both heavy and light chain subunits. In skeletal muscles fast and slow types of myosin isoforms have been shown to change according to developmental states and activity patterns (9). In heart ventricles of rodents two types of myosin heavy chains (HC) have been described forming homodimeric and heterodimeric isoenzymes, V-1 = $(HC\alpha)_2$, V-2 = $(HC\alpha HC\beta)$ and V-3 = $(HC\beta)_2$ (8). V-1 myosin has the highest and V-3 the lowest ATPase activity (7). The population of these isoenzymes varies according to hormonal (thyroxine) and developmental state (1) as well as in response to mechanical heart overloading (11). In addition to these ventricular isoenzymes, a distinct form of myosin HC has been observed in atrial tissue of chicken (5), bovine (6) and rabbit (4, 15). The light chain (LC) subunits also differ in mammalians between atrial and ventricular tissues and in the ventricle their complement undergoes developmental transitions (14, 15, 17).

In normal human ventricle the main isoenzyme is thought to be V-3 with its low ATPase activity (2, 12). No changes in the ventricular HC composition was observed in obstructive hypertrophic cardiomyopathies (13). The ventricular LC complement undergoes analogous developmental transitions (3) as in bovine, rat, and rabbit (14, 15, 17). In pressure overload-induced hypertrophies of moderate to severe degrees the appearance of ventricular VLC-2 and to a lesser extent, VLC-1 was found in atrial tissues (3). We examined the LC complement in both atrial and ventricular tissues from patients with pressure-induced heart hypertrophies. In addition, the myosin HC from both types of tissues were studied.

Methods

Autopsy samples of ventricular and atrial myocardium from 55–79-year-old patients with pressure overload-induced moderate to severe hypertrophy were provided by Dr. J. Schneider from the Dept. of Pathology and from infants with congenital malformation (Tetralogy of Fallot) we obtained biopsies during operations from Prof. M. Turina from the Dept. of Surgery of the University Hospital of Zürich. For comparison, autopsy samples of patients in the same age group without heart disorders were used.

Total tissue homogenates were prepared for direct application on electrophoresis without prior washing. Samples were examined in 2-dimensional acrylamide gel electrophoresis (isoelectrofocusing followed by electrophoresis in sodium dodecyl sulfate = SDS) for evaluation of the myosin light chain complement as described earlier (15). Isolation of myosin HC from total tissue homogenates by electrophoretic means, using the chemically cleavable cross-linker, bis-acrylylcystamine, and subsequent partial digestion of the isolated HC in 0.23 % SDS at pH 6.5 and 37 °C for 30 min. with proteinase from Staphylococcus aureus V-8 (EC 3.4.21.19) and papain (EC 3.4.22.2) was performed exactly as described earlier (15). The molar ratio of both proteinases to myosin HC of 200 000 molecular weight ranged from 0.001 up to 0.05. The protein digests were resolved in 1-dimensional SDS electrophoresis (15). Electrophoretic patterns were all stained by Coomassie Brilliant Blue R-250 (15), and in many instances they were, after destaining in 40 % methanol plus 10 % acetic acid, stained again with silver (18) in order to increase sensitivity for visualization of peptides occurring in small amounts.

Results

1 Light chain complement in atrium

In support of the findings by Cummins (3) we also observed in 2-dimensional electrophoresis the occurrence of the ventricular VLC-2 in atrial tissues of hypertrophied hearts due to pressure overload. In hearts with severe hypertrophy even the ventricular VLC-1 started to appear in the atrium. VLC-2 in general occurs as a double spot due to partial phosphorylation. Occasionally a faint, slightly more acidic, third spot appears at the level of VLC-2. This third spot was more prominent in severly hypertrophied atrium where VLC-2 is visible. This third spot was considered to represent a second type of VLC-2 and occurs in several vertebrate species beside man (3, 16).

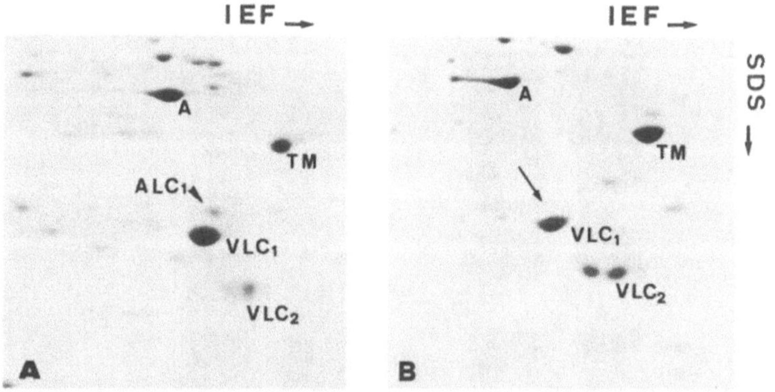

Fig. 1. Two-dimensional electrophoresis of total tissue homogenates from hypertrophic (A) and normal (B) adult left ventricular myocardium. Gels are presented with the basic pH range to the left and decreasing molecular weight from top to bottom. A, actin; TM, tropomyosin; myosin light chains, ALC-1, VLC-1 and VLC-2. Coomassie staining.

2 Light chain complement in ventricle

On the other hand, in ventricles of hypertrophied hearts we observed the occurrence of an additional peptide, which migrated above the VLC-1 (fig. 1A). This peptide was even more prominent in cases of tetralogy of Fallot (fig. 2A). Co-electrophoresis of both these cases with normal atrial tissue revealed that this peptide exhibits identical electrophoretic properties as the atrial ALC-1. This additional ALC-1 is not seen in normal adult ventricles (fig. 1B), but is present as a faint spot in normal ventricle of infants 7–8 months old (fig. 2B). While in normal and hypertrophied ventricles of infants as well as in normal ventricles of adults the ratio of LC-1 to LC-2 was around 1, it was consistently found higher, 3–6, in hypertrophied ventricles of adults (fig. 1A).

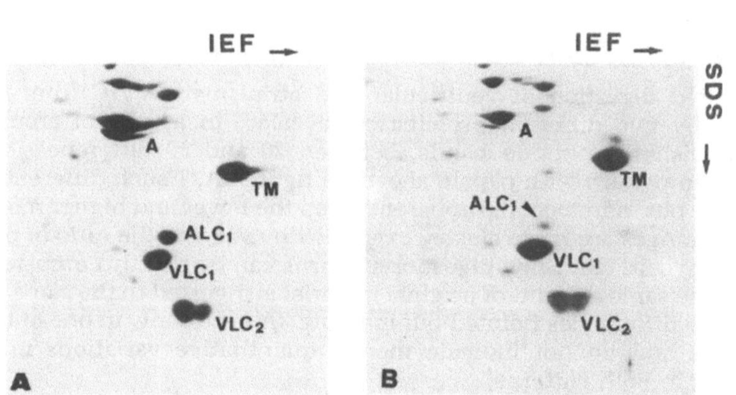

Fig. 2. Two-dimensional electrophoresis of hypertrophic (A) and normal (B) right ventricle of 7–8-month-old infants. Presentation of gels and abbreviations are the same as in figure 1.

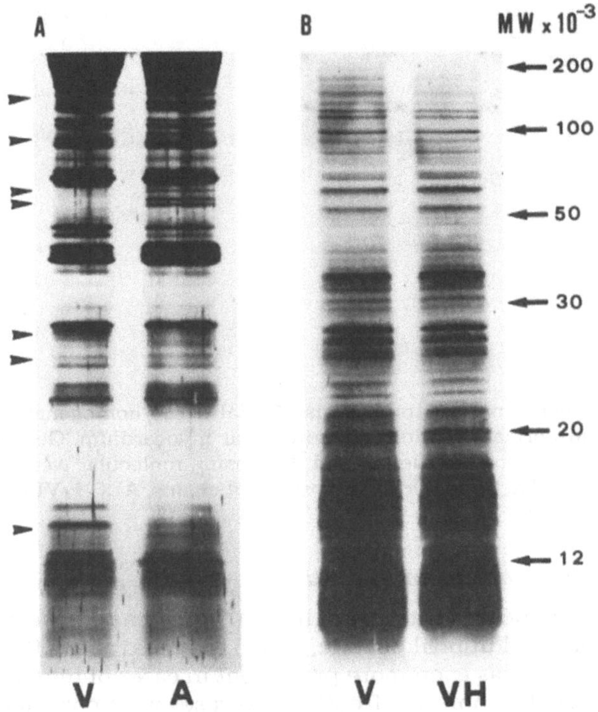

Fig. 3. SDS gel electrophoresis of peptides obtained by digestion with papain of myosin heavy chains isolated from adult normal ventricle and atrium (A) and from adult normal and hypertrophic left ventricles (B). The molar ratio of papain to myosin heavy chains was 0.006 (A) and 0.020 (B). A, normal atrium; V, normal ventricle; VH, hypertrophic ventricle. Arrowheads on left side indicate peptide bands which are present only in one of the two patterns. Numbers given indicate apparent molecular weights. Silver staining.

3 Heavy chain structure in atrium and ventricle

Limited digestion of ventricular and atrial myosin HC from normal hearts by two different proteinases revealed, in a total of around 180 distinguishable peptide bands, between 20 and 30 differences. In the digestion pattern with papain shown in figure 3A, 7 such differences can be seen, but more become apparent when the lower and higher molecular weight ranges are more closely examined by varying the ratio of proteinase to myosin HC. Such digestion patterns can be strictly compared only when the same amount of original material is digested to the same degree (15). The differences pointed out in figure 3A occur only in one of the two patterns and do not indicate merely quantitative variations in bands existing in both patterns.

In contrast, no peptide differences could be detected in digestions of myosin HC from normal and hypertrophied ventricles. In figure 3B is shown a digestion pattern from normal and hypertrophied left ventricle with a higher ratio of papain to myosin HC than in the case of normal ventricle and atrium in figure 3A. Furthermore, no differences were visible in the peptide patterns of myosin HC from normal right and left heart chambers.

Conclusion

Myosin light chain complement and structure of heavy chains were examined in total tissue homogenates of ventricle and atrium in 4 cases with pressure overload-induced hypertrophy of the left chambers and in two cases affecting the right chambers as well as in two cases affecting the right heart of infants with malformation (tetralogy of Fallot). We describe the occurrence of atrial ALC-1 in hypertrophied ventricular tissue and the occurrence of the ventricular VLC-1 and VLC-2 in hypertrophied atrial tissue as well as a stoichiometric imbalance involving an excess of LC of type 1 in hypertrophied heart chambers. The occurrence of atrial ALC-1 in hypertrophied ventricles of adult or old patients was small, around 2–10 % of LC of type-1. This may explain why Klotz et al. (10) failed to detect variations in primary structure of LC of type 1 and type 2 derived from myosin of hypertrophied left ventricles. Our results were the same in right and left hypertrophied heart chambers.

In ventricle of infants the disappearance of the atrial ALC-1 represents a developmental feature (3). With tetralogy of Fallot pathological effects only develop after birth, so the strong presence of ALC-1 in the right ventricle must represent an abnormal persistence in expression of this LC.

While the myosin HC differ in primary structure between atrium and ventricle as judged from their peptide maps, no further variants occurred in hypertrophy of either right or left heart ventricles. These latter findings concerning ventricular tissue support those already published by Schier and Adelstein (13).

Acknowledgments

This work was supported by the Swiss National Science Foundation Grant No. 3.535.79, the Swiss Foundation for Cardiology, and the Fritz Hofmann-La Roche Foundation.

References

1. Chizzonite, R. A., A. W. Everett, W. A. Clark, S. Jakovcic, M. Rabinowitz, R. Zak: Isolation and characterization of two molecular variants of myosin heavy chain from rabbit ventricle. Change in their content during normal growth and after treatment with thyroid hormone. J. Biol. Chem. **257,** 2056–2065 (1982).
2. Clark, W. A., R. A. Chizzonite, A. W. Everett, M. Rabinowitz, R. Zak: Species correlations between cardiac isomyosins. A comparison of electrophoretic and immunological properties. J. Biol. Chem. **257,** 5449–5454 (1982).
3. Cummins, P.: Transitions in human atrial and ventricular myosin light chain isoenzymes in response to cardiac-pressure-overload-induced hypertrophy. Biochem. J. **205,** 195–204 (1982).
4. Dalla Libera, L., S. Sartore: Immunological and biochemical evidence for atrial-like isomyosins in thyrotoxic rabbit ventricle. Biochim. Biophys. Acta **669,** 84–92 (1981).
5. Dalla Libera, L., S. Sartore, S. Schiaffino: Comparative analysis of chicken atrial and ventricular myosins. Biochim. Biophys. Acta **581,** 283–294 (1979).

6. Flink, I. L., J. H. Rader, S. K. Banerjee, E. Morkin: Atrial and ventricular cardiac myosins contain different heavy chain species. FEBS Letters **94,** 125–130 (1978).
7. Hoh, J. F. Y., P. A. McGrath, P. T. Hale: Electrophoretic analysis of multiple forms of rat cardiac myosin. Effects of hypophysectomy and thyroxine replacement. J. Molec. Cell. Cardiol. **10,** 1053–1076 (1978).
8. Hoh, J. F. Y., G. P. S. Yeoh, M. A. W. Thomas, L. Higginbottom: Structural differences in the heavy chains of rat ventricular myosin isoenzymes. FEBS Letters **97,** 330–334 (1979).
9. Jolesz, F., F. A. Sreter: Development, innervation and activity-pattern induced changes in skeletal muscle. Ann. Rev. Physiol. **43,** 531–552 (1981).
10. Klotz, C., J. J. Leger, M. Elzinga: Comparative sequence of myosin light chains from normal and hypertrophied human hearts. Circulat. Res. **50,** 201–219 (1982).
11. Klotz, C., B. Swinghedauw, H. Mendes, F. Marotte, J. J. Leger: Evidence for new forms of cardiac myosin heavy chains in mechanical heart overloading and in ageing. Europ. J. Biochem. **115,** 415–421 (1981).
12. Lompre, A. M., J. J. Mercadier, C. Wisnewsky, P. Bouveret, C. Pantaloni, A D'Albis, K. Schwartz: Species- and age-dependent changes in the relative amounts of cardiac myosin isoenzymes in mammals. Develop. Biol. **84,** 286–290 (1981).
13. Schier, J. J., R. S. Adelstein: Structural and enzymatic comparison of human cardiac muscle myosins isolated from infants, adults and patients with hypertrophic cardiomyopathy. J. Clin. Invest. **69,** 816–825 (1982).
14. Srihari, T., C. R. Tuchschmid, H. O. Hirzel, M. C. Schaub: Electrophoretic analyses of atrial and ventricular cardiac myosins from foetal and adult rabbit Comp. Biochem. Physiol. **72B,** 353–357 (1982).
15. Srihari, T., C. R. Tuchschmid, M. C. Schaub: Isoforms of heavy and light chains of cardiac myosins from rat and rabbit. Basic Res. Cardiol. **77,** 599–609 (1982)
16. Westwood, S. A., S. V. Perry: Two forms of the P light chain of myosin in rabbit and bovine hearts. FEBS Letters **142,** 31–34 (1982).
17. Whalen, R. G., S. M. Sell, A. Eriksson, L. E. Thornell: Myosin subunit types in skeletal and cardiac tissues and their developmental distribution. Develop Biol **91,** 478–484 (1982).
18. Wray, W., T. Boulikas, V. P. Wray, R. Hancock: Silver staining of proteins in polyacrylamide gels. Anal. Biochem. **118,** 197–203 (1981).

Authors' address:

C. R. Tuchschmid, T. Srihari, H. O. Hirzel and M. C. Schaub, Institute of Pharmacology, University of Zürich, Gloriastraße 32, CH-8006 Zürich, Switzerland

Cardiac Adaptation to Hemodynamic Overload, Training and Stress
Dr. D. Steinkopff Verlag 129–133 (1983)

Myosin isozymes in normal and pathological human cardiac muscle

F. A. Sreter, K. Mabuchi, and E. Somogyi, P. Sotonyi

Dept. of Muscle, Boston Biomedical Research Institute, Dept. of Anesthesia and Neurology, Mass. General Hospital and Harvard Medical School, Boston, MA. (U.S.A.) and
Dept. of Forensic Medicine, Semmelweiss Medical School, Budapest (Hungary)

Summary

Differences between human foetal, atrial and ventricular myosins were confirmed with the use of gel electrophoresis under native (pyrophosphate) and dissociating (SDS) conditions. In biopsies taken from the left ventricle of patients with severe congestive cardiomyopathy additional bands were found in the LC_1 region. The slowest moving LC_{1a} band showed a mobility similar to the foetal LC_1 band; however, this band was missing in biopsy samples taken from patients with glycogen storage disease.

Key words: cardiac biopsy, congestive cardiomyopathy, cardiac myosin isozymes, cardiac myosin light chains, glycogen storage disease, foetal cardiac myosin

Introduction

The presence of myosin isozymes in fast and slow skeletal muscles – differing either in the heavy chain or light chain composition – is well established (1–3). In cardiac myosins, species and age dependent isozyme differences have been reported (4). In rat and rabbit ventricles three isozymes termed V_1, V_2 and V_3 in order of their decreasing electrophoretic mobilities in a non-dissociating medium are present (5, 6). Only one form, the V_3, was reported in adult dog and human ventricles (4). The existence of isozymes in fast twitch skeletal muscle differing in the alkali light chain complement [$(LC_1)_2$ or $LC_3)_2$], has been known for some time. We have recently reported that other isoenzymes, containing variants of the heavy chains, distinguishable by their mobility on PP_i-gels, also exist (8).

The light chain complement of human atrial and ventricular cardiac muscle myosin was investigated in detail by Price et al. (7) using SDS-gel electrophoresis in the presence of urea, two-dimensional gel electrophoresis and limited proteolytic digestion. They reported no differences between right and left ventricular myosin light chains, but light chains of atrial and ventricular myosins differed. They also reported that the foetal ventricular myosin contained a characteristic light chain disappearing shortly after birth. This band could not be distinguished from the adult atrial LC_1 band by SDS-gel electrophoresis.

In the present paper, we are introducing some evidence showing that the light chains of human cardiac ventricular myosin obtained from biopsy samples taken during catheterization might be altered in some pathological cases.

Materials and methods

Normal human cardiac muscle (atrial and ventricular) was obtained from accident victims selected as renal transplant donors with the informed consent of the relatives and by special permit of the Hungarian Ministry of Health. Samples from six patients with various medical histories (3 severe congestive cardiomyopathies, 2 glycogen storage diseases and 1 child with Fallot tetralogy) were taken by left ventricle endomyocardial biopsy. The biopsy was carried out at the Central Heart Institute of Hungary (Budapest) with the consent of the patients, either at the same time when routine cardiac catheterization and angiography was carried out or as a separate procedure. The samples were immediately frozen, stored and transported in liquid N_2. Foetal human hearts were dissected from 4-week-old foetuses obtained during legal abortions.

The biopsy sample (weighing only ~2–4 mg) was used in toto for myosin extraction as described for single fiber preparations (8). Briefly, thawed samples were kept in a solution containing 50 % glycerol, 1 % β-mercaptoethanol, 5 mM DTT and 50 mM sodium pyrophosphate, pH 8.8 at 5–8 °C for 16 hrs. The residue was removed by a fine needle and the solution used as a crude myosin extract. An aliquot was used for pyrophosphate gel electrophoresis carried out according to Hoh (9) with some modifications (8). For light chain and limited proteolysis studies the crude myosin was first purified by a short pyrophosphate gel electrophoresis (120 V, 2 hr, 0 °C, pH 8.3, inner diameter of tubes 2.6 mm, length 5 cm). Gels were briefly (2–3 min) stained in Coomassie blue (10), washed in cold running buffer for 30 min at 0 °C, and the myosin bands cut out and frozen. The gel slices containing pure myosin were subjected to SDS-gel electrophoresis either directly or after limited proteolytic digestion. For the latter, gel slices were kept at 4 °C overnight in a solution containing 0.11 μg each of trypsin (Sigma Chemical, Type 3) and papain (2× crystallized, Sigma Chemical Co, 11.1 BAEE units per mg), dissolved in the myosin extraction medium. Under these mild conditions the digested myosin remains in the gel slices, which were then transferred into the wells of the SDS gel slab. About 30 min after adding 10 μl of solution containing 0.5 % SDS and 1 % β-mercaptoethanol, electrophoresis was started according to Laemmli (11) using a 13 running gel. The gels were stained with Coomassie blue R-250 (10) in 50 % methanol and 10 % acetic acid. After adequate destaining the gels were restained by the silver method (12).

Results and discussion

Human ventricular muscle myosin contains two light chains. The faster moving LC_2, M_r ~19–20,000 dalton, has a mobility which is slightly less than that of the LC_2 from fast-twitch muscle myosin of rabbit. The mobility of the slower moving LC_1 doublet is slightly faster than that of the atrial LC_1, the difference between the two clearly showing up on coelectrophoresis (not shown). Atrial LC_2 was definitely slower than ventricular LC_2. The mobility of the foetal LC_1 was identical with that of adult atrial

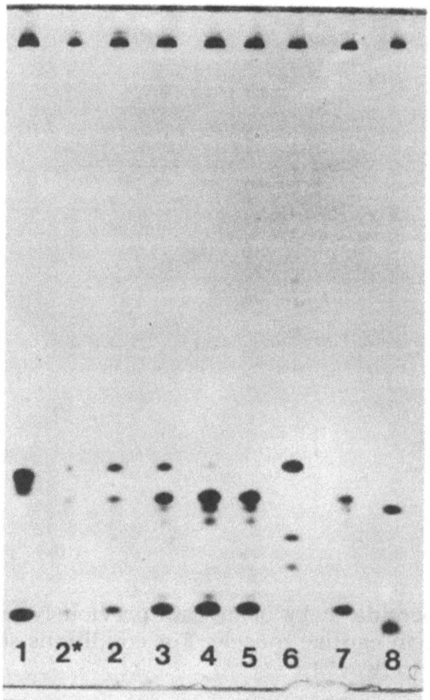

Fig. 1. SDS-gel electrophoretogram of PP_i-gel-purified human cardiac myosins. Key: 1 – adult ventricular myosin, normal control; 2-2* – human foetal cardiac myosin; one slice (2*) and 3 slices (2) were electrophorised. Note relative intensity of bands. 3-4 – biopsy samples taken from two patients with severe congestive cardiomyopathy; 5 – biopsy sample of glycogen storage disease; 6 – adult atrial myosin, normal control; 7-8 – rabbit skeletal muscle myosin for comparison, fast-twitch, and slow-twitch muscle myosins, respectively.

LC_1 and the LC_2 has a mobility slightly slower than the adult ventricular LC_2.

In biopsy samples (fig. 1: #3–5) we found additional band(s) showing mobilities faster than LC_1 seen in adult atrial or ventricular myosin. We labeled them according to the order of their increasing mobilities as LC_{1a}, 1_b, 1_c, and 1_d. LC_{1a} shows the same mobility as the LC_1 band of foetal myosin. This band is clearly present in biopsy #3 while only minimally present in biopsy #4 (both taken from patients suffering from severe congestive cardiomyopathy), and it is absent in biopsy #5 (glycogen storage disease). However, LC_{1b}, LC_{1c} and LC_{1d} are all present in various amounts in the six biopsy samples thus far examined (only three of which are shown in fig. 1), but only LC_{1b} is present in the foetal myosin. None of these bands (LC_{1b-d}) are present in atrial myosin. The question arises whether these bands are genuine light chain bands or result from proteolytic digestion. The latter case, however, is unlikely since no bands are present between the heavy chain (top) band and the putative light chain bands.

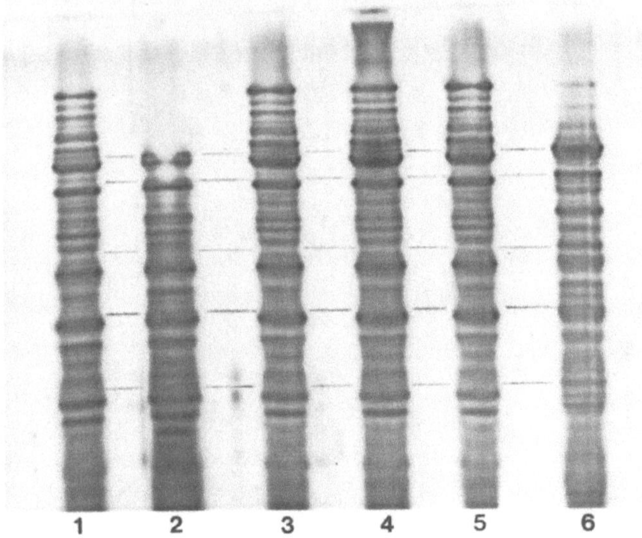

Fig. 2. SDS-gel 1-D peptide maps of myosin previously purified by PP_i-gel electrophoresis from human cardiac muscle. For conditions see Methods. Key is the same as in the legend to fig. 1.

When the proteolytic fragments (one dimensional peptide maps) of these myosins were compared after a limited digestion with trypsin and papain we found that the maps of adult atrial and ventricular myosins were different (fig. 2). The map of foetal myosin differed from both. The maps of the three ventricular biopsy samples are indistinguishable from normal ventricular maps. The first two biopsies were obtained from patients with severe congestive cardiomyopathy while #5 is a biopsy sample from a patient suffering from glycogen storage disease. In the latter, the slower moving band – with a mobility similar to that of the embryonic 28,000 dalton chain – is completely missing.

In conclusion, we found differences between normal adult left ventricular myosin and those of biopsy samples obtained from cardiac patients with respect to the LC_1 light chain band(s). These differences indicate that further studies are needed to evaluate the role and presence of these myosin light chains in cardiac pathology. In contrast no differences were found between normal and pathological samples in the peptide band pattern of the digested myosin. The latter finding is in agreement with the report of Schier and Adelstein (13).

References

1. Hoh, J. F. Y., G. P. S. Yeoh: Rabbit skeletal myosin isoenzymes from fetal, fast-twitch and slow-twitch muscle. Nature (Lond.) **280**, 321–322 (1979).
2. Lowey, S., P. A. Benfield, L. Silberstein, L. M. Lang: Distribution of light chains in fast skeletal myosin. Nature (Lond.) **282**, 522–524 (1979).

3. Jolesz, F., F. A. Sreter: Development, innervation and activity-pattern induced changes in skeletal muscle. Ann. Rev. Physiol. **43,** 531–552 (1981).
4. Lompre, A. M., J. J. Mercadier, C. Wisnewsky, P. Bouveret, C. Pantaloni, A. D'Albis, K. Schwartz: Species and age-dependent changes in the relative amounts of cardiac myosin isoenzymes in mammals. Dev. Biol. **84,** 286–290 (1981).
5. Hoh, J. F. Y., P. A. McGrath, P. T. Hale: Electrophoretic analysis of multiple forms of rat cardiac myosin. Effect of hypophysectomy and thyroxine replacement. J. Mol. Cell Cardiol. **11,** 1053–1076 (1978).
6. Litten, R. Z. III., B. J. Martin, R. B. Low, N. R. Alpert: Altered myosin isozyme patterns from pressure-overloaded and thyrotoxic hypertrophied rabbit hearts. Circulat. Res. **50,** 856–864 (1982).
7. Price, K. M., W. A. Littler, P. Cummins: Human atrial and ventricular myosin light chain subunits in the adult and during development. Biochem. J. **191,** 571–580 (1980).
8. Mabuchi, K., D. Szvetko, K. Pinter, F. A. Sreter: Type IIB to IIA fiber transformation in intermittently stimulated rabbit muscles. Amer. J. Physiol. **242** (Cell Physiol. 11) C373–C381 (1982).
9. Hoh, J. F. Y., P. A. McGrath, R. T. White: Electrophoretic analysis of multiple forms of myosin in fast-twitch and slow-twitch muscles of the chick. Biochem. J. **157,** 87–95 (1976).
10. Laemmli, U. K.: Cleavage of structural proteins during the assembly of the head of bacteriophage T4, Nature (Lond.) **227,** 680–685 (1970).
11. Oakley, B. R., D. R. Kirsch, N. R. Morris: A simplified ultrasensitive silver stain for detecting proteins in polyacrylamide gels. Anal. Biochem. **105,** 361–363 (1980).
12. Schier, J. J., R. S. Adelstein: Structural and enzymatic comparison of human cardiac muscle myosin isolated from infants, adults and patients with hypertrophic cardiomyopathy. J. Clin. Invest. **69,** 816–825 (1982).

Authors' address:

Dr. F. A. Sreter, Dept. of Muscle, Boston Biomedical Research Institute, Dept. of Anesthesia and Neurology, Mass. General Hospital and Harvard Medical School Boston, Ma. 02114, U.S.A.

Cardiac Adaptation to Hemodynamic Overload, Training and Stress
Dr. D. Steinkopff Verlag 134–138 (1983)

Structural and enzymatic alterations of cardiac contractile proteins under chronic pressure overload

M. Nagano, N. Takeda, H. Maeno, K. Noma, and T. Ohkubo

Department of Internal Medicine, Jikei University, Tokyo (Japan)

Summary

Heart muscles obtained from human left ventricles at autopsies and from hypertrophied hearts of SHR were homogenized in Weber's solution and the crude actomyosin was extracted. Crude extract was designed as sample I. Natural actomyosin (sample II) was purified from sample I.

The Ca^{++}-activated ATPase activity of sample II from SHR was lower than that of the control rats. The superprecipitation of sample II from SHR decreased with the increasing heart weight. The proportion of myosin heavy chains in sample I was higher in hypertensive hypertrophied human and rat hearts. The myosin HC amount in sample II of a human heart correlated positively with the content of myosin HC from sample I of the equal heart. In a failing heart, the yield of myosin HC in sample II from sample I was diminished. In SHR, the ratio of myosin HC in sample II to that in sample I correlated negatively with heart weight.

Key words: actomyosin, Ca^{++}-activated ATPase activity, myosin heavy chains, human myocardium, cardiac failure, spontaneously hypertensive rats

Introduction

In this study, structural and enzymatic properties of actomyosin of left ventricle of human hearts and hypertrophied hearts of SHR are described and discussed in relation to pathogenesis of heart failure.

Methods

Human hearts

Transmural samples were taken from the free wall of the left ventricle at autopsies from 66 patients at Tokyo Jikei University Hospital. The cardiac muscles were taken 3 hours after death from macroscopically non-infarcted and non-scarred areas.

The cardiac muscle was homogenized in Weber solution, and contractile proteins were extracted for 24 hours at 0~4 °C. The crude actomyosin was separated at 20,000 g for 60 min.

This fraction was referred to sample I. Natural actomyosin was further purified by changing ionic strength and was referred to as sample II (4). Samples I and II were analyzed on SDS polyacrylamide gel electrophoresis (7).

Hearts from SHR

SHR (Okamoto-Aoki B strain) were obtained from Shimane University, Department of Pathology. Male Wistar rats were used as controls. Hearts were removed under Nembutal anesthesia. Superprecipitation of the actomyosin was carried out by the modified Ebashi method (6), and final concentrations were 0.04 M Tris-maleate buffer (pH 6.8), 0.2 mM EGTA, 0.01 M KCl, 0.1 mM $MgCl_2$, 1.0 mM $CaCl_2$, 1.0 mM ATP and 0.5 mg/ml actomyosin. The extent of superprecipitation was expressed as the plateau level of the turbidity after addition of ATP. The slope at the point of half-maximal superprecipitation was considered a measure of superprecipitation rate.

Results

Human hearts

Figure 1a shows the correlation between heart weight and myosin heavy chain (HC) in sample I. The content of myosin HC in the heart correlated positively with the heart weight.

The amount of myosin HC from non-infarcted areas of the ischemic heart and from the heart with hypertension were significantly higher than that in the non-ischemic heart. In cardiac hypertrophy, which was caused by valvular disease, the myosin HC content was less than that from the equivalent hypertrophied heart with coronary sclerosis.

Figure 2 shows the correlation between heart weight and myosin HC content of sample II. The myosin HC from the non-diabetic heart was correlated positively with the heart weight. But the myosin HC content from the diabetic heart was disconnected from this regression line. The myosin HC in the diabetic heart, which was influenced in general by metabolic and ischemic disorders, was independent of the heart weight.

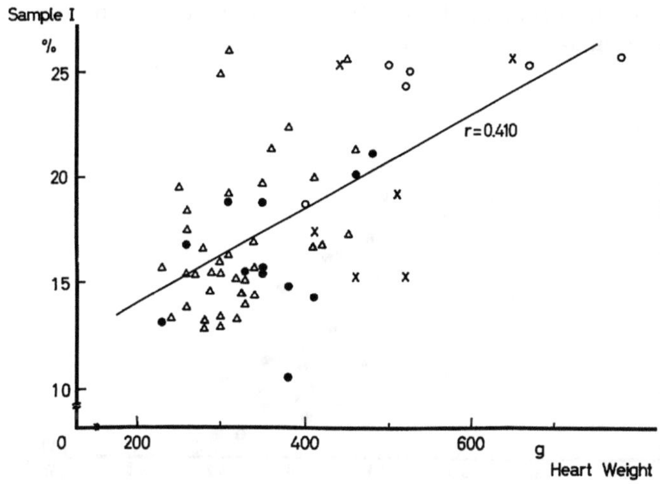

Fig. 1. Relationship between heart weight and myosin HC (sample I).
× Diabetes mellitus with heart failure
● Diabetes mellitus without heart failure
○ Non-diabetics with heart failure
△ Non-diabetics without heart failure

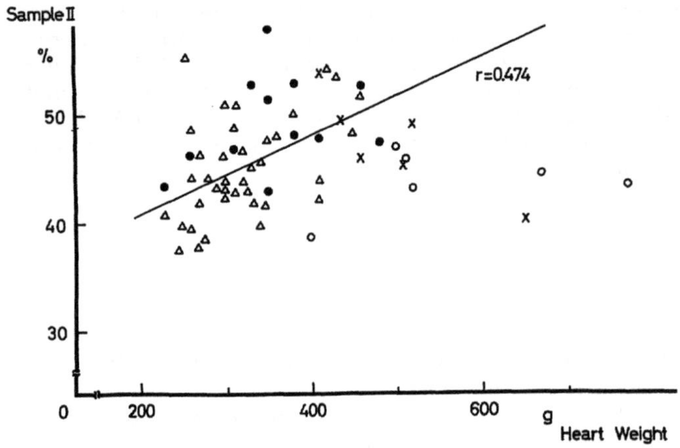

Fig. 2. Relationship between heart weight and myosin HC (sample II).
× Diabetes mellitus with heart failure
● Diabetes mellitus without heart failure
○ Non-diabetics with heart failure
△ Non-diabetics without heart failure

Hearts from SHR

The ratio of heart weight to body weight was higher in SHR than that of control rats. This ratio increased with advancing age. The average blood pressure of SHR was 185 mm Hg, that of control rats was 105 mm Hg. Ca^{++}-activated ATPase of cardiac natural actomyosin of SHR was significantly lower than that of the control rat heart and gradually decreased with advancing age (not shown).

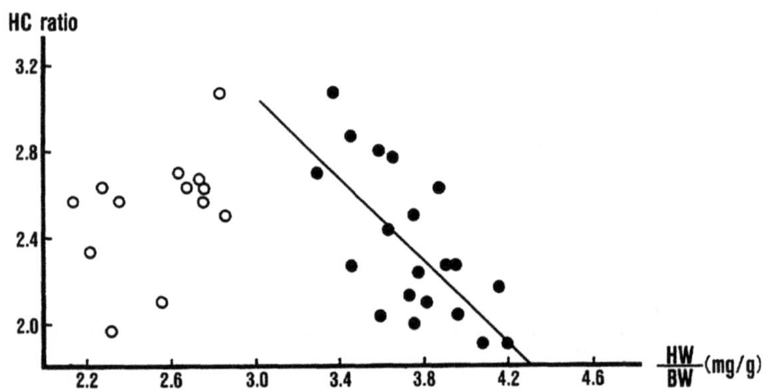

Fig. 3. Relation between HC ratio (sample II/sample I) and the ratio of heart weight to body weight.
○ NWR (n = 13)
● SHR (n = 20)
r = −0.680

We have examined further the biological activity of actomyosin by the method of superprecipitation of actomyosin. The extent and the rate of superprecipitation of actomyosin from SHR heart decreased with the increasing ratio of heart weight to body weight.

Figure 3 shows the correlation between the myosin HC ratio of samples II to I to the ratio of heart weight to body weight of SHR. In the control rats, there was no correlation between both ratios, whereas in the SHR, a significant negative correlation was observed.

Discussion

The Ca^{++}-activated ATPase activity of SHR was approximately twothird that of normal control rats at about 10 weeks after birth and decreased linearly with advancing age.

There have been many studies about ATPase activity of actomyosin, the majority of the studies show that ATPase activity decreases when the heart is pressure-overloaded (5).

Cardiac myosin has two classes of light chains (LC), and these chains are known to be essential for myosin to show ATPase activity. Katagiri and Morkin (2), and other observers have not discovered any alteration in the ratios of myosin LC to HC in cardiac hypertrophy. Recently, Medugorac (3) reported that the ratio of myosin HC to LC decreased in the case of SHR.

The myosin HC ratio, sample II to sample I, in the heart decreased in hypertensive hypertrophied human and rat hearts. The turnover rate of myosin HC measured by isotope increased about 20 % (Yazaki and Raben [9]) and increased twice as much as myosin LC (Wikman-Coffelt et al.) (8). Evans et al. (1) reported that when the heart was overloaded the myosin turnover rate increased 3 times. So it can be assumed that in overloaded cardiac muscles, there is an increase in myosin HC degeneration and regeneration. Through this process, the biochemical non-functional myosin HC, similar in form to functional myosin HC, is probably not recovered in the purification process, causing a decrease in the myosin HC ratio.

The decrease of superprecipitation and Ca^{++}-activated ATPase of actomyosin suggests a reduced energy utilization in cardiac muscle. The change of myosin HC ratio, we believe, indicates the existence of degenerative myosins.

References

1. Evans, C., S. S. Schreiber, M. Oratz, M. A. Rothschild: Synthesis of myosin heavy and light chains in the afterloaded guinea pig ventricle. Cardiovasc. Res. **12,** 731–743 (1978).
2. Katagiri, T., E. Morkin: Studies on the substructure of myosin in cardiac hypertrophy. Biochim. Biophys. Acta. **342,** 262–274 (1974).
3. Medugorac, I.: The myofibrillar ATPase activity and the substructure of myosin in the hypertrophied left ventricle of the rat. Basic Res. Cardiol. **75,** 163–170 (1980).

4. Ohkubo, T., K. Takahashi, N. Takeda, K. Kaito, K. Noma, M. Nagano: Study on the pathophysiology of heart failure. Cardiac Structure and Metabolism, Vol. 2, edt. Nagano, M. et N. Yamazaki, 143–151 (1979).
5. Scheuer, J., A. K. Bahn: Cardiac contractile proteins. Adenosine triphosphatase activity and physiological function. Circulat. Res. **45,** 1–12 (1979).
6. Watanabe, S.: Relation between superprecipitation and ATPase of myosin B. J. Biochem. **68,** 913–921 (1970).
7. Weber, K., M. Osborn: The reliability of molecular weight determination by dodecyl-sulfate-polyacrylamide gel electrophoresis. J.B.C. **244,** 4406–4412 (1969).
8. Wikmann-Coffelt, J., C. Fenner, J. McPherson, R. Zelis, D. T. Mason: Studies on the synthesis and degradation of light and heavy chains of cardiac myosin. J.B.C. **248,** 5206–5207 (1973).
9. Yazaki, Y., M. S. Raben: Comparison of the synthesis of light and heavy chains of cardiac myosin. Recent Advances in Studies on Cardiac Structure and Metabolism, Vol. **12,** 39–45 (1978).

Authors' address:

Dr. M. Nagano, Department of Internal Medicine, Jikei University, Tokyo, Japan

Cardiac Adaptation to Hemodynamic Overload, Training and Stress
Dr. D. Steinkopff Verlag 139–143 (1983)

The phosphorylation of cardiac contractile proteins

P. J. England, D. Mills, S. A. Jeacocke, and H. T. Pask

Department of Biochemistry, University of Bristol Medical School, University Walk, Bristol (UK)

Summary

Two contractile proteins, troponin-I and C-protein, are rapidly phosphorylated in perfused heart in response to stimulation by catecholamines. Both are phosphorylated only in response to increases in intracellular cyclic AMP, and are good substrates for cyclic AMP-dependent protein kinase *in vitro*. The phosphorylation of troponin-I decreases the affinity of the troponin complex for Ca^{2+} by increasing the off-rate for Ca^{2+} dissociation. This is probably part of the mechanism whereby catecholamines increase the rate of relaxation in heart. C-protein is phosphorylated *in vivo* and *in vitro* on 4–5 sites, but the function of both C-protein and its phosphorylation are unknown. Myosin P-light chain (phosphorylated by a Ca^{2+}-dependent kinase) is approximately 50 % phosphorylated in control perfusions, and this is unchanged during acute inotropic interventions. However, perfusions with $32P_i$ indicate an active kinase/phosphatase couple, which may be fully active under control conditions.

Key words: protein phosphorylation, troponin-I, C-protein, myosin light chain

Introduction

Cardiac contractility may be regulated acutely either by changes in intracellular Ca^{2+}, or by reversible changes in the properties of the contractile proteins. The first of these is probably the primary regulatory mechanism, with modifcation of contractile proteins playing an important, but secondary role. Reversible modification of proteins by phosphorylation is a widespread phenomenon, and a number of contractile proteins in the heart are known to be modified in this way. Phosphorylated proteins may be divided into two categories: those in which phosphorylation and dephosphorylation can occur rapidly; and those in which the phosphate group may be permanently attached to the protein. Obviously only proteins in the first category can have any role in the acute regulation of contraction, and this article will focus on the contractile proteins belonging to this group.

Phosphorylation of troponin-I

Troponin, the protein which confers Ca^{2+}-sensitivity on striated muscle actomyosin, is composed of three subunits, troponin-C, troponin-I and troponin-T. Troponin-I is rapidly phosphorylated *in vitro* by cyclic-AMP-dependent protein kinase (cAMP-PK) when present either in the isolated troponin complex (1) or on intact myofibrils (2). The phosphate is incorporated mainly into Ser-20 (3), and the rate of incorporation is comparable to other physiological substrates.

In control-perfused hearts from several species, troponin-I contains only low levels of phosphate (<0.2 moles phosphate per mole troponin-I), but following stimulation with catecholamines there is a rapid increase to >1 mole phosphate per mole within 30 sec (4–7). This occurs over a very similar time course to the increase in contraction induced by the hormone. Agents which increase contractility without increasing intracellular cyclic AMP do not cause phosphorylation of troponin-I (6, 8), indicating that it is not obligatory for increased contraction.

Dephosphorylation of troponin-I in perfused heart following a pulse of catecholamine is very slow, in contrast to phosphorylase, which is dephosphorylated rapidly (9, 10). We have recently isolated a number of phosphoprotein phosphatases from rat heart with different specificities to physiological phosphoproteins (11). Thus there are two phosphatase activities which will dephosphorylate phosphorylase but not troponin, and at least two general phosphatases which will dephosphorylase most phosphoproteins, including troponin-I. If the phosphorylase phosphatase activities are under different controls to the general phosphatases, this could give an explanation for the differential dephosphorylation of these proteins. However, it is still not clear why the dephosphorylation of troponin-I is slow, although cholinergic control has been implicated (9).

Phosphorylation of troponin-I causes a decrease in Ca^{2+} affinity of troponin (12), which is manifest as a decreased Ca^{2+} sensitivity of myofibrillar ATPase (13) and tension development in skinned fibres (13). This is a consequence of increased dissociation rate for the troponin-Ca complex (12). This effect is probably of importance in the action of catecholamines in increasing the rate of relaxation of cardiac muscle. Thus catecholamines increase the rate of Ca^{2+} removal from the cytoplasm during relaxation. However, if the rate of release of Ca^{2+} from troponin is slow, this may become the rate-limiting step for relaxation following catecholamine stimulation. Therefore an increase in the rate of dissociation of the Ca^{2+}-troponin complex by phosphorylation could prevent it becoming rate-limiting and allow a more rapid rate of relaxation.

Phosphorylation of C-protein

C-protein is a protein of the thick filament which occurs every 43 nm along the filament (14) and had a molecular weight of 150,000 in heart (15). Both structural and regulatory roles have been proposed, (16, 17), although its true function is unknown. When cardiac myofibrils were incubated with cAMP-PK and [γ-^{32}P] ATP, ^{32}P was covalently bound to troponin-I and a protein of molecular weight 150,000 (2). This latter protein was subsequently indentified as C-protein. There were approximately equal amounts of ^{32}P incorporated into troponin-I and C-protein and this was increased by prior treatment with phosphoprotein phosphatase, indicating endogenously-bound phosphate. Subsequent work has shown that C-protein is a very good substrate for cAMP-PK *in vitro,* having a higher

Vmax than troponin-I. As isolated, C-protein from both rat and beef heart contains 2–3 mole phosphate per mole C-protein, and an additional 1–1.5 moles can be incorporated with cAMP-PK. This indicates the presence of 4–5 phosphorylation sites per mole C-protein.

C-protein is phosphorylated in perfused rat heart in response to catecholamines over the same time course as troponin phosphorylation (18). In control perfusions there is approximately 1 mole phosphate per mole C-protein, and this is increase to 4–5 mole during the 30 sec following catecholamine administration. The maximum level of phosphorylation is thus very similar *in vivo* and *in vitro*. Phosphorylation of C-protein has also been reported in frog atria (19), and shows very similar characteristics to the mammalian systems.

Phosphorylation of C-protein and troponin-I have several features in common. Thus both are phosphorylated *in vitro* by cAMP-PK but not by Ca^{2+}-dependent kinases and are both phosphorylated *in vivo* only in response to increases in cytoplasmic cAMP. Both proteins are phosphorylated in heart, but not in skeletal muscle. It would thus appear that phosphorylation of both proteins is a specific adaptation in the heart to the control of contraction by catecholamines. Although the effect of phosphorylation on C-protein and its role in the control of contraction are not understood at present, the highly specific nature of the phosphorylation indicates an important function.

Phosphorylation of myosin light chains

The P-light chain of myosin is phosphorylated in all vertebrate muscle and non-muscle cells by a specific, Ca^{2+}-activated light chain kinase (20, 21). In fast skeletal muscle, phosphorylation of the P-light chain causes a decrease in the rate of ATP hydrolysis at any given tension (22, 23) and is equivalent to a decrease in the rate of cross-bridge cycling. Recently, this effect of phosphorylation has also been reported in cardiac muscle (24).

A number of studies measuring myosin phosphorylation in perfused heart have found that the P-light chain contains 0.4–0.5 mole phosphate per mole P-light chain in control conditions, and that this value is unchanged during acute inotropic interventions (25–28). There also appears to be little change under a number of chronic conditions such as cardiac hypertrophy or hyperthyroidism (29). The lack of change during acute increases in contraction can be explained by the observation that myosin light chain kinase is rapidly activated in the presence of Ca^{2+}, but only slowly inactivated when the Ca^{2+} is removed (11). Thus in control hearts, the constant cycling of Ca^{2+} during each beat will fully activate the kinase, and any increase in the concentration of cytoplasmic Ca^{2+} cannot cause a further increase in its activity. Evidence for this scheme has come from measurement of the turnover of the phosphate on the light chain by perfusions with $^{32}P_i$ (27). These results show a rate of phosphate turnover of 3–6 nmoles/min/g heart, which is comparable to the measured myosin light chain kinase activity of 5 nmoles/min/g heart (30). The lack of any changes on the level of P-light chain phosphorylation during inotropic intervention strongly suggests that it can play no part in the acute regulation of contraction. There may be a long-term regulatory role for this phosphorylation system, but further study is clearly required.

References

1. Reddy, Y. S., D. Ballard, N. Y. Giri, A. Schwartz: Phosphorylation of cardiac native tropomyosin and troponin: inhibitory effect of actomyosin and the possible presence of endogenous myofibrillar-located cyclic AMP-dependent protein kinase. J. Mol. Cell. Cardiol. **5,** 461–71 (1973).
2. Ray, K. P., P. J. England: Phosphorylation of the inhibitory subunit of troponin and its effect on the calcium dependence of myofibril adenosine triphosphatase. FEBS Lett. **70,** 11–16 (1976).
3. Moir, A. J. G., R. J. Solaro, S. V. Perry: The site of phosphorylation of troponin-I in the perfused rat heart. Biochem. J. **185,** 505–13 (1980).
4. England, P. J.: Correlation between contraction and phosphorylation of the inhibitory subunit of troponin in perfused rat heart. FEBS Lett. **50,** 57–60 (1975).
5. England, P. J.: Phosphorylation of the inhibitory subunit of troponin in perfused hearts of mice deficient in phosphorylase kinase. Biochem. J. **168,** 307–10 (1977).
6. Solaro, R. J., A. J. G. Moir, S. V. Perry: Phosphorylation of troponin-I and the inotropic affect of adrenaline in perfused rabbit heart. Nature **262,** 615–616 (1976).
7. Stull, J. T.: Phosphorylation of contractile proteins in relation to muscle function. Adv. Cyclic. Nucleotide Res. **13,** 39–93 (1980).
8. Ezrailson, E. G., J. D. Potter, L. Michael, A. Schwartz: Positive inotropy induced by ouabain, by increased frequency, by X573A (R02-2985), by calcium and by isoproterenol: The lack of correlation with phosphorylation of Tn-I. J. Mol. Cell. Cardiol. **9,** 693–698 (1977).
9. England, P. J.: Studies on the phosphorylation of the inhibitory subunit of troponin during modification of contraction in perfused rat heart. Biochem. J. **160,** 295–304 (1976).
10. Stull, J. T., C. F. Sanford, D. R., Manning, D. K. Blumenthal, C. W. High: Phosphorylation of myofibrillar proteins in striated muscle. Cold. Spring Harbor Conf. Prolif. **8,** 823–840 (1981).
11. England, P. J.: Cardiac function and contractile protein phosphorylation. Proc. Royal Soc. Lond., Ser. B, in press (1983).
12. Robertson, S. P., J. D. Johnson, M. J. Holroyde, E. G. Kranais, J. D. Potter, R. J. Solaro: The effect of troponin-I phosphorylation on the Ca^{2+} binding properties of Ca^{2+}-regulatory site of bovine cardiac troponin (1982).
13. Herzig, J. W., G. Kohler, G. Pfizer, J. C. Ruegg, G. Woffle: Cyclic AMP inhibits contractility of detergent treated, glycerol extracted cardiac muscle. Pflügers Arch. **391,** 208–212 (1981).
14. Craig, R., G. Offer: The localisation of C-protein in rabbit skeletal muscle. Proc. Roy. Soc. Lond. Ser. B. **192,** 451–461 (1976).
15. Yamamoto, K., C. Moos: A comparative study of C-proteins from heart and skeletal muscle. Biophys. J. **33,** 237a (1981).
16. Moos, C., G. Offer, R. Starr, P. Bennett: Interaction of C-protein with myosin, myosin rod and light meromyomyosin. J. Mol. Biol. **97,** 1–9 (1975).
17. Starr, R., G. Offer: The interaction of C-protein with heavy meromyosin and subfragment-2. Biochem. J. **171,** 813–816 (1978).
18. Jeacocke, S. A., P. J. England: Phosphorylation of a myofibrillar protein of Mr 150,000 in perfused rat heart, and the tentative identification of this as C-protein. FEBS Lett., **122,** 129–132 (1980).

19. Hartzell, H. C., L. Titus: Effects of cholinergic and adrenergic agonists on phosphorylation of a 165,000-dalton myofibrillar protein in intact cardiac muscle. J. Biol. Chem. **257,** 2111–2120 (1982).
20. Pires, E., S. V. Perry, M. A. W. Thomas: Myosin light chain kinase a new enzyme from striated muscle. FEBS Lett. **41,** 292–296 (1974).
21. Frearson, N., S. V. Perry: Phosphorylation of the light chain components of myosin from cardiac and red skeletal muscles. Biochem. J. **151,** 99–107 (1975).
22. Crow, M., M. J. Kushmerick: Light chain phosphorylation and muscle energetics. Biophys. J. **33,** 236a (1981).
23. Cooke, R., K. Franks, J. T. Stull: Myosin phosphorylation regulates the ATPase activity of permeable skeletal muscle fibres. FEBS Lett. **144,** 33–37 (1982).
24. Ruegg, J. C., G. Pfitzer, F. Hofmann: Contractility of skinned cardiac fibres: Modification by phosphorylation on contractile proteins. Basic Res. Cardiol. in press (1983).
25. Holroyde, M. J., D. A. P. Small, E. Howe, R. J. Solaro: Isolation of cardiac myofribils and myosin light chains with in vivo levels of light chain phosphorylation. Biochem. Biophys. Acta **587,** 628–637 (1979).
26. Perry, S. V., H. A. Cole, N. Frearson, A. J. G. Moir, A. C. Nairn, R. J. Solaro: Phosphorylation of the myofibrillar proteins. Proc. 12th FEBS Meeting **54,** 147–159 (1979).
27. Jeacocke, S. A., P. J. England: Phosphorylation of myosin light chains in perfused rat heart. Biochem. J. **188,** 763–768 (1980).
28. High, C. W., J. T. Stull: Phosphorylation of myosin in perfused rabbit and rat hearts. Amer. J. Physiol. **239,** H756–H764 (1980).
29. Litten, R. Z., B. J. Martin, E. R. Howe, N. R. Alpert, R. J. Solaro: Phosphorylation and adenosine triphosphatase activity of myofribrils from thyrotoxic rabbit hearts. Circulat. Res. **48,** 498–501 (1981).
30. Hofmann, F., H. Wolf: Basic properties of myosin light chain kinase from bovine cardiac muscle. Cold Spring Harbor Conf. Prolif. **8,** 841–848 (1981).

Authors' address:

Dr. P. J. England, Department of Biochemistry, University of Bristol, Medical School, University Walk, Bristol BS8 1TD, UK

Morphological and functional aspects of adaptation or damage

Cardiac Adaptation to Hemodynamic Overload, Training and Stress
Dr. D. Steinkopff Verlag 147–157 (1983)

Isoenzyme contribution to economy of contraction and relaxation in normal and hypertrophied hearts

N. R. Alpert, L. A. Mulieri, and R. Z. Litten
with the technical assistance of R. P. Goulette and B. J. Martin

Department of Physiology & Biophysics, University of Vermont, College of Medicine, Burlington, Vermont (U.S.A.)

Summary

In heart muscle, substantial sarcomere shortening and lengthening occurs during the rise and fall of isometric tension (6–9 %). If heart muscle behaves like skeletal muscle, then energetically the contraction phase should be less economical than the relaxation phase. Experiments we carried out on normal (N), pressure overload hypertrophied (P), and thyrotoxic hypertrophied (T) heart muscle using rapid myothermal techniques and isolated papillary muscles to test this hypothesis.

Economy is defined as the ∫Pdt/TDH where ∫Pdt is the tension time integral and TDH is the tension-dependent heat. The economy for the contraction (E_c) and relaxation (E_R) phases of the isometric twitch for P and T were: 1) P, E_c = 5.79 ± 0.82, E_R = 8.91 ± 1.14; 2) T, E_c = 1.80 ± 0.82, E_R = 4.52 ± 1.14. In both preparations relaxation was more economical than contraction. We were surprised to find that for the N hearts the contraction and relaxation phases had the same economy (E_c = 7.15 ± 1.29 while E_R = 6.89 ± 0.75). This difference is explained in terms of the different myosin isoenzyme profiles where the V_1 isoenzyme content was 12, 0 and 90 % in the N, P and T heart preparations, respectively.

Key words: myosin isoenzymes, tension-dependent heat, crossbridge cycling, isometric contraction, isometric relaxation, hypertrophy, pressure overload, L-thyroxine, myothermal techniques, economy

Introduction

When an activated skeletal muscle is stretched during a twitch or short tetanus, less heat appears than would be expected from the muscle force present and the work put into the muscle during the lengthening (1, 2). Consistent with this finding are the results obtained when cyclists pedal two bicycle ergometers placed back to back and coupled by a chain so that when one cyclist pedals in the forward direction the other has the pedalling muscles driven backwards (3). Under these circumstances the oxygen cost of negative work is significantly less than the oxygen cost of identical quantities of positive work (3). The evidence for suppression of heat releasing or oxygen demanding reactions during stretch is supported by the chemical finding that during slow stretch of activated skeletal muscle the tension is always greater than during shortening while the rate of ATP

Supported in part by USPHS PHS R01 17592 and HL28001

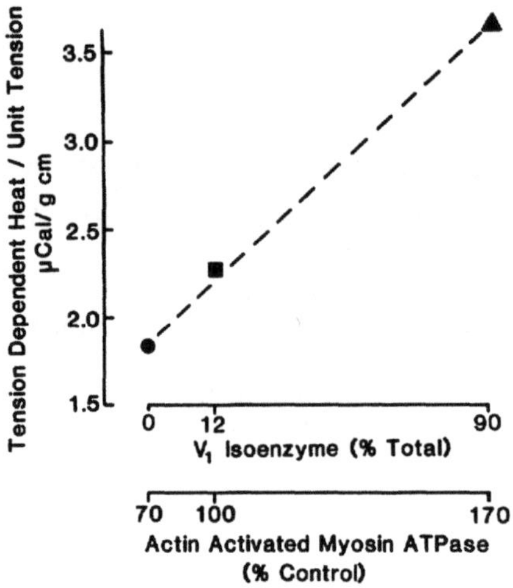

Fig. 1. The relationship of tension-dependent initial heat to actin activated myosin ATPase and V_1 myosin isoenzyme content. The results presented are the average of a series of experiments previously described (6, 7). The symbols used signify the following: ■ = control; ● = pressure overload hypertrophy; ▲ = thyrotoxic hypertrophy.

breakdown is less and approaches base line levels (4). Thus for activated skeletal muscle, force is developed more economically when the muscle is lengthened than when it is allowed to shorten.

Visualization of the sarcomere pattern during isometric contraction and relaxation in heart muscle indicates the presence of significant sarcomere shortening and lengthening during the rise and fall of isometric tension, respectively (5). If heart muscle exhibits energetic behavior similar to skeletal muscle, one would expect that isometric contraction would be less economical than isometric relaxation. To evaluate this hypothesis, myothermal experiments were carried out on rabbit right ventricular papillary muscles. We had previously observed that tension-dependent initial heat (TDH) liberated during an isometric twitch is a function of the type of myosin present in the heart and its intrinsic ATPase activity (6, 7) (fig. 1). In pressure overload hypertrophy (P), where the myosin ATPase is low and the primary myosin isoenzyme present is the V_3 variety, the TDH is low. Conversely, in thyrotoxic hypertrophy (T), where the myosin ATPase is high and the primary myosin isoenzyme present is the V_1 variety, the TDH is high. Hence use of P and T preparations further allows assessment of the contribution of myosin isoenzyme profile to the economy of isometric contraction and relaxation.

Methods

Animal models. Experiments were carried out on right ventricular papillary muscles from male albino rabbits weighing 1.8–2.0 kg. Pressure overload hypertrophy was induced by constricting the pulmonary artery by 66 % with a spiral monel metal spring using the method previously described (8, 10). The animals were used in experiments four weeks after the initial surgical procedure. The stress produced a substantial hypertrophy which is stable for two to ten weeks following the banding. Thyrotoxic hypertrophy was produced by 14 daily intramuscular injections of 0.2 mg/kg of L-thyroxine (9). The daily injection of L-thyroxine was omitted if the body weight fell below 80 % of the weight at the start of the 14-day period.

Papillary muscle preparation. The detailed procedures for preparing right ventricular rabbit papillary muscles for mechanical and myothermal measurements have been previously described (10). The thinnest papillary muscle with a length greater than 3.5 mm was excised and mounted on planar, vacuum-deposited thermopile with the tendinous end anchored to a stationary hook while the cut end was attached to the isometric force transducer (11, 12). The conical shape of the muscle was compensated for by pulling the thinner, tendon end into contact with the thermopile surface with an adjustable tether (11).

Mechanical measurements. Isometric force was measured using a capacitance force transducer which had a compliance of 0.4 μm/g and a resonant frequency of 3 kHz (12). The measurements described below were made at lo, which was established by gradually increasing the muscle length in 0.05-mm increments during continuous pacing at 0.2 Hz until stable twitch tension exhibited a plateau. Muscles were rejected when the active to passive tension ratio was less than 4:1.

Stimulation. End-to-end stimulation was carried out with monophasic, 10 % supra maximal rectangular wave stimuli of 2 msec duration and 0.2 Hz frequency through 25-μm diameter annealed platinum wires (11).

Myothermal measurements. Temperature measurement were made using vacuum-deposited, bismuth and antimony, Hill-type, planar thermopiles (11). The advantage of this system is the low thermal capacity, high sensitivity and low electrical resistance, which can be matched to a Kipp galvanometer recording system and provides a high signal-to-noise ratio. The frequency response of the system is 60 Hz and the thermal delay about 6.5 msec so that the relatively slow response of heart muscle can be analyzed without correction for thermal-lag time. The heat output of a muscle may be divided into initial, recovery and resting phases.

Separating the initial heat into a contraction phase was accomplished by measuring the temperature rise up to the moment when peak tension was reached; the initial heat associated with relaxation is obtained from the remaining temperature rise attained by the end of the twitch. The contraction and relaxation times, respectively, for the normal, pressure overload and thyrotoxic preparations were in msec: 1) normal 652 ± 25, 1088 ± 64; 2) pressure overload 838 ± 32, 1048 ± 124; and 3) thyrotoxic 348 ± 9, 1103 ± 149. Thermal conduction delays in the system were evaluated by electrically heating a 1 % agar Krebs cylinder, mounted on the thermopile in place of the papillary muscle, by passing a 3 MHz sine wave current through the ends of the agar rod (11). The temperature change in the agar rod can be detected 1.6 ms after the heating current begins. In actual measurements on papillary muscles we found the delay to be about 6.5 msec. Thus, under worst-case conditions, in measuring the initial heat for the contraction phase of the thyrotoxic muscles, the error would be less than 2 % and thus can be neglected. The vacuum-deposited bismuth-antimony thermopile system is ideally suited for resolving the differences between the thermal output during isometric contraction and relaxation.

The temperature changes measured in this study are associated with heat liberated by crossbridge cycling during isometric contraction (tension-dependent heat for contraction, TDH_c) and relaxation (tension-dependent heat for relaxation, TDH_R). The sum of tension-dependent heat for contraction and relaxation ($TDH_c + TDH_R$) is equal to the tension-dependent initial heat (TDH_I). The tension dependent heat is obtained by first measuring the initial heat (I) in normal Krebs-

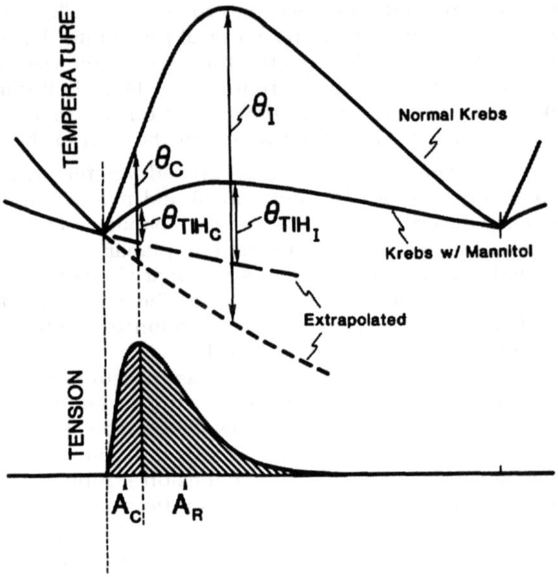

Fig. 2. A record of isometric force (below) and temperature change (above) for an isometric twitch at lo in normal and hyperosmotic mannitol Ringers. A_C and A_R are the tension time integrals for contraction and relaxation phases of the isometric twitch. θ_I is the temperature change associated with initial heat (I) in normal Krebs. The temperature change (θ_{TIH_I}) associated with tension-independent heat (TIH_I) is the triggerable temperature change in hyperosmotic Krebs with mannitol. (θ_I–θ_{TIH_I}) is the temperature change associated with tension-dependent heat (TDH_I). θ_C is the temperature change associated with the contraction phase of the twitch. θ_{TIH_C} is the temperature change associated with tension-independent heat liberated during the contraction phase of the twitch. θ_C–θ_{TIH_C} is the temperature change associated with tension-dependent heat (θ_{TDH_C}) liberated during the contraction phase of the twitch. $\theta_{TDH_I}-\theta_{TDH_C} = \theta_{TDH_R}$, the tension-dependent heat of relaxation. Temperature changes were corrected for heat loss graphically and then converted to heat units by multiplication with corresponding thermal capacitance and heat loss coefficient (see 10, 11).

Ringer solution and then measuring the triggerable heat after eliminating force development (tension-independent heat, TIH) by incubating the muscle in 2.5 × hyperosmotic mannitol solution (13). The tension-dependent initial heat (TDH_I) is the difference between I and TIH. These methods for measuring I, TIH and TDH_I and the rationale for their use have been described in detail elsewhere (6, 10, 13, 14, 15). The methods are extended to partition the tension-dependent initial heat (TDH_I) into the contraction (TDH_c) and relaxation (TDH_R) components as described in figure 2.

Obtaining a reliable answer to the question posed in this set of experiments depends on our ability to measure initial heat without significant contamination from recovery heat and to separate the heat associated with contraction from relaxation. We convinced ourselves that recovery metabolism did not contaminate our measurements of initial heat by evaluating the change in the ratio of initial heat to tension in muscles whose recovery metabolism was partially blocked by 0.1 mM iodoacetic acid and oxygen lack (10). Under these conditions the ratio of initial heat-to-peak twitch tension was 95 ± 4 % of the mean value before blockade. A paired t test failed to show a significant difference between the values before and after blockade. Accordingly no correction need be made for contamination of initial heat by recovery heat.

Economy of isometric contraction and relaxation. The economy of isometric contraction (E) is defined as the tension time integral (∫Pdt) divided by the tension-dependent heat (TDH). Thus E = ∫Pdt/TDH. The economy of the contraction phase of the isometric twitch is the ratio of the tension time integral of contraction (A_c fig. 2) to TDH_c. The economy of the relaxation phase is the ratio of the tension time integral of relaxation (A_R fig. 2) to TDH_R.

Separation and quantification of myosin isoenzymes. The right ventricular free wall was removed from the heart and placed in extraction buffer (100 mM sodium pyrophosphate, pH 8.8, 5 mM EGTA and 2 mM 2-mercaptoethanol). In some instances the left ventricle was also used from the thyrotoxic hearts. Both right and left ventricles gave similar results. The tissue was then homogenized using a motor-driven Potter-Elvehjem teflon glass homogenizer. The homogenate was centrifuged at 48,000 g for 3 hours and the supernatant mixed with an equal volume of cold (0 °C) glycerol. Each pyrophosphate gel was loaded with 1–2 µg of protein and the electrophoresis was carried out at 60 V for 22 hours at 2 °C using an electrophoresis chamber (Pharmacia GE-2/4), which circulates the upper and lower chamber buffers (7, 16). The gels were scanned using a laser-beam densitometer. The percent V_1 isoenzyme was calculated from the densitometer trace using the following formula: $(A_{V1}/A_T) \times 100$ where A_{V1} is the area under the V_1 peak and A_T is the sum of the areas under the V_1, V_2 and V_3 peaks. The V_1 peak area (A_{V1}) was determined by weighing the paper which makes up half the V_1 peak (side away from V_2 peak) and multiplying by two. To obtain the half area, a line was drawn from the V_1 peak through two points midway between the two sides of the upper portion of the peak where contamination from V_2 and V_3 peaks was judged to be minimal. A_T was obtained by weighing the paper making up the total scan (V_1, V_2, and V_3 peaks). The percent V_3 was calculated as described above for percent V_1. Percent V_2 was calculated by subtracting the areas of V_1 and V_3 from the total area. The V_2 myosin isoenzyme was not greater than 5 % in the control and thyrotoxic preparations and was 0 % in the pressure overload preparations, hence it was not separated from V_3.

Statistics. Values presented in this paper represent the mean ± standard error of the mean. Values are compared by a paired Student's t-test. A two-tailed P value of 0.05 or less was considered significant.

Results

Mechanical measurements. The tension time integral for the normal preparations was 6.120 ± 0.570 gsec/mm². In the P and T preparations the tension time integrals were 5.644 ± 0.570 and 4.832 ± 0.862 gsec/mm²,

Table 1. Tension time integral (g sec/mm²).

Preparation	Contraction (A_c)	Relaxation (A_R)	A_c/A_R	
N (10)*	2.107 ± 0.236	4.013 ± 0.352	0.523 ± 0.025	$P < 0.001$
P (8)	2.234 ± 0.769	3.416 ± 0.602	0.703 ± 0.051	$P < 0.01$
T (5)	0.761 ± 0.122	4.071 ± 0.391	0.198 ± 0.039	$P < 0.005$

* The number in the parentheses indicates the number of experiments carried out in each group; N, P and T represent the normal, pressure overload and thyrotoxic groups.

Table 2. Tension-dependent heat (m cal/g).

Preparation	Contraction (TDH_c)	Relaxation (TDH_R)	THD_c/TDH_I	
N (10)*	0.350 ± 0.037	0.629 ± 0.069	0.588 ± 0.067	$P < 0.001$
P (8)	0.463 ± 0.085	0.486 ± 0.141	1.265 ± 0.253	NS
T (5)	0.457 ± 0.080	1.043 ± 0.224	0.491 ± 0.124	$P < 0.05$

* The number in the parentheses indicates the number of experiments carried out in each group; N, P and T represent the normal, pressure overload and thyrotoxic groups.

respectively. The contraction phase tension time integral was significantly shorter than the relaxation phase with the A_c to A_R ratio being 0.52, 0.70 and 0.20 for the normal, pressure overload and thyrotoxic preparations (table 1).

Tension-dependent heat measurements. The tension-dependent initial heat (TDH_I) for normal muscle is 0.979 ± 0.094 m cal/g. For the pressure overload and thyrotoxic preparations it is 97 (NS) and 154 ($p < .02$) percent of normal, respectively. The ratios of TDH_c to TDH_R for normal, pressure overload and thyrotoxic hearts are given in table 2.

Partitioned economy of the isometric twitch. The goal of these experiments was to compare the economy of isometric contraction and relaxation. In the normal muscle the economy for the contraction phase is 7.15 ± 1.29 gcm sec/μcal. This is unchanged during the relaxation phase of the twitch (table 3). In the pressure overload and thyrotoxic hearts the economy of force maintenance during the relaxation phase of the isometric twitch is 45 and 46 percent greater than during the contraction phase (table 3).

Table 3. Economy of isometric contraction (g cm sec/μcal).

Preparation	Contraction (E_C)	Relaxation (E_R)	E_C/E_R
N (10)	7.15 ± 1.29	6.89 ± 0.75	1.00 ± 0.11 (NS)
P (8)	5.79 ± 0.82	8.91 ± 1.14	0.69 ± 0.09 ($p < .02$)
T (5)	1.80 ± 0.23	4.52 ± 0.84	0.51 ± 0.14 ($p < .05$)

* The number in the parentheses indicates the number of experiments carried out in each group; N, P and T represent the normal, pressure overload and thyrotoxic groups.

Table 4. Right ventricular myosin isoenzyme composition.

	Control	Pressure overload	Thyrotoxic
Percent V_1	12 ± 4 (6)*	0 ± 0 (5)	90 ± 2 (3)

* The number in the parentheses indicates the number of rabbit hearts for each group.

Isoenzyme composition. The V_1 myosin isoenzyme content of the free wall of the right ventricle from normal hearts was 12 percent. This was significantly reduced in the pressure overloaded (0 %) and increased in the thyrotoxic hearts (90 %) (table 4). Isoenzyme composition was measured in the right ventricular free wall whereas the thermomechanical measurements were made on the right ventricular papillary muscles. In a series of experiments with control rabbits we determined that there was a slightly greater V_1 content in the papillary muscle than in the right ventricular free wall (19 vs. 12 %). However, we do not consider this small difference important to the results of this study.

Discussion

In activated skeletal muscle the economy of contraction is lower than during lengthening (1, 2, 3, 4). Since it is known that heart muscle and especially isolated papillary muscle exhibits substantial sarcomere shortening during isometric tension development and sarcomere lengthening during relaxation of tension (6–9 %) (5), the hypothesis was proposed that isometric force development would be less economical than isometric relaxation. This was confirmed in the pressure overload and thyrotoxic hearts. We were surprised to find that in normal hearts the contraction and relaxation phases of the isometric twitch exhibited identical economy.

In pressure overload, normal and thyrotoxic muscle the V_1 myosin isoenzyme makes up 0, 12 and 90 percent of the total myosin (table 4). How do these differences in isoenzyme profile contribute to the observed economy of contraction and relaxation? Some information about this problem can be gained by analyzing the contractile behavior in terms of modern kinetic schemes of the actomyosin crossbridge cycle (14, 15, 17, 18). In this scheme when the muscle is activated and developing force, actomyosin exists in two states: A) dissociated non-force producing; B) associated force producing. The dissociated non-force producing steps of the cycle are listed below: 1) ATP combines with actomyosin AM causing a dissociation (ATP + AM → A + M*ATP); 2) M*ATP is transformed to $M^{**}ADPP_i$, an energized but refractory state; 3) a slow rate limiting conformation change then occurs ($M^{**}ADPP_i \rightarrow M{+}ADPP_i$) which then permits the binding of actin (A) to the energized myosin. The associated, force-producing steps follow: 1) the energized myosin combines with actin ($M{+}ADPP_i + A \rightarrow AM{+}ADPP_i$) with a contact angle of 90°; 2) the contact angle rotates from 90° to 45° stretching the flexible portion of the bridge and producing tension ($AM{+}ADPP_i \rightarrow AM\,ADPP_i$), 3) the subsequent loss of hydrolysis products (ADP and P_i) and the binding of the ATP molecule to AM starts the cycle again. Thus force generation in activated muscle can be divided into a power step which occurs during the associated or "on" phase of the cycle and a rate-limiting step which occurs in the dissociated or "off" phase of the cycle. Thermal and mechanical measurements can be used to assess the contribution of each of these phases to the economy of force production during contraction and relaxation. An estimate of the average crossbridge cycling frequency (f) is calculated as follows:

$$f = N/D \quad (1)$$

Where N is the number of crossbridge cycles and D is the duration of the total period of cycling.

$$N = TDH/K \quad (2)$$

Where TDH is the tension-dependent heat and K is the enthalpy of ATP hydrolysis. By combining (1) and (2) one gets:

$$f = TDH/KD \quad (3)$$

The "on" time (τ) for force development can be estimated as follows:

$$\int Pdt = N\tau S \quad (4)$$

Where $\int Pdt$ is the tension time integral, N is the number of crossbridge cycles, τ is the duration each bridge is "on" in the force producing state, and S is the average force produced by the crossbridge during the "on" time. For this analysis, S is assumed to be unity.

$$\tau = \int Pdt/NS \quad (5)$$

Or combining equations (2) and (5):

$$\tau = (K/S) \int Pdt/TDH \quad (6)$$

It is interesting to note that τ is proportional to the economy ($E = \int Pdt/TDH$). Calculations of f (assuming 35 mg of myosin per gram of muscle and total activation of all the myosin molecules) and τ for contraction and relaxation are presented in table 5. In the pressure overload model, which is pure V_3, it is possible to interpret the increased economy of relaxation as a decrease in the average crossbridge cycling frequency (19 %) and a substantial increase in the "on" time (54 %). These changes may be attributed to the effect of lengthening the sarcomeres during the relaxation on the kinetic properties of actomyosin. Similarly, larger changes in f and τ could account for the increased economy of relaxation in the thyrotoxic preparations. It is not clear why there is no change in economy during relaxation in the control hearts especially considering that the myosin isoenzyme mixture (88 % V_3 and 12 % V_1) is not substantially more heterogeneous than in the thyrotoxic hearts (10 % V_3 and 90 % V_1).

Failing to consistently explain these economy differences on the basis of alterations in f and τ, we would like to advance a speculative hypothesis that increased economy during sarcomere lengthening may be related to the "give" phenomenon described by Flitney, Hirst, and Jones (19). They changed crossbridge cycling rate in contracting skeletal muscle by changing the temperature at which the experiments were carried out. The activated muscles were subjected to steady-state stretches. The force P_s during lengthening was above P_o and was a function of the velocity of stretch. The force P_s rose rapidly as the velocity was increased to a critical point, and then it ceased to rise. Similar "give" in response to stretch of

Table 5. Crossbridge cycling rate (f, Hz) and relative "on" time ($\tau = \tau_{exp}/\tau_C$) in control (C), pressure overload (P), and thyrotoxic (T) hypertrophied hearts.

	Contraction		Relaxation	
	f	τ	f	τ
P	.65	.81	.53	1.25
T	1.55	.25	1.16	.63
C	.65	1.00	.71	.96

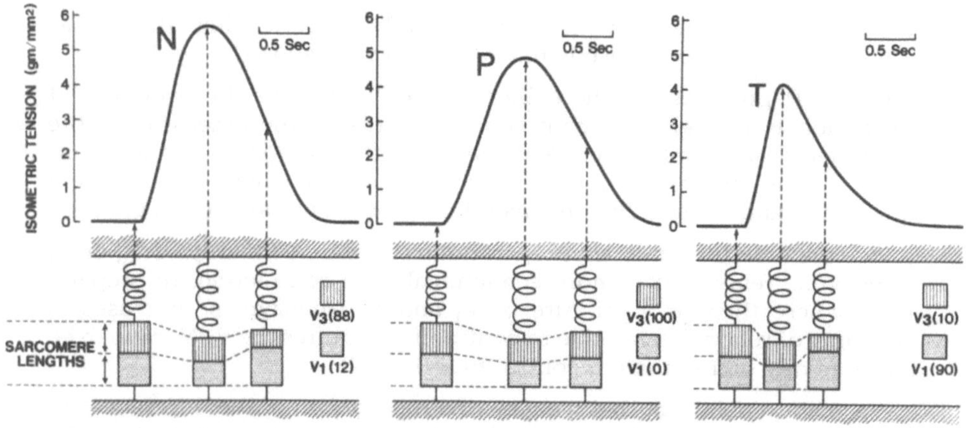

Fig. 3. Proposed differences in sarcomere motion during relaxation in normal and hypertrophied papillary muscle. Above: Isometric twitch myograms from normal (N), pressure overload (P), and thyrotoxic (T) hypertrophied papillary muscles. Below: Two-element muscle model showing proposed changes in sarcomere lengths during contraction and during relaxation when the series elastic element (coiled element) re-extends the sarcomeres (rectangular elements). The sarcomeres are composed of two series connected populations, one containing the slower myosin isoenzyme population, V_3 (vertical hatching) and the other containing the faster, V_1 isoenzyme (dotted). See text for explanation.

rabbit papillary muscle has been observed by Moss et al. (20). This represents a new mode of crossbridge behavior in which high forces are maintained with little or no ATP consumption (4) and possibly no "cycling" in the conventional sense. For the slowly cycling crossbridge (low temperature) the critical velocity (V_c) was lower, and P_s/P_o was higher than for the more rapidly cycling crossbridges (higher temperature). During the rise of tension in a muscle composed of slow and fast sarcomeres connected in series both fast and slow sarcomeres are shortening against series compliance. During the relaxation phase, energy stored in the passive, compliant elements extends the sarcomeres (fig. 3). The fast sarcomeres are extended preferentially over the slow sarcomeres because they have a lower P_s/P_o at critical velocity. For the normal muscle (N, fig. 3), which has 88 % V_3 myosin, during relaxation only 12 % of the sarcomeres would undergo the economical "give" phenomenon, and the increase in economy for this small fraction of V_1 containing sarcomeres will be masked by the unchanged economy in the 88 % of the sarcomeres containing V_3 which do not experience the "give" phenomenon during relaxation. In addition to "give" induced by the passive recoil of the series compliance during relaxation, muscles with a low ratio of V_1/V_3 would also undergo "give" in the minority population (V_1) of sarcomeres as a result of "give-and-take" interaction with the majority population (V_3) of sarcomeres. Hence not only would increased economy during relaxation be small due to the small fraction of sarcomeres undergoing "give", but it would be counteracted by the extra heat expected to be liberated by the V_3

containing sarcomeres which are actually experiencing the lower economy, contraction phase behavior during relaxation (N, fig. 3).

In the P preparation where there is no V_1 present the economy of relaxation is greater than contraction because of the extension of the sarcomeres during relaxation. As expected in the T preparation, the majority of the sarcomeres (90 %) undergo the economical lengthening reaction during relaxation, and thus the overall economy of relaxation is greater.

We conclude that in heart preparations made up primarily of V_3 or V_1 isoenzyme, relaxation is more economical than contraction. In preparations where there is a mixture of V_1 and V_3 isoenzymes, increases in economy of relaxation relative to contraction requires the V_1/V_3 ratio to be substantially higher than in control muscles (12).

We wish to point out that we view the mechanism of the differences in economy between contraction and relaxation in a given muscle to be different than the one we previously proposed to account for differences in economy of isometric force production between different forms of cardiac hypertrophy (6, 10, 13). In the latter case, the change from one particular isoenzyme complement to a different one brings about a new set of kinetics for the crossbridge cycle. In the former case, differences in economy between contraction and relaxation are attributed to different *modes* of interaction of a given crossbridge population with actin.

References

1. Abbott, B. C., X. M. Aubert, A. V. Hill· The absorption of work by muscle stretched during a single twitch or a short tetanus. Proc. Roy. Soc. B **139,** 86–104 (1951).
2. Abbott, B. C., X. M. Aubert: Changes in energy in a muscle during very slow stretches. Proc. Roy. Soc. Lond. B **139,** 104–117 (1951).
3. Abbott, B. C., B. Bigland, J. M. Ritchie: The physiological cost of negative work. J. Physiol. **117,** 380–390 (1952)
4. Curtin, N., R. E. Davies: Very high tension with very little ATP breakdown by active skeletal muscle. J. Mechanochem. Cell. Motility **3,** 147–154 (1975)
5. Krueger, J. W., G. H. Pollack: Myocardial sarcomere dynamics during isometric contraction. J. Physiol. **251,** 627–643 (1975).
6. Alpert, N. R., L. A. Mulieri, R. Z. Litten: Functional significance of altered myosin adenosine triphosphatase activity in enlarged hearts. Amer. J. Cardiol. **44,** 947–953 (1979).
7. Litten, R. Z., B. J. Martin, R. B. Low, N. R. Alpert: Altered myosin isoenzyme patterns from pressure overload and thyrotoxic hypertrophied hearts. Circulat. Res. **50,** 856–864 (1982).
8. Hamrell, B. B., N. R. Alpert· The mechanical characteristics of hypertrophied rabbit cardiac muscle in the absence of congestive heart failure: the contractile and series elastic elements. Circulat. Res. **40,** 20–25 (1977).
9. Banerjee, S. K., I. L. Flink, E. Morkin: Enzymatic properties of native and N-Ethylmaleimide-modified cardiac myosin from normal and thyrotoxic rabbits. Circulat. Res. **39,** 319–326 (1976).
10. Alpert, N. R., L. A. Mulieri: Increased myothermal economy of isometric force generation in compensated cardiac hypertrophy induced by pulmonary artery

constriction in the rabbit. A characterization of heat liberation in normal and hypertrophied right ventricular papillary muscles. Circulat. Res. **50,** 491–500 (1982).

11. Mulieri, L. A., G. Luhr, J. Trefry, N. R. Alpert: Metal film thermopiles for use with rabbit right ventricular papillary muscles. Amer. J. Physiol. **233,** C146–156 (1977).
12. Hamrell, B. B., R. Panaanen, J. Trono, N. R. Alpert: A stable, sensitive, low-compliance capacitance force transducer. J. Appl. Physiol. **38,** 190–193 (1975).
13. Alpert, N. R., L. A. Mulieri: Heat mechanics and myosin ATPase in normal and hypertrophied heart muscle. Fed. Proc. **41,** 192–198 (1982).
14. Alpert, N. R., L. A. Mulieri: The utilization of energy by the myocardium hypertrophied secondary to pressure overload. In: *The Heart in Hypertension,* edited by B. E. Strauer, pp. 153–163. Springer Verlag (Berlin 1981).
15. Alpert, N. R., L. A. Mulieri: The functional significance of altered tension dependent heat in thyrotoxic myocardial hypertrophy. Basic Res. Cardiol. **75,** 179–184 (1980).
16. Hoh, J. F. Y., P. A. McGrath, P. T. Hale: Electrophoretic analysis of multiple forms of rat cardiac myosin: Effect of hypophysectomy and thyroxine replacement. J. Mol. Cell Cardiol. **10,** 1053–1076 (1977).
17. Eisenberg, E., T. L. Hill: A crossbridge model of muscle contraction. Prog. Biophys. Mol Biol. **33,** 55–82 (1978).
18. Lymm, R. W., E. W. Taylor: Mechanism of adenosine triphosphate hydrolysis by actomyosin. Biochemistry **10,** 4617–4624 (1971).
19. Flitney, F. W., D. G. Hirst, D. A. Jones: Effects of temperature and velocity of stretch on the maximum tension borne by the sarcomeres in contracting muscle. J. Physiol. **256,** 127–128P (1976).
20. Moss, R. L., M. R. Sollins, F. J. Julian: Calcium activation produces a characteristic response to stretch in both skeletal and cardiac muscle. Nature **260,** 619–621 (1976).

Authors' address:

Norman R. Alpert, Ph.D., Department of Physiology and Biophysics, University of Vermont, College of Medicine, Burlington, Vermont 05405, U.S.A.

Cardiac Adaptation to Hemodynamic Overload, Training and Stress
Dr. D. Steinkopff Verlag 158–166 (1983)

Heat liberation in experimentally induced tetanic contractions of myocardium from normal and Goldblatt rats

Ch. Holubarsch*, R. P. Goulette, L. A. Mulieri**, and N. R. Alpert****

* Institute of Physiology II, University of Tübingen, Tübingen (FRG)
**Dept. of Physiology and Biophysics, College of Medicine, University of Vermont, Burlington, Vermont (USA*)

Summary

We induced hypertension in Wistar Kyoto rats by constricting the left renal artery according to the method of Goldblatt (GOP). Five weeks after the surgery, papillary muscle preparations of the left ventricle from normal and GOP rats were tetanized by incubation in Krebs-Ringer solution containing 11 mM calcium and 7.5 mM caffeine and stimulated with various numbers of stimuli (frequency 3.0 Hz). Using antimony-bismuth planar thermopiles, total activity-related heat (T_A) and the developed tension-time integral ($\int \sigma \cdot t$) were measured during isometric tetani of normal and GOP myocardium. For each preparation, a linear regression equation was fitted to the plot of T_A versus $\int \sigma \cdot t$. The slope of this function was significantly ($P < 0.01$) steeper in the control than in the GOP preparations. The present data demonstrates that less heat is liberated per unit $\int \sigma \cdot t$ in GOP compared to control myocardium, i.e., economy of force generation is higher in GOP myocardium. This finding can be interpreted in terms of altered cross-bridge cycling mechanisms in the GOP myocardium.

Key words: hypertension, pressure-overload hypertrophy, heat, cross-bridges, excitation-contraction coupling, adaptation

Introduction

In the last 15 years, many authors have reported that compensated pressure-overload cardiac hypertrophy is accompanied by a decrease in maximum shortening velocity (Spann et al., 1967; Bing et al., 1971; Alpert et al., 1974; Jacob et al., 1977). Interpreted in light of the concept of contractility, this decrease in v_{max} would be considered as a malfunction of the pressure-overloaded myocardium. This view was supported by findings of Gunning and Coleman (1973) and Cooper et al. (1973) who showed an increase in oxygen consumption per peak developed tension in hypertrophied myocardium.

Recently, however, the myothermal method was used to study cardiac energetics in papillary muscles of the pressure-overloaded right ventricle (Alpert and Mulieri, 1982). In contrast to the mentioned oxygen consumption measurements, less heat liberation was found per peak developed tension in the hypertrophied myocardium. This finding reflects an

*) The experimental part of the present study was performed in this laboratory.

increase in economy of force generation due to a fundamental change in the contractile event. The purpose of the present study was to expand myothermal investigations to another model of hypertrophy, i.e., left ventricular hypertrophy due to experimental renal hypertension in the rat (Goldblatt). Tetanic contractions were induced according to Gibbs and Loiselle (1978) in left ventricular papillary muscles of control and Goldblatt myocardium.

Methods

Rationale

Tetanic responses were used to minimize the possible effect of internal shortening on heart generation and tension production. Tetanization was made possible using solutions containing high calcium and caffeine, and stimuli at 3.0 Hz (Gibbs

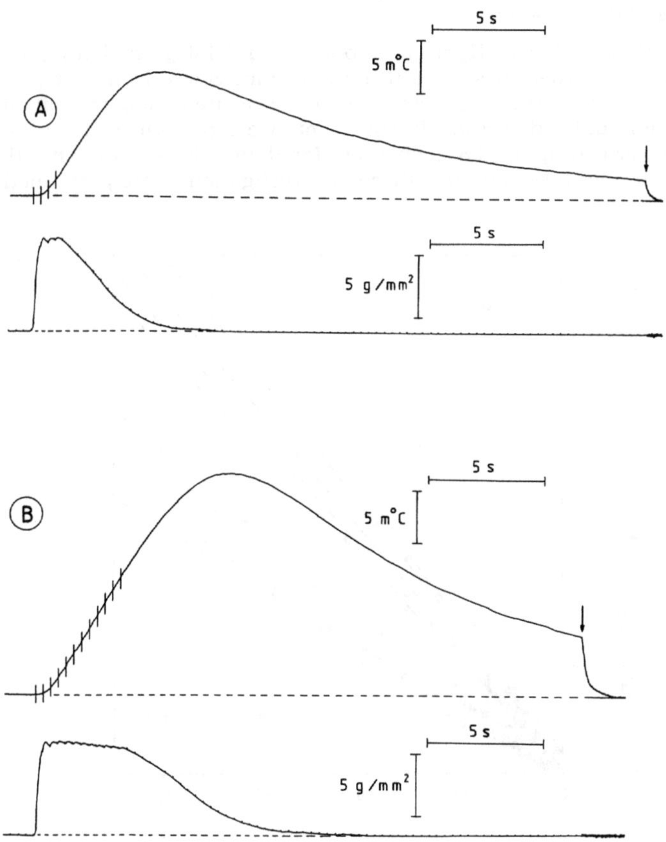

Fig. 1. Original records of experimental tetanic contractions: A: 4 stimuli were applied; B: 12 stimuli were applied. The number of stimuli can be counted from the capacitively coupled stimulus artifact in the temperature signal. Temperature trace: Top in A and B; Tension trace: Bottom in A and B. The arrows indicate that the paper speed was slowed down by a factor of 100.

and Loiselle, 1978; Holubarsch et. al., 1983). In such a tetanic contraction internal shortening occurs only at the beginning of a contraction followed by steady isometric tension maintenance (fig. 1). Thus, heat liberated as a result of shortening during the initial phase of tension development is relatively small compared to the heat from tension maintenance in a long duration tetanus.

Contraction duration was varied by applying various numbers of stimuli thus allowing the relation between total activity-related heat versus developed tension-time integral to be investigated.

Total activity-related heat (T_A) can be divided into tension-dependent total heat (TDT_A) associated with cross-bridge cycling and tension-independent total heat (TIT_A) resulting from calcium cycling using the method proposed by Gibbs and Loiselle (1978). With this method, the initial and recovery heat processes are combined.

When the muscle length is reduced 1.0 to 1.5 mm below its optimum length, very little or no active tension is developed. A heat signal occurs, however, representing activation heat, i.e., the energy necessary for calcium turnover.

Animals and instruments

In normotensive Wistar Kyoto rats (body weight 130 g) the left renal artery was narrowed under ether anesthesia using a 0.2-mm Ø silver clip. At three and five weeks after surgery, the blood pressure was measured using the tail-cuff method and a volume pulse detector. Measurements were performed in awake rats after they were warmed up in a 38 °C chamber for 15 min. Five weeks after the surgery, the rats were sacrificed, and myothermal investigations were performed.

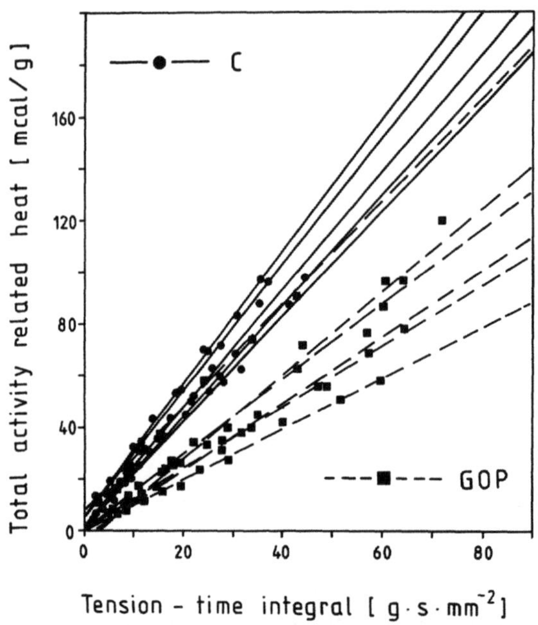

Fig. 2. Total activity-related heat versus tension-time integral. Each linear regression line represents one papillary muscle. Data from 5 control (C, solid lines) and 6 Goldblatt (GOP, broken lines) preparations. The slopes are significantly ($p < 0.01$) lower in the GOP myocardium.

Detailed descriptions of the thermopile and the instruments, as well as the procedure of papillary muscle preparation have been published previously (Mulieri et al., 1977; Alpert and Mulieri, 1982; Holubarsch et al., 1982; 1983). For this study, two different thermopiles were used which had temperature sensitivities of 1.325 and 1.206 mV/°C and heat loss coefficients of 0.590 and 0.564 mcal/°C · s.

Experimental protocol

All experiments were carried out at 21 °C. After an equilibration period of 2 hours during which time the muscles contracted isometrically at 12/min, the muscles were stretched to l_{max} in 0.05 to 0.10 mm increments. The preparations were incubated in Krebs-Ringer solution containing 11 mM calcium and 7.5 mM caffeine for 15 min. No stimulus was applied during this period. Tetanic contractions were induced by stimulating the preparations with various numbers of stimuli (1, 2, 3, 4, 5, 8, 12, 16, 20) at a frequency of 3.0 Hz (fig. 1). Subsequently, the muscle preparation was shortened to a length at which no or very little tension development was induced by stimulation, although a considerable temperature signal was obtained. We interpret this temperature change to be a reflection of activation heat plus a small definable portion of TDT_A (see Appendix for detailed method of analysis).

Data analysis

Total activity-related heat (T_A) was obtained as follows: The area between the temperature baseline (resting temperature) and the temperature signal excursion due to tetanic contraction (fig. 1) was evaluated by a planimeter and converted into heat by multiplication with the heat loss coefficient. The heat was then normalized per g muscle tissue. In contrast to paced or single twitches (Alpert and Mulieri, 1982; Holubarsch et al., 1982; 1983), separation of initial and recovery heat is not possible because of the long duration of tetanic contraction. The force-time integral was also analyzed with a planimeter, and the obtained value was divided by the cross-sectional area for normalization.

For each preparation, the measured heat data was related to the corresponding tension-time integral. A linear regression equation was determined from the data by least squares regression analysis (fig. 2).

Tension-independent total heat (TIT_A) was evaluated from the temperature signal at short muscle length in the same way as total activity-related heat at l_{max}. In some preparations, the developed tension-time integral at short muscle length was not negligible. In such cases, we corrected the evaluated TIT_A for the tension-dependent heat due to tension generation (see Appendix).

TIT_A was subtracted from T_A yielding TDT_A. These values were also correlated with the corresponding tension-time integrals. A linear regression equation was determined from the data (fig. 3).

Results

Blood pressure and degree of hypertrophy

Systolic blood pressure was increased from a control value of 119 ± 8 mm Hg to 220 ± 21 mm Hg in the Goldblatt animals. The left-ventricular-to-body-weight ratio was 3.40 ± 0.32 in GOP and 2.14 ± 0.10 mg/g in control rats (C; $P < 0.01$).

Myothermal measurements

As shown in figure 1, application of multiple stimuli to a rat papillary muscle preparation pretreated with caffeine and high calcium resulted in relatively smooth tetanus. Figure 2 shows the relation between T_A and tension-time integral. The correlation coefficients of the linear regression equations fit to the plot of the observed total activity-related heat versus the corresponding tension-time integral were between 0.98 and 0.99. There was a significant ($P < 0.01$) difference between the slope of the linear regression equations from normal (2.21 ± 0.24 mcal $\cdot$ $g^{-1}/g \cdot s \cdot mm^2$) and GOP myocardium ($1.38 \pm 0.36$ mcal $\cdot$ $g^{-1}/g \cdot s \cdot mm^{-2}$).

The intercepts of the functions were significantly different (2.82 ± 2.20 (C) versus -0.77 ± 4.23 (GOP) mcal $\cdot$ g^{-1}; fig. 2). There was a significant ($P < 0.01$) difference between normal and GOP myocardium when the slopes of the TDT_A versus $\int \cdot \sigma \cdot t$ functions were analyzed (1.52 ± 0.16 (C) versus 0.90 ± 0.31 (GOP) mcal $\cdot$ $g^{-1}/g \cdot s \cdot mm^{-2}$; fig. 3).

Discussion

Myothermal data

Figure 2 reveals a linear relationship between total-activity related heat and tension-time integral for data obtained from individual preparations. The intercept is close to zero for control and GOP myocardium. This data indicates that in rat papillary muscles the economy of force generation remains constant throughout the duration of a tetanic contraction. This observation supports the view of adequate oxygenation of rat papillary

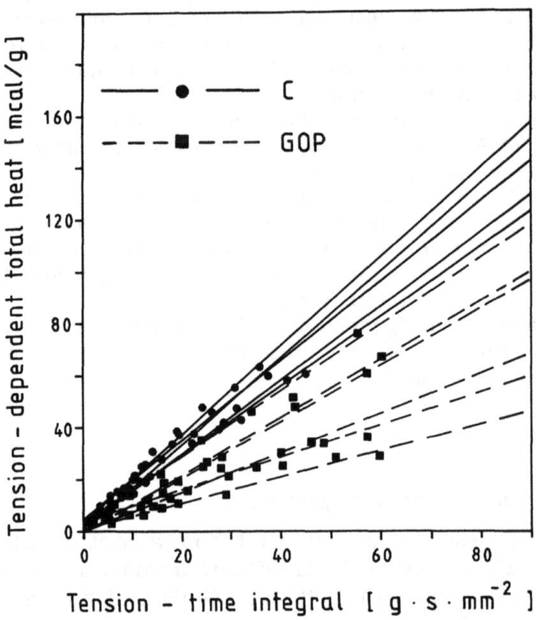

Fig. 3. Tension-dependent total heat (TDT_A) versus tension-time integral. TDT_A was analyzed by the shortening method (see text). Each linear regression line represents one papillary muscle. Data from 5 control (C, solid lines) and 6 Goldblatt preparations (GOP, broken lines). TDT_A is significantly ($p < 0.01$) lower in GOP than in normal rat myocardium.

muscles under conditions of the present study and makes intracellular ATP deficiency unlikely.

The method used for assessment of activation heat was described by Gibbs and Loiselle (1978) for tetanic contractions in cardiac muscle. When shortening the muscle preparation to a length at which very little or no tension is developed, a considerable amount of heat is liberated which represents tension-independent heat, i.e., activation heat. In those preparations which developed small but not negligible tension at short muscle length, we corrected for the heat associated with this tension (Appendix). Nevertheless, there are two potential problems associated with this method: (1) At short length, muscle shortening might occur without tension development but with considerable heat due to shortening. The present study was performed to eliminate the influences of internal shortening on heat output. In a twitch contraction, internal shortening may contribute a significant portion of the T_A at optimum and the shorter length. In tetanic contractions, however, internal shortening occurs only in the very beginning of the contraction. Therefore, the longer the contractions the smaller the relative effect of internal shortening on the heat output. This applies to tetanic contractions at optimum length as well as at shorter muscle length. (2) As indicated by Fabiato (1980), the degree of activation may be dependent on muscle length itself in rat ventricular myocardium. We assume that in the presence of high extracellular calcium and caffeine activation is maximum and similar at optimum length as well as at the short muscle length (see also Fabiato and Fabiato, 1975). The amount of activation heat was about 30% of T_A which is considerably higher than in twitch contractions (Holubarsch et al., 1982). This finding is consistant with the assumption that activation is maximum under these conditions.

Model of hypertrophy

The systolic blood pressure values in this study were considerably higher than those previously reported (Kissling et al., 1977; Kämmereit and Jacob, 1979; Holubarsch et al., 1982). This discrepancy may be attributed to differences in the conditions used during the measurements (use of ether, warming up the rats). In comparing the earlier studies with the present one, lower blood pressure values were found in the control as well as the GOP rats. This supports the view that the differences are mainly due to differences in the blood pressure measurement protocol. The degree of hypertrophy is comparable in all of the studies.

The time-course of the pressure-overload imposed upon the myocardium is a factor which is held to be important for changes of intrinsic properties of the hypertrophied myocardium. With respect to the abruptly induced pressure-overload (Alpert et al., 1974; Cooper et al., 1973) and the slowly developing pressure-overload in spontaneous hypertension of the rat (Pfeffer et al., 1979; Bing et al., 1983), the GOP model shows an intermediate time-course (fig. 2 in Kämmereit and Jacob, 1979).

Interpretation of myothermal economy

Before interpreting the results of control and GOP myocardium, a comparison between the present data and that of Gibbs and Loiselle is instructive. For normal rat myocardium they found the slope of T_A versus $\int \sigma \cdot t$ in tetanic contractions to be 2.54 mcal $\cdot$ $g^{-1}/g \cdot s \cdot mm^{-2}$; for guinea pig and cat myocardium the mean values were 1.46 and 1.22 mcal $\cdot$ $g^{-1}/g \cdot s \cdot mm^{-2}$, respectively. (For the purpose of comparison, the values and dimensions used by Gibbs and Loiselle were transformed to those used in this paper.) The value of 2.54 is very close to the present value of 2.21 for normal rat myocardium, especially, if one considers that Gibbs and Loiselle used an experimental temperature of 27 °C, whereas the temperature in the present study was 21 °C.

In the GOP myocardium, this slope is decreased to 1.38, which indicates an increase in economy of force generation and maintenance. Interestingly, the 1.38 value is close to that reported for the guinea pig and cat myocardium (Gibbs and Loiselle, 1978). Moreover, the myothermal data of the present study is in agreement with the myothermal measurements on pressure-overloaded myocardium from the rabbit (Alpert and Mulieri, 1982) as well as oxygen consumption measurements on isovolumic whole heart preparations of control and GOP rats (Kissling et al., 1982).

In contrast to the paper of Cooper et al. (1973), the present myothermal data indicates that the slow GOP myocardium (Jacob et al., 1977; 1980) exhibits an increased economy of force generation when compared to control rat myocardium. This similarity to the slower and more economic guinea pig and cat myocardium (Henderson et al., 1970; Gibbs and Loiselle, 1978) as well as to the slower and more economic hypothyrotic rat myocardium (Ebrecht et al., 1982; Holubarsch et al., 1983) suggests that decreases in the mechanical and biochemical rate parameters (mechanical v_{max} and actomyosin ATPase) are associated with an increase in economy of force maintenance. Therefore, the observed decrease in the rate of myocardial contraction and associated actomyosin ATPase per se cannot be considered to be pathological or even detrimental as has been suggested by others (Wikman-Coffelt, 1979; Scheuer et al., 1982), because it has been demonstrated that this change is accompanied by an increase in economy of force generation in two different models of hypertrophy. This interpretation of velocity *and* energetic parameters should be taken into account when discussing the term "contractility" (see also Katz, 1973).

As shown by the analysis of activation heat, the change in economy of force generation in GOP myocardium has to be attributed mainly to the TDT_A, and thus indicates a change in the basic mechanism of the contractile event, i.e., cross-bridge cycling. Although Rupp (1981) has demonstrated a shift of the myosin isoenzyme pattern towards the slow V_3 in GOP myocardium, it remains to be seen whether alterations in economy of force generation of papillary muscles correlate directly to changes in the isoenzyme pattern of papillary muscles and free wall myocardium, as has been shown for hypothyrotic rat myocardium (Holubarsch et al., 1983).

Appendix

Assuming a linear relationship of TDT_A versus tension-time integral between optimum length (l_{max}) and short length (l_s), the following equations can be developed:

(TIT_A = tension-independent heat; $T_{Al_{max}}$ = total activity-related heat l_{max}; $T_{A_{ls}}$ = total activity-related heat at short muscle length; $TDT_{Al_{max}}$ = tension-dependent total heat at l_{max}; $TDT_{A_{ls}}$ = tension-dependent total heat at short length; $\int \sigma \cdot t_{lmax}$ = tension-time integral at l_{max}; $\int \sigma \cdot t_{ls}$ = tension-time integral at short length).

(1) $T_{A\,l_{max}} - TIT_A = TDT_{A\,l_{max}}$

(2) $T_{A\,l_s} - TIT_A = TDT_{A\,ls}$

(3) $TDT_{A\,l_s} : TDT_{A\,l_{max}} = \int \sigma \cdot t_{l_s} : \int \sigma \cdot t_{l_{max}} = k$

Substituting the values from equation (1) and (2) into equation (3) we obtain

$$\frac{TDT_{A\,l_s}}{TDT_{A\,l_{max}}} = k = \frac{T_{A\,ls} - TIT_A}{T_{A\,l_{max}} - TIT_A}$$

$$TIT_A = \frac{T_{A\,l_s} - k \cdot T_{A\,l_{max}}}{(1-k)} \text{ when } k = \frac{\int \sigma\, t_{l_s}}{\int \sigma \cdot t_{l_{max}}}$$

Acknowledgement

Ch. Holubarsch greatly appreciates the support and advice of Prof. Dr. R. Jacob, Chairman, Institute of Physiology II, University of Tübingen.

References

Alpert, N. R., B. B. Hamrell, W. Halpern: Mechanical and biochemical correlates of cardiac hypertrophy. Circulat. Res. **34/35** II, 71–82 (1974).

Alpert, N. R., L. A. Mulieri: Increased myothermal economy of isometric force generation in compensated cardiac hypertrophy induced by pulmonary artery constriction in the rabbit. Circulat. Res. **50,** 491–500 (1982).

Bing, O. H. L., S. Matsushita, B. L. Fanburg, H. J. Levine: Mechanical properties of rat cardiac muscle during experimental hypertrophy. Circulat. Res. **28,** 234–245 (1971).

Bing, O. H. L., A. W. Wiegner: Myocardial mechanics in the spontaneously hypertensive rat: Changes with age. In: Perspectives in Cardiovascular Research. Vol. 7. Myocardial Hypertrophy and Failure. pp. 281–291. Ed.: N. R. Alpert. Raven Press, New York 1983.

Cooper, G. IV, R. M. Satava, C. E. Harrison, H. N. Coleman: Mechanism for abnormal energetics of pressure-induced hypertrophy of cat myocardium. Circulat. Res. **33,** 213–223 (1973).

Ebrecht, G., H. Rupp, R. Jacob: Alterations of mechanical parameters in chemically skinned preparations of rat myocardium as a function of isoenzyme pattern of myosin. Basic Res. Cardiol. **77,** 220–234 (1982).

Fabiato, A., F. Fabiato: Dependence of the contractile activation of skinned cardiac cells on the sarcomere length. Nature **256,** 54–56 (1975).

Fabiato, A.: Sarcomere length dependence of calcium release from the sarcoplasmic reticulum of skinned cardiac cells demonstrated by differential microspectrophotometry with Arsenazo III. J. Gen. Physiol. **76,** 15a (1980).

Gibbs, C., D. Loiselle: The energy output of tetanized cardiac muscle: Species differences. Pflügers Arch. **373,** 31–38 (1978).

Gunning, J. F., H. N. Coleman: Myocardial oxygen consumption during experimental hypertrophy and congestive heart failure. J. Mol. Cell. Cardiol. **5,** 25–38 (1973).

Henderson, A. H., R. J. Craig, E. H. Sonnenblick, C. W. Urschel: Species differences in intrinsic myocardial contractility. Proc. Soc. Exp. Biol. Med. **134,** 930–932 (1970).

Holubarsch, Ch., N. R. Alpert, R. Goulette, L. A. Mulieri: Heat production during hypoxic contracture of rat myocardium. Circulat. Res. **51,** 777–786 (1982).

Holubarsch, Ch., Th. Holubarsch, R. Jacob, I. Medugorac, K. U. Thiedemann: Passive elastic properties of rat myocardium in different models of hypertrophy. In: Perspectives in Cardiovascular Research, Vol. 7, Myocardial Hypertrophy and Failure. Ed. N. R. Alpert. Raven Press. New York 1983, pp. 323–336.

Holubarsch, Ch., R. P. Goulette, R. Z. Litten, B. J. Martin, L. A. Mulieri, N. R. Alpert: Changes in mechanical energetic, and biochemical parameters of left ventricular myocardium of hypothyrotic rats. Submitted to Circulat. Res.

Jacob, R., G. Ebrecht, A. Kämmereit, I. Medugorac, M. F. Wendt-Gallitelli: Myocardial function in different models of cardiac hypertrophy. An attempt at correlating mechanical, biochemical, and morphological parameters. Basic Res. Cardiol. **72,** 160–167 (1977).

Jacob, R., B. Brenner, G. Ebrecht, Ch. Holubarsch, I. Medugorac: Elastic and contractile properties of the myocardium in experimental cardiac hypertrophy of the rat. Methodological and pathophysiological considerations: Basic Res. Cardiol. **75,** 253–261 (1980).

Kämmereit, A., R. Jacob: Alterations in myocardial mechanics under Goldblatt hypertension and experimental aortic stenosis. Basic Res. Cardiol. **74,** 389–405 (1979).

Katz, A.: Biochemical "defect" in the hypertrophied and failing heart: Deleterious or compensatory? Circulation **47,** 1076–1079 (1973).

Kissling, G. T., M. F. Gassenmaier, Wendt-Gallitelli, R. Jacob: Pressure-volume relations, elastic modulus, and contractile behavior of the hypertrophied left ventricle of rats with Goldblatt II hypertension. Pflügers Arch. **269,** 213–221 (1977).

Kissling, G., H. Rupp, R. Jacob: Alterations in cardiac oxygen consumption under chronic pressure overload. Significance of the isoenzyme pattern of myosin. Basic Res. Cardiol. **77,** 255–269 (1982).

Mulieri, L. A., G. Luhr, J. Trefry, N. R. Alpert: Metal-film thermopiles for use with rabbit right ventricular papillary muscles. Amer. J. Physiol. **233** (5), C146–C156 (1977).

Pfeffer, J. M., M. A. Pfeffer, M. C. Fishbein, E. D. Frohlich: Cardiac function and morphology with aging in the spontaneously hypertensive rat. Amer. J. Physiol. **237** (4), H 461–H468 (1979).

Scheuer, J., A. Malhotra, C. Hirsch, J. Capasso, T. F. Schaible: Physiologic cardiac hypertrophy corrects contractile protein abnormalities associated with pathologic hypertrophy of rats. J. Clin. Invest. **70,** 1300–1305 (1982).

Spann, J. F., R. A. Buccino, E. H. Sonnenblick, E. Braunwald: Contractile state of muscle obtained from cats with experimentally produced ventricular hypertrophy and heart failure. Circulat. Res. **21,** 341–354 (1967).

Wikman-Coffelt, J., W. W. Parmley, D. T. Mason: The Cardiac Hypertrophy Process. Analyses of factors determining pathological versus physiological development. Circulat. Res. **45,** 697–707 (1979).

Authors' address:

Doz. Dr. Ch. Holubarsch, Physiologisches Institut, Lehrstuhl II d. Univ. Tübingen, Gmelinstr. 5, 7400 Tübingen, FRG

Cardiac Adaptation to Hemodynamic Overload, Training and Stress
Dr. D. Steinkopff Verlag 167–173 (1983)

Energetics of the rat heart in chronic pressure overload*) **)

G. Kissling, L. Malloy*) and H. Rupp**

Physiologisches Institut II der Universität Tübingen (FRG)

Summary

Myocardial oxygen consumption and efficiency were evaluated in Goldblatt rats 24 weeks after operation and in age-matched controls. The myosin isoenzyme pattern of each heart was determined with pyrophosphate gel electrophoresis.

The pressure-overloaded hearts revealed reduced oxygen consumption and improved myocardial efficiency which could be attributed to a redistribution of myosin isoenzymes in favour of VM-3. The results can be interpreted such that the redistribution of myosin isoenzymes reflects an adaptive process, which transforms the myocardium into a slower but more efficiently working muscle.

Key words: left ventricular hypertrophy, pressure overload, myocardial energetics, myocardial oxygen consumption, myocardial efficiency, myosin isoenzymes

Introduction

The myocardium of the rat includes three different isoenzymes of myosin (2, 4). The distribution of the isoenzymes may change in consequence of age, hormonal state, and hemodynamic load. In all cases the isoenzyme pattern correlates with myofibrillar ATPase activity and shortening velocity (3, 4, 5, 9, 10, 11).

Chronic pressure load of the myocardium leads to a redistribution of myosin isoenzymes in favour of VM-3, the isoenzyme with the lowest ATPase activity. Both the reduced heat release for a given amount of developed tension, measured in the isolated preparation of pressure-hypertrophied myocardium (1), as well as the diminished oxygen consumption per g ventricular weight and per unit of developed tension, measured in the whole heart preparation of the pressure-overloaded rat heart (7, 8), indicate that the efficiency of tension development is increased as a consequence of the redistribution of myosin isoenzymes.

However, in our previous in situ heart-lung preparation the left ventricle worked under nearly isovolumetric conditions. Therefore ejection fraction and calculated myocardial efficiency were low; and accordingly, differences in efficiency were not accessible to direct measurement. With the

*) Prof. Dr. E. Bauereisen, Würzburg, dedicated on the occasion of his 70th birthday

**) Supported by the Deutsche Forschungsgemeinschaft

***) Department of Physiology, University of Virginia, Charlottesville, Virginia 22908/USA aid of a rubber balloon, which was placed at the aortic root and which works like an additional "windkessel", it was possible to enhance left ventricular ejection fraction and efficiency in our preparation such that differences in efficiency became detectable.

Materials and methods

Left ventricular hypertrophy was produced in young male Wistar rats by narrowing of one renal artery (Goldblatt II). Experiments were performed 24 weeks after operation on Goldblatt rats and age-matched controls.

After opening the chest under urethane anesthesia (1.2–1.5 g/kg b.w.), an electromagnetic flow probe was placed around the pulmonary artery trunk. The left ventricle was pierced with a cannula at the apex for pressure measurement and withdrawal of arterial blood samples. The superior and inferior venae cavae were ligated and the inferior vena cava was cannulated for measurement of central venous pressure, withdrawal of venous blood samples, and blood infusion. The ascending aorta was ligated and cannulated directly above the aortic valve for measurement of aortic pressure. An additional "windkessel" in the form of a rubber balloon was repeatedly connected to the aortic trunk with the aid of a three-way valve.

The above ligatures cut off the entire systemic circulation with the exception of coronary circulation, whereas pulmonary circulation remains intact (fig. 1).

Left ventricular wall stress was calculated assuming a thick-walled sphere (12). Internal ventricular volume was evaluated from enddiastolic pressure-volume relationships, which were measured from each heart at the end of the experiment (6).

Oxygen concentrations were measured in arterial and venous blood samples (Lex O_2 Con-TL). Cardiac oxygen consumption was calculated from the arteriovenous oxygen concentration difference and pulmonary flow.

The isoenzyme pattern of each individual heart was determined using polyacrylamide gel electrophoresis in the presence of sodium pyrophosphate.

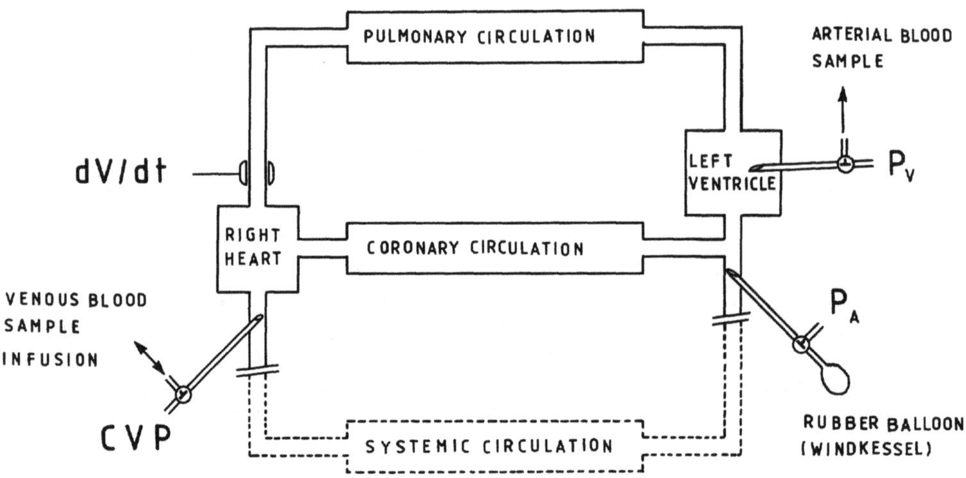

Fig. 1. Schematic diagram of the modified in-situ heart-lung preparation. For explanation, see the text.

Table 1. Mean values and standard error ($\bar{x} \pm s_{\bar{x}}$) of body weight, left ventricular weight, and isoenzyme pattern of myosin.

	Body weight (g)	Left ventricular weight (mg)	VM-1 (%)	VM-2 (%)	VM-3 (%)
Controls (n=4) (age-matched)	449 ± 22	869 ± 32	33.5 ± 2.1	33.0 ± 0.6	33.5 ± 2.0
Goldblatt (n=4) (24 weeks after operation)	388 ± 21	1168 ± 45	22.6 ± 1.3	33.1 ± 0.4	44.3 ± 1.2
Δ%	−14	+34	−33	±0	±32
p <	0.05	0.0025	0.0025	n.s.	0.0025

Results and discussion

Left ventricular hypertrophy and isoenzyme pattern of myosin

Body weight, left ventricular weight, and isoenzyme pattern of myosin of the operated animals and the age-matched controls are summarized in table 1.

Effects of the artificial "windkessel" on the hemodynamic parameters

Connection of the artificial "windkessel" leads to a distinct increase in stroke volume and ejection fraction. Left ventricular peak pressure is diminished. Mean pressure during the ejection period, however, is largely unchanged. Mean pressure over the whole heart cycle is even increased as a result of the marked elevation of aortic pressure during diastole. Stroke work is enhanced whereas left ventricular mean wall stress during the ejection period is only slightly diminished. The changes in the hemodynamic parameters are summarized in table 2.

Cardiac oxygen consumption

In the present preparation no influence of the artificial "windkessel" on cardiac oxygen consumption was detected. The hypertrophied hearts, however, consume less oxygen than the age-matched controls at a given left ventricular mean wall stress during the ejection period (fig. 2a).

In order to be able to compare the effect of the isoenzyme pattern of myosin on the oxygen consumption data, the various levels of oxygen consumption measured under various mechanical loads in each individual experiment were normalized to the wall stress of 1 N/cm^2, and mean oxygen consumption values were calculated for each animal.

In figure 2b this calculated oxygen consumption per g left ventricular weight and beat under mean wall stress of 1 N/cm^2 is plotted against the percent proportion of VM-3. Cardiac oxygen consumption decreases with enhanced concentration of VM-3.

Table 2. Mean values and standard error ($\bar{x} \pm s_{\bar{x}}$) of heart rate; left ventricular enddiastolic volume (V_d); stroke volume (V_s); ejection fraction; left ventricular peak pressure ($P_{ventr\ max}$); mean aortic pressure during the ejection period ($\bar{P}_{ET}$), during diastole ($\bar{P}_{diast}$), and over the whole heart cycle ($\bar{P}_{cycl}$); stroke work; and left ventricular mean wall stress during the ejection period ($\bar{\sigma}_{ET}$) measured on Goldblatt rats and age-matched controls before and after connection of an artificial windkessel.

	Controls (n=12)				Goldblatt (n=20)			
	without windkessel	with windkessel	Δ(%)	p	without windkessel	with windkessel	Δ(%)	p
Heart rate (min^{-1})	138 ± 10	139 ± 9	+ 1	n.s.	122 ± 6	121 ± 6	− 1	n.s.
V_d (cm^3)	0.403 ± 0.031	0.397 ± 0.036	− 1	n.s.	0.398 ± 0.021	0.391 ± 0.018	− 2	n.s.
V_s (cm^3)	0.067 ± 0.005	0.084 ± 0.006	+ 25	< 0.0005	0.054 ± 0.004	0.086 ± 0.006	+ 59	< 0.0005
Ejection fraction (%)	17.6 ± 1.8	22.4 ± 2.1	+ 28	< 0.0005	14.9 ± 1.7	23.5 ± 2.3	+ 58	< 0.0005
$P_{ventr\ max}$ (mm Hg)	174 ± 14	159 ± 11	− 9	< 0.01	208 ± 10	185 ± 9	− 11	< 0.0005
$\bar{P}_{ET}$ (mm Hg)	142 ± 15	132 ± 10	− 7	n.s.	174 ± 7	175 ± 10	+ 1	n.s.
$\bar{P}_{diast}$ (mm Hg)	59 ± 5	100 ± 7	+ 69	< 0.0005	79 ± 3	145 ± 9	+ 84	< 0.0005
$\bar{P}_{cycl}$ (mm Hg)	90 ± 9	110 ± 8	+ 22	< 0.0005	122 ± 5	155 ± 9	+ 27	< 0.0005
Stroke work (erg)	12,686 ± 1,614	14,981 ± 1,574	+ 18	< 0.05	12,633 ± 1,027	21,011 ± 2,375	+ 66	< 0.005
$\bar{\sigma}_{ET}$ (dyn/cm^2)	148,948 ± 13,895	134,182 ± 12,408	− 10	n.s.	150,538 ± 11,654	138,242 ± 9,664	− 8	< 0.01

Substrate uptake and efficiency

Previous studies under comparable experimental conditions have shown that the energy supply of the control hearts as well as of the Goldblatt hearts consists of 80 % carbohydrates and 20 % fat (7).

This combination of utilized substrates yields a respiratory quotient of 0.94 and a respiratory equivalent of 4970 cal/l O_2. Since 1 cal is equivalent to 4.1855 Joules, one can calculate the mechanical equivalent of the consumed oxygen. Under our experimental conditions: 1 cm^3 O_2 is equivalent to 20.8019 Joules.

$$\text{Efficiency (\%)} = \frac{\text{external work/beat (Joule)}}{\text{mechanical equivalent of oxygen consumption/beat (Joule)}} \cdot 100$$

Without the artificial "windkessel" the left ventricle ejects a small stroke volume. Due to the small stroke volume, the external work of the left ventricle is low despite high afterload, and thus efficiency of the left ventricle is low. The connection of the artificial "windkessel" to the aorta leads to a marked increase in stroke volume. External work is increased due to enhanced ejection fraction and, consequently, efficiency is improved. Furthermore, the Goldblatt hearts show improved efficiency at a given ejection fraction, in comparison to the controls (fig. 3a).

In order to be able to estimate the effect of the isoenzyme pattern of myosin on left ventricular efficiency, the latter was normalized to an

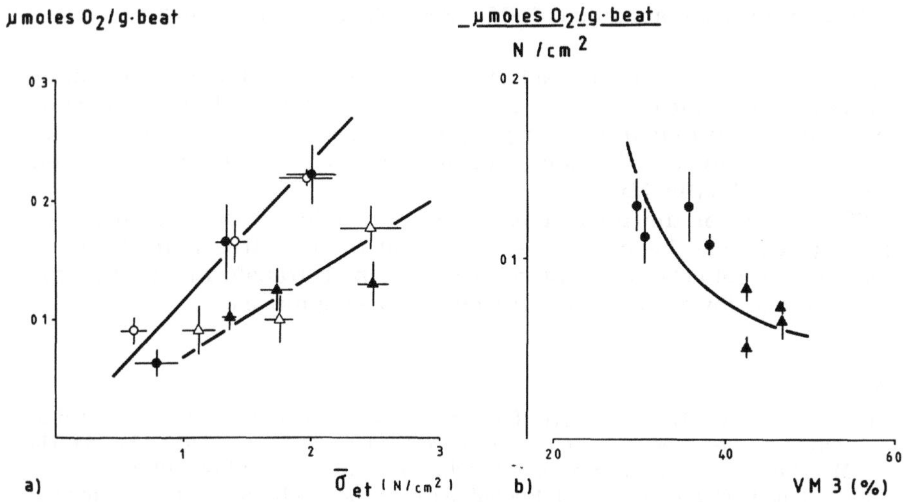

Fig. 2. a) Relationship between the myocardial oxygen consumption per g left ventricular weight and beat, and left ventricular mean wall stress during the ejection period. Mean values ($\bar{x} \pm s_{\bar{x}}$) of ▲ Goldblatt hearts without windkessel, △ Goldblatt hearts with an artificial windkessel, ● age-matched controls without windkessel, and ○ controls with an artificial windkessel. b) Correlation of myocardial oxygen consumption per g left ventricular weight and beat, normalized to the mean wall stress of 1 N/cm^2 during the ejection period with the percentage proportion of VM-3. ▲ Goldblatt hearts, ● age-matched controls.

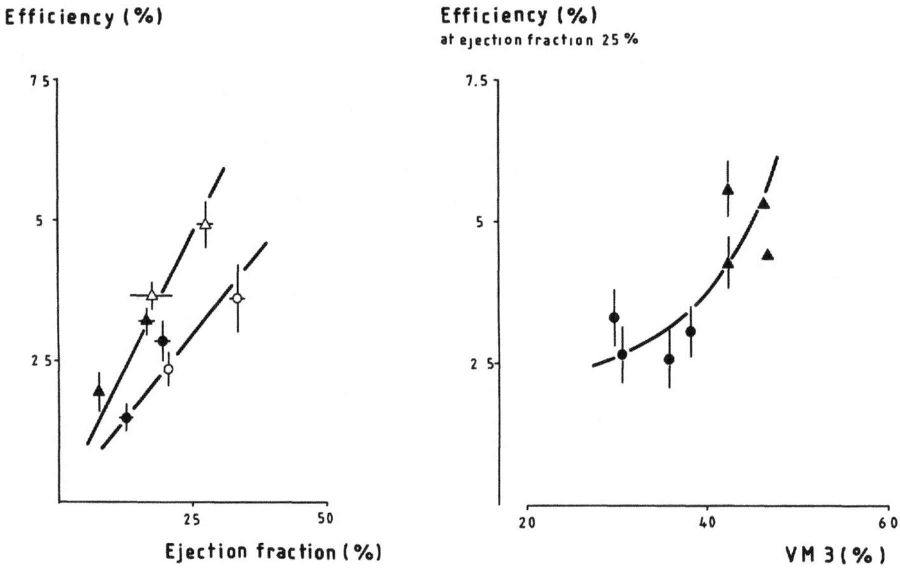

a) b)

Fig. 3. a) Relationship between left ventricular efficiency and ejection fraction. b) Correlation of left ventricular efficiency, normalized to an ejection fraction of 25 %, with the percentage proportion of VM-3. Symbols same as in figure 2.

ejection fraction of 25 % in each individual experiment, and mean values of normalized efficiency were calculated for each animal. When this normalized left ventricular efficiency is plotted against the percent proportion of VM-3, it is obvious that the efficiency increases with enhanced concentration of VM-3 (fig. 3b).

The results of the present paper on energetics of the pressure-overloaded heart can be interpreted such that the redistribution of myosin isoenzymes reflects an adaptive process, which transforms the myocardium into a slower but more efficiently working muscle.

References

1. Alpert, N. R., L. A. Mulieri: The utilization of energy by the myocardium hypertrophied secondary to pressure overload. In: B. Strauer (ed.), 153–163. The Heart in Hypertension, Springer (Berlin–Heidelberg–New York 1981).
2. d'Albis, A., C. Pantaloni, J. J. Bechat: An electrophoretic study of native myosin isoenzymes and of their subunits content. Europ. J. Biochem. **99,** 261 (1979).
3. Ebrecht, G., H. Rupp, R. Jacob: Alterations of mechanical parameters in chemically skinned preparations of rat myocardium as a function of isoenzyme pattern of myosin. Basic Res. Cardiol. **77,** 220–234 (1982).
4. Hoh, J. F. Y., P. A. McGrath, P. T. Hale: Electrophoretic analysis of multiple forms of rat cardiac myosin: effects of hypophysectomy and thyroxine replacement. J. Molec. Cell. Cardiol. **10,** 1053–1076 (1978).
5. Jacob, R., G. Ebrecht, Ch. Holubarsch, H. Rupp, G. Kissling: Mechanics and energetics in cardiac hypertrophy as related to the isoenzyme pattern of myosin.

In: Alpert, N. R. (ed.), Biology of myocardial hypertrophy and failure. Raven Press (1982), in press.
6. Kissling, G., T. Gassenmaier, M. F. Wendt-Gallitelli, R. Jacob: Pressure volume relations, elastic modulus, and contractile behaviour of the hypertrophied left ventricle of rats with Goldblatt II hypertension. Pflügers Arch. **269,** 213–221 (1977).
7. Kissling, G.: Oxygen consumption and substrate uptake of the hypertrophied rat heart in situ. Basic Res. Cardiol. **75,** 185–192 (1980).
8. Kissling, G., H. Rupp, L. Malloy, R. Jacob: Alterations in cardiac oxygen consumption under chronic pressure overload. Significance of the isoenzyme pattern of myosin. Basic Res. Cardiol. **77,** 255–269 (1982).
9. Lompré, A. M., J. J. Mercadier, C. Wisnewsky, P. Bouveret, C. Pantaloni, A. d'Albis, K. Schwartz: Species and age-dependent distribution of mammalian cardiac myosin isoenzymes. J. Muscle Res. Cell. Motility **1,** 479 (1980).
10. Mercadier, J. J., A. M. Lompré, C. Wisnewsky, J. L. Samuel, J. Berovici, B. Swynghedauw, K. Schwartz: Myosin isoenzymic changes in several models of rat cardiac hypertrophy. Circulat. Res. **49,** 525–532 (1981).
11. Rupp, H.: The adaptive changes in the isoenzyme pattern of myosin from hypertrophied rat myocardium as a result of pressure overload and physical training. Basic Res. Cardiol. **76,** 79–88 (1981).
12. Sandler, H., H. T. Dodge: Left ventricular tension and stress in man. Circulat. Res. **13,** 91–104 (1963).

Authors' address:

Prof. Dr. G. Kissling, Physiol. Institut II d. Univ. Tübingen, Gmelinstraße 5, 7400 Tübingen, FRG

Cardiac Adaptation to Hemodynamic Overload, Training and Stress
Dr. D. Steinkopff Verlag 174–181 (1983)

Alterations in electrical properties of rat myocardium accompanying different models of cardiac hypertrophy*)

R. W. Gülch and J. Mohrmann

Physiologisches Institut II, Universität Tübingen (FRG)

Summary

Comparison of the action potentials of hypertrophied and control rat hearts reveals the following for all types of hypertrophy: depending on the degree of hypertrophy, there is a variously pronounced prolongation of the action potential with nearly unchanged amplitude, resting potential and maximum upstroke velocity. In pressure-hypertrophied myocardium of spontaneously hypertensive rats as well as in the myocardium of swimming-trained and crotalaria-treated rats, the prolongation equally affects the entire repolarization phase. In contrast, substantially hypertrophied hearts of rats subjected to thyrotoxicosis produce action potentials hardly distinguishable from controls up to the middle of the repolarization phase. Thereafter the second portion of the repolarization phase is clearly prolonged.

Despite the formally different time-course of the repolarization phase of the thyrotoxic model, the cause of the prolongation may still be sought in changed inactivation kinetics of the slow transmembrane inward current, as also applies to the other models of hypertrophy mentioned above. This is suggested by experiments performed under K^+ depolarization, 4-aminopyridine, or Cs^+. Supplementary investigation of the interval-strength relations of rat myocardium in the present study supports the notion that intracellular recirculation of activator Ca^{++} plays the dominant role in excitation-contraction coupling, both in the hypertrophied and nonhypertrophied myocardial cell.

Key words: cardiac hypertrophy, action potential, crotalaria, thyrotoxicosis, interval-strength relation

Introduction

The hypertrophied rat heart is undoubtedly the most popular model of cardiac hypertrophy, particularly in investigation of the accompanying alterations in cardiac morphology, biochemistry and mechanics. Full understanding of cardiac hypertrophy would not be possible, however, without knowledge of the electrophysiological changes as well. Earlier investigations of our group on hypertrophied myocardium of hypertensive rats revealed that pressure-hypertrophied myocardium consistently shows prolongation of its action potential (3, 4).

The aim of the present study has been to investigate whether corresponding changes in membrane potential also accompany hypertrophy of

*) This work has been supported by grant from the Deutsche Forschungsgemeinschaft

different genesis. Thus action potential recordings will be compared from swimming-trained rats, thyroxine-treated rats, and rats having solely pulmonary hypertension induced by ingestion of crotalaria spectabilis. In order to permit interpretation of the relevance of the observed electrophysiological changes in light of cardiac performance, a series of "interval-strength" experiments was devoted to the question of the intracellular recirculation of the activator Ca^{++}

Methods and materials

All measurements in the individual experiments were performed simultaneously on isolated left and right ventricular papillary muscles of the same heart of male Wistar rats at L_{max}. The action potentials of isometrically contracting muscle preparations were detected intracellularly from different muscle areas using KCl-filled glass microelectrodes with a tip diameter < 0.5 µm. In addition, isometric mechanograms were recorded. All experiments were conducted under the following conditions: 25 °C bath temperature, 0.25 s^{-1} stimulation frequency, 1 ms stimulus duration, 10 % suprathreshold strength. The horizontal muscle bath was continuously perfused with oxygenated (95 % O_2 and 5 % CO_2) solution of the following composition (mmoles/l): NaCl 130, $NaHCO_3$ 20, NaH_2PO_4 1.2, KCl 4.1, $CaCl_2$ 1.1, glucose 23.6. The pH was maintained between 7.3 and 7.4.

The present study is based on the following four models of hypertrophy:

(1) Whole-heart hypertrophy of spontaneously hypertensive rats *(SHR)*.

(2) Whole-heart hypertrophy of swimming-trained rats *(STR)*. The animals underwent 90 minutes of swimming training twice daily over a period of 9 weeks.

(3) Whole-heart hypertrophy of thyroxine-treated rats *(TTR)*. The animals received daily intraperitoneal thyroxine injections of 5 mg/kg body weight over a period of 17 days (2, 7).

(4) Right ventricular hypertrophy of crotalaria spectabilis-treated rats *(CTR)*. The animals were fed ad libitum solely with dry rat food specially prepared with the alkaloid crotalaria (9) at a concentration of 0.05 %.

The age of the animals is stated in the legend to figure 1. For statistical analysis Student's t-test was used and a $p < 0.05$ was considered significant.

Results

The macroscopic manifestation of cardiac hypertrophy can be seen in myocardial mass increase. When left ventricular weight (W_{LV}) and body weight (W_B) of control rats are correlated, data from animals of all ages can be plotted on a straight line through the origin, which is described by the equation:

$$W_{LV}(g) = 0.002\ W_B(g) \qquad (n = 34,\ r = 0.83)$$

The regression is based on all control hearts of table 1.

All data of hypertrophic ventricles lay well above this regression line. If one uses the common procedure for calculating the degree of hypertrophy (h), as used in table 1, by comparison of left ventricular weight of the hypertrophied hearts to the left ventricular weight of control animals of the same body weight, then the resulting degree of hypertrophy is likely to be overestimated, because the body weight of the animals with hypertrophy lags behind that of age-matched controls.

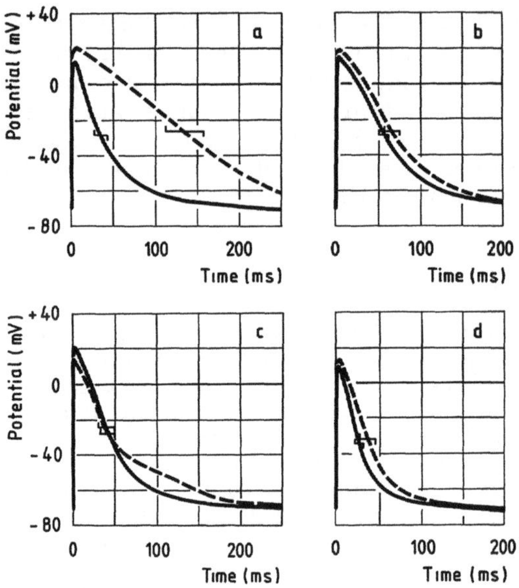

Fig. 1. Mean time course of the action potential of hypertrophied myoardium (---) as compared to the control time course (——). The horizontal bars calculated at half-width ($T_{1/2}$) indicate (±) standard deviation. The hypertrophy data stem from experiments on: a) left ventricular papillary muscles of 26-week-old spontaneously hypertensive rats (SHR); b) left ventricular papillary muscles of 17-week-old swimming-trained rats (STR); c) left ventricular papillary muscles of 12-week-old thyroxine-treated rats (TTR); d) right ventricular papillary muscles of 12-week-old crotalaria-treated rats (CTR).

A more accurate indication of the age and maturity of the animals is provided by skeletal size (14). So the hyperthyrotic animals reveal the same tibial length as controls of the same age. Exemplarily, we plotted the left ventricular weight (W_{LV}) of the thyroxine animal group as a function of tibial length (L_{TIB}). Again the following satisfactory linear regression:

$$W_{LV}(g) = 0.018\ L_{TIB}(mm) \qquad (n = 9,\ r = 0.92)$$

is found in the control group. A more realistic degree of hypertrophy can thus be calculated from the ratio of the left ventricular weights of animals with the same tibial length.

For all four hypertrophy models, figure 1 demonstrates that action potentials of hypertrophied left or right ventricles are consistently prolonged compared to control action potentials. With the exception of thyrotoxic myocardium, the prolongation is detectable during the entire repolarization phase. Hypertrophied hearts of thyrotoxic rats produce action potentials, which are hardly distinguishable from those of controls up to the middle of the repolarization phase. Only the second part of the repolarization phase is markedly prolonged and leads to a hump in the time-course.

As shown in table 1, the most important action potential parameters were analyzed statistically; with the exception of the thyrotoxic group the

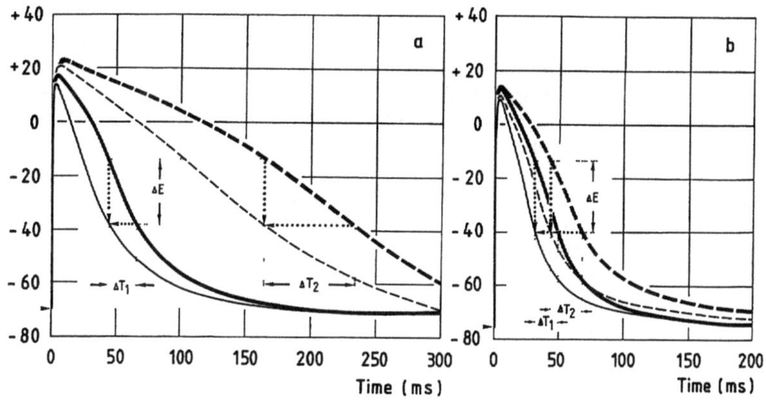

Fig. 2. Mean action potentials of the SHR model in a) and the CTR model in b) under normal conditions (thin lines) and after blocking the repolarizing outward K^+ current with 0.5 mmoles/l 4-aminopyridine (thick lines). Note the more pronounced prolongation of the repolarization phase in the case of hypertrophy (ΔT_2) in comparison to the control case (ΔT_1) under this blocking intervention. Nevertheless, the potential shift (ΔE) is the same in both cases.

half-width ($T_{1/2}$) is quite suitable for characterization of the action potential duration. The prolongation in this group is best quantified by ($T_{1/4}$), the "quarter-width" of the action potential, which is measured as the time required for 75 % repolarization. The time to isometric peak tension (T_p) is also shown in the table. The marked broadening of the action potential is more pronounced in the models with severe hypertrophy. While the extreme prolongation of the action potential in the SHR model is accompanied by a significant increase in the time to peak tension, this parameter is nearly unchanged or even shortened in the other models.

When correlating the action potential duration with the degree of hypertrophy within each experimental group, a linear regression line with a positive slope can be fitted to the data. This means that the higher the degree of hypertrophy, the broader are the corresponding action potentials.

Experiments under depolarization in the presence of 12.3 mmoles/l KCl, conditions which suppress the early sodium inward current, reveal that the differences in duration of the so-called slow response action potentials of hypertrophied and normal myocardium are similar to those prior to blocking.

To estimate the role of the K^+ outward currents in repolarization, action potentials were recorded under 0.5 mmoles/l 4-aminopyridine (8) or 20 mmoles/l Cs^+ (6), conditions which block the K^+ outward current. The results are demonstrated in the form of mean action potentials in figure 2. In both cases, which are also representative of the other models, repolarization is strongly slowed subsequent to administration of 4-aminopyridine. Cs^+ causes similar prolongation in addition to its depolarizing effect. The broadening of the repolarization phase which is attributed to the inhibition of the repolarizing K^+ effect is more pronounced in the case of hypertrophy (ΔT_2) than in the control case (ΔT_1). Assuming that a

Table 1. The most important action potential parameters, the degree of hypertrophy (h) and the time to isometric peak force (T_p) of the four presented models of hypertrophy in comparison to the respective controls. For the CTR group, the time required for 75% repolarization ($T_{1/4}$) has been used in place of the half-width ($T_{1/2}$) to accommodate the humped time-course of the action potential (see ■). E_A indicates the amplitude, E_R the resting potential and $(dE/dt)_{max}$ the maximum upstroke velocity. All values are expressed as mean ± standard error. ⊛ indicates significant differences between the control group (CR) and the respective group of hypertrophy, each consisting of n samples. All measurements were performed on either left (LV) or right (RV) ventricular papillary muscles.

	n	h	T_p (ms)	$T_{1/2}$ (ms)	E_A (mV)	E_R (mV)	$(dE/dt)_{max}$ (V/s)
SHR	10	1.88	182 ± 6.7	135 ± 6.9	84 ± 4.5	75 ± 1.9	47 ± 5.6
LV			⊛	⊛			
CR	7	1.0	149 ± 5.8	36 ± 2.9	96 ± 1.9	71 ± 1.6	47 ± 6.0
STR	8	1.32	237 ± 6.5	66 ± 3.9	89 ± 2.3	70 ± 2.2	48 ± 4.0
LV			⊛	⊛			
CR	8	1.0	256 ± 4.7	57 ± 2.6	85 ± 2.1	71 ± 1.5	41 ± 4.7
				■			
TTR	9	1.85	135 ± 9.0	111 ± 6.4	83 ± 1.0	71 ± 2.0	59 ± 4.1
LV			⊛	⊛	⊛		⊛
CR	9	1.0	182 ± 6.6	67 ± 3.3	92 ± 1.3	73 ± 1.5	79 ± 3.0
CTR	10	1.35	175 ± 4.6	36 ± 3.3	83 ± 1.6	71 ± 2.1	60 ± 2.9
RV				⊛			
CR	10	1.0	176 ± 40	26 ± 1.5	83 ± 1.6	68 ± 1.7	63 ± 2.5

considerable fraction of the repolarizing current is conducted through K^+ channels that only display strong voltage-dependence, and not significant time-dependence (11) the same shift in potential ΔE due to the K^+ outward current would lead to a greater shortening of the repolarization phase (ΔT_2) in the hypertrophy model than in the controls (ΔT_1). Thus one may conclude that the repolarizing K^+ current is probably not affected by the process of hypertrophy.

Remarkably, comparison of the action potential duration with the time to peak tension (T_p) in table 1 shows that the isometric rising phase is hardly changed, or even shorter despite substantial prolongation of the action potential. The only exception was in the case of SHRs with the enormeous broadening of the action potential. Furthermore, isometric tension development of hypertrophied myocardium is almost unchanged in comparison to control myocardium. The apparent inconsistency of the above findings is substantially due to the dominating intracellular recirculation of the activator calcium which greatly reduced the importance of the transmembrane Ca^{++} currents. According to Ragnarsdottir (12), interval-strength experiments, such as those shown schematically in the inset of figure 3, can be used to estimate the recirculating Ca^{++} fraction. Subsequent to a priming period with a stimulation frequency of 0.5 s^{-1}, during which the peak isometric tension amounts to F_o, stimulation is interrupted

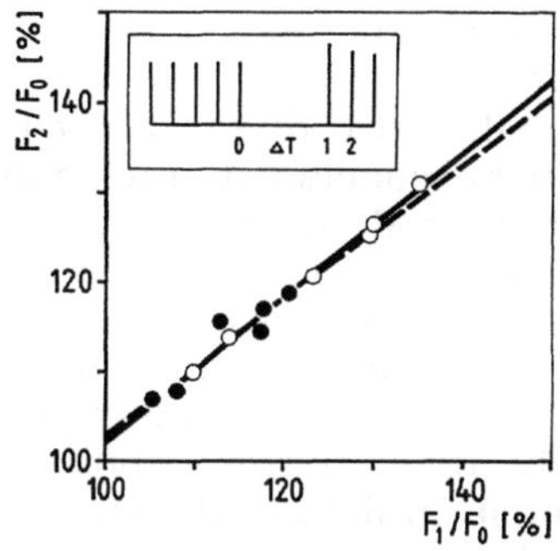

Fig. 3. Interval-strength relations of rat myocardium of normotensive rats (——○——) and SHR (---●---). Peak isometric force of test contraction (2) is related to peak force of test contraction (1) after normalization with respect to steady-state contraction (0). Regression lines were fitted to data obtained after variable stimulation intervals (ΔT). The pacing sequence is shown schematically in the inset.

for a varied period of time ΔT and both mechanograms 1 and 2 of amplitudes F_1 and F_2 are analyzed immediately after renewed stimulation. When plotting F_2 as a function of F_1, both normalized with respect to F_o, for all different resting intervals ΔT a linear relationship results, the slope of which is a direct measure of the recirculation fraction. This concept is based on the assumption that the action potentials of the rat are hardly dependent on the stimulation pause (12). In the control case the slope amounts to 0.81, in the case of hypertrophy 0.75.

Discussion

The action potentials of hypertrophied myocardium of the left or right ventricle display significantly slowed repolarization, which is reflected in prolongation of the action potential in all four models of hypertrophy under consideration. While hypertension, thyroxine, or cardiac overload by physical training lead to hypertrophy of both ventricles, solely right ventricular hypertrophy was found in the course of the pure pulmonary hypertension induced by ingestion of crotalaria spectabilis. As only the right ventricular action potentials of the CTRs were affected, this model nicely proves that the described alterations in the action potentials constitute a property specific to the hypertrophied heart cell. In a given model of hypertrophy the prolongation of the action potential is more pronounced, the greater the degree of hypertrophy. Whereas the entire repolarization process proceeds more slowly in the pressure-induced hypertrophy of spontaneously hypertensive or crotalaria-treated rats, as well as in the training-induced hypertrophy of swimming-trained rats, only the second half of repolarization is delayed in the thyroxine-treated rats. Unlike the first three models, the maximum upstroke velocity is significantly reduced in the hypertrophied myocardium of thyroxine-treated rats. Other action potential parameters such as resting potential and amplitude are either unchanged or not significantly altered in all four cases.

Despite the qualitatively different time-course of the action potentials in the thyrotoxic model compared to the other forms of hypertrophy, the prolongation is most probably also due to altered kinetics of the slow inward current. This can be concluded from experiments conducted under inhibition of the early sodium inward current through selective KCl-induced depolarization or under blockade of the repolarizing K^+ outward current using 4-aminopyridine or Cs^+. The maximum upstroke velocity of the so-called slow response action potentials is significantly reduced in the thyrotoxic case (10), which means that the slow inward current interferes with the other transmembrane currents in the later course of an action potential. In light of the fact that inactivation of the slow inward current is delayed similar to the case in other hypertrophy models it alone may well be responsible for the humped repolarization phase.

The significantly slowed maximum upstroke velocity in thyrotoxicosis is an indication that hypertrophy-induced alterations in the rapid inward current kinetics have to be considered in addition. This interpretation is supported by experiments under Mn^{++} which still showed somewhat broader action potentials in the hypertrophy case than in the control case after suppression of the slow inward current (5).

The studies of Antoni (1) have shown that an action potential broadening leads to a prolonged mechanical activity which, on its part, might cause a prolonged time to peak force and an increase in isometric force production. Apart from the SHR model showing a significant increase in the time to peak force (T_P) and a small augmentation of isometric peak force (F_P), all other hypertrophied heart muscles under consideration reveal either no change, or even a reduction in T_P as well as minor nonsignificant alterations in F_P. When dealing with the rat heart one certainly must consider changes in the activity of the sarcoplasmic reticulum which, for example, is enhanced in thyrotoxicosis (13) and thus leads to a shorter period of activity; the great fraction of activator Ca^{++} recirculating within the myocardial cell also should be taken into account. Under the assumption that action potentials of rat myocardium are hardly affected by a variable stimulation pause (12), interval-strength experiments indicated a recirculation fraction of almost 80 %. This means that the transmembrane Ca^{++} fluxes are only of subordinate importance in the mechanical activity of the rat heart. Thus such a strong interdependence between excitation and mechanical performance as is known in the myocardium of other species cannot be proposed for the hypertrophied and nonhypertrophied rat heart.

We would like to thank Miss Sigrid Schultheiss for excellent technical assistance.

References

1. Antoni, H., R. Jacob, R. Kaufmann: Mechanische Reaktionen des Frosch- und Säugetiermyokards bei Veränderungen der Aktionspotentialdauer durch konstante Gleichstrompulse. Pflügers Arch. **306,** 33–75 (1969).
2. Beznak, M.: Cardiovascular effects of thyroxine treatment in normal rats. Can. J. Biochem. Physiol. **40,** 1647–1654 (1962).

3. Gülch, R. W.: Alterations in excitation of mammalian myocardium as a function of chronic loading and their implications in the mechanical events. Basic Res. Cardiol. **75,** 73–80 (1980).
4. Gülch, R. W.: The effects of elevated chronic loading on the action potential of mammalian myocardium. J. Mol. Cell. Cardiol. **12,** 415–420 (1980).
5. Gülch, R. W.: Electrophysiological properties of hypertrophied myocardium. In: Myocardial Hypertrophy and Failure (Ed. N. R. Alpert) Raven Press N. Y. 1983 (in press).
6. Isenberg, G.: Cardiac purkine fibers: Cesium as a tool to block inward rectifying potassium currents. Pflügers Arch. **365,** 99–106 (1976).
7. Jacob, R., G. Kissling, G. Ebrecht, Ch. Holubarsch, I. Medugorac, H. Rupp: Adaptive and pathological alterations in experimental cardiac hypertrophy. Advanc. Myocardiol. **4,** 55–77 (1983).
8. Kenyon, J. L., W. R. Gibbons: 4-aminopyridine and the early outward current of sheep cardiac purkinje fibers. J. Gen, Physiol. **73,** 139–157 (1979).
9. Meyrick, B., L. Reid: Development of pulmonary arterial changes in rats fed crotalaria spectabilis. Amer. J. Pathol. **94,** 37–50 (1979).
10. Mohrmann, J.: Elektrophysiologische Untersuchungen an hypertrophierten Myokardzellen von crotalaria- und thyroxin-vorbehandelten Ratten. Diplomarbeit Tübingen (1982).
11. Noble, D.: The repolarization process of heart cells. In: Electrical Phenomena in the Heart. (Ed.: W. C. De Mello) Academic Press N.Y. (1972).
12. Ragnarsdottir, K., B. Wohlfart, M. Johannsson: Mechanical restitution of the rat papillary muscle. Acta Physiol. Scand. **115,** 183–191 (1982).
13. Suko, J.: The calcium pump of cardiac sarcoplasmic reticulum. Functional alterations at different levels of thyroid state in rabbits. J. Physiol. **228,** 563–582 (1973).
14. Yin, F. C. P., H. A. Spurgeon, M. L. Weisfeldt, E. G. Lakatta: Mechanical properties of myocardium from hypertrophied rat hearts. A comparison between hypertrophy induced by senescence and by aortic banding. Circulat. Res. **46,** 292–300 (1980).

Authors' address:

Prof. Dr. R. W. Gülch, Physiologisches Institut II der Universität Tübingen, Gmelinstraße 5, 7400 Tübingen, FRG

Cardiac Adaptation to Hemodynamic Overload, Training and Stress
Dr. D. Steinkopff Verlag 182–188 (1983)

Calcium binding and Na-Ca exchange in cardiac sarcolemma in experimental hypertension

M. Kawamura, S. Watari, T. Nagata, T. Iimura, T. Ohkubo, M. Kawanishi, and M. Nagano

Dept. Int. Med., Aoto Hospital, Jikei University School of Medicine, Tokyo (Japan)

Summary

Abnormalities of cation permeability, sodium pump activity and Ca^{2+} binding were reported on the sarcolemma of vascular smooth muscle in various forms of experimental hypertension. Recent evidences indicate that the myocardial sarcolemma bears important roles in the excitation-contraction coupling as well as the regulation of intracellular cation concentration of myocardium. In this study, Na^{+}-K^{+} ATPase activity, Ca^{2+} binding, and Na^{+}-Ca^{+} exchange in the cardiac sarcolemma of Goldblatt rats and spontaneously hypertensive rats (SHR) were studied.

Cardiac sarcolemma was isolated by the method described by Bers. Ca^{2+} binding and Na^{+}-Ca^{2+} exchange were estimated by the dual wavelength spectrophotometer employing Ca^{2+}-sensitive dye arsenazo III.

Ouabain-sensitive Na^{+}-K^{+} ATPase activity in SHR was reduced while in Goldblatt rats it was slightly elevated as compared to normal Wistar rats. Ca^{2+} binding of sarcolemma representing high affinity site was 7.13 ± 0.96 nM/mg in normal rats, however, it was significantly reduced to 4.18 ± 1.24 and 3.16 ± 1.92 in SHR and Goldblatt rats, respectively. Rates of Na^{+}-Ca^{2+} exchange were also reduced in both types of hypertensive rats.

These results, suggesting the impaired Ca^{2+} extrusion, would contribute to explain the functional alteration of hypertensive hearts.

Key words: sarcolemma, spontaneously hypertensive rats, Goldblatt rats, Na^{+}-K^{+} ATPase, Ca^{2+} binding, Na^{+}-Ca^{2+} exchange

Introduction

Though the biochemical basis of altered cardiac contractility is primarily the abnormality of contractile protein, functional alterations of membrane systems which regulate cyclic fluctation of the cytoplasmic calcium concentration must also be considered. Indeed, diminished calcium accumulating activity of cardiac sarcoplasmic reticulum was reported in spontaneously hypertensive rats (1). Studies on the cation fluxes of the vascular smooth muscle and erythrocytes indicate the existence of altered calcium transport and altered sodium-potassium pump activity in the plasma membrane of several kind of cells in various types of experimentally hypertensive animals (2–9). For this reason, biochemical study on myocardial sarcolemma, which is one of the most important organelles for the excitation-contraction coupling and regulation of intracellular cation concentration, will be interesting for the understanding of the functional deterioration as well as adaptation of hypertensive heart. In 1981 we have reported the diminished Na^+-K^+ATPase activity and diminished calcium binding of sarcolemma from SHR (9). Devynck also reported the decrease in calcium binding of the sarcolemma from SHR in 1982 (8).

Several mechanisms or channels are postulated for the calcium transport of sarcolemma, for example, sodium-calcium exchange. Binding of calcium to the respective binding site on the sarcolemma constitutes the first step in the operation of such transport machinery. Calcium extrusion from myocardial cells, by which calcium load of myocardial organelles will be regulated, is thought to be mainly facilitated by the sodium-calcium exchange mechanism (11).

In this report, calcium binding and sodium-calcium exchange of isolated myocardial sarcolemma were estimated in two types of experimentally hypertensive rats.

Methods

Spontaneously hypertensive rats were bred in our laboratory from the Okamoto Aoki strain rats, which were kindly supplied from Shimane University. Two-kidney Goldblatt-hypertensive rats were produced by constricting the right renal artery. Blood pressures were estimated by the tail plethysmography.

Rats were killed by decapitation under nembutal anaesthesia and the hearts were immediately excised. After the trimming, ventricular weight was estimated. Preparation of the cardiac sarcolemmal fraction was performed by the method described by Bers (12). This procedure involves homogenization, brief treatment with 0.3 M potassium chloride containing 25 μM pyrophosphate to remove contractile protein and subsequent sucrose gradient centrifugation to separate sarcolemmal fraction. Membrane fractions residing in the sucrose concentration from 30 to 32 % were identified as sarcolemma from the study on the marker enzyme activity as is shown in figure 1.

Calcium binding and Na^+-Ca^{++} exchange were estimated by the dual-wavelength spectrophotometric assay as originally described by Mela (13), monitoring the change of ionized calcium concentration. For the calcium concentration ranging from 0 to 40 μM, using arsenazo III as a calcium indicator dye, the differential light absorbance changes were measured at a wavelength pair of 660–680 nm and for the calcium concentration ranging from 100 to 500 μM, using murexide as calcium indicator dye, the differential light absorbance changes were estimated at a wavelength pair of 540 and 507 in a Hitachi UW 300 spectrophotometer.

ATP-independent calcium binding of sarcolemma was estimated in the incubation mixture containing 20 mM Tris-Malate, 40 μM arsenazo III or murexide, 20 to 500 μM calcium chloride, and 30 to 60 μg sarcolemmal protein at pH 7.6.

To estimate sodium-calcium exchange, sarcolemmal vesicles were preincubated in the Mops-Tris buffer containing 140 mM NaCl for 20 minutes to preload vesicles with sodium and diluted 40-fold into 140 mM KCl medium containing 40 μM calcium and 20 mM Mops-Tris buffer at zero time. Calcium uptake was monitored with metachromic dye arsenazo III as described above.

Tris ATP, arsenazo III, and murexide were purchased from Sigma Chemical Company. Student's t-test was used for the statistical analysis of the results.

Results and discussion

Blood pressure of SHR rose to 150 mmHg about 10 weeks after birth and was maintained at this level. Average weight of cardiac ventricles from SHR was 1.4 times that from age-matched normal Wistar rats. Two-kidney one-clip Goldblatt hypertensive rats of approximately the same level of blood pressure were also utilized. After 12 weeks duration of high blood pressure, animals were sacrificed.

Yield of sarcolemmal protein from rat cardiac vesicles was 0.7 mg/g wet weight. There was essentially no difference in the yield of sarcolemma between normal Wistar rats and hypertensive rats. G-6-Phase activity of the sarcolemma from normal Wistar rats was 0.096 μM/mg/h and that from SHR was 0.107 μM/mg/h. There again was no difference between normal Wistar rats and hypertensive rats. Succinate reductase activity was not detectable in sarcolemmal fractions. These results indicate minimal contamination of both sarcoplasmic reticulum and mitochondrial fragments in this preparation.

Sodium potassium ATPase activity of sarcolemma from normal Wistar rats was 13.41 + 2.00 μM/mg/h and that from SHR was 3.96 + 1.52 μM/mg/h. The difference between these two values was significant. Sodium potassium ATPase activity of the sarcolemma from Goldblatt-hypertensive rats showed slightly higher values than normal, but the difference was not significant.

Depressed sodium pump activity was proposed by Mendonca (5) who observed the decreased sodium efflux in the erythrocytes of SHR. Jones (14) also demonstrated the decreased ability to accumulate potassium and to extrude sodium in the vascular smooth muscle of SHR. Urry et al. (6) reported the decrease in the intracellular sodium binding of erythrocyte

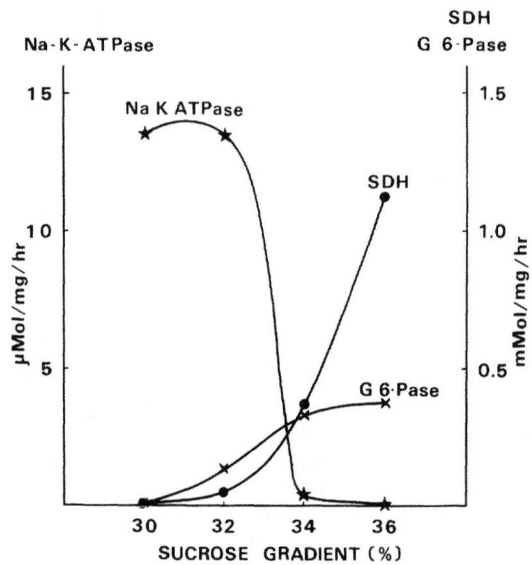

Fig. 1. Estimation of marker enzyme activity indicates that the sarcolemma reside in the fraction of 30–32 % sucrose concentration.

membrane, which they had presumed to be the binding site of sodium-potassium ATPase in essential hypertensive patients. On the contrary, Friedman (15) presumed that the ouabain-sensitive sodium pump activity was increased in the vascular smooth muscle of SHR based on the analysis of cation fluxes. Postonov reported the increased flux of sodium and potassium on the erythrocyte of SHR possibly due to the increased passive diffusion. Though these investigators did not clearly characterize the transport mechanisms affected, Friedman concluded the increase in the activity of sodium-potassium ATPase by the interpretation of indirect evidences. In this regard it must also be considered that the ouabain-sensitive sodium flux through the plasma membrane does not solely depend on the maximum activity of sodium-potassium ATPase. Estimation of sodium-potassium ATPase activity on the vascular smooth muscle sarcolemma has not been reported. On the myocardium, Godfraind and Neol (16) reported that the affinity of microsomal sodium-potassium ATPase for sodium was low in SHR although maximum activity was higher in SHR. It is conceivable that a more purified sarcolemmal fraction than that isolated in this experiment could unmask the difference in the ATPase activity which was not revealed by the estimation with microsomal fraction. In the two-kidney Goldblatt hypertension, sodium pump activity was postulated to be increased on the basis of studies on sodium efflux (17). Sodium-potassium ATPase activity of microsomal fraction from several tissues was reported to be increased when assayed in the presence of angiotensin II (18, 19). However, Brock (20) reported that sodium-potassium ATPase activity of smooth muscle membrane was not stimulated by angiotensin II.

Calcium binding curve and its Scatchard plot of sarcolemma in the calcium concentration range from 20 μM to 500 μM are indicated in figure 2.

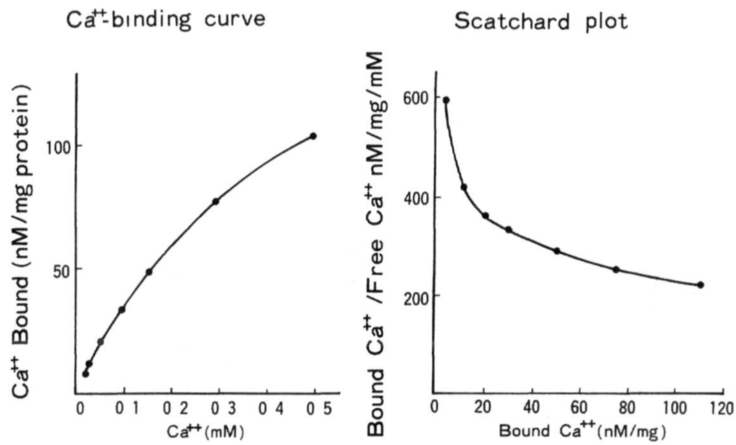

Fig. 2. Calcium binding curve and Scatchard plot of sarcolemma indicate that the amount of calcium bound to sarcolemma at the medium calcium concentration of 20 μM will roughly reflect the amount of high-affinity binding sites of calcium.

From this curve and the documentation of Bers (22), who resolved Scatchard plot of the essentially identical calcium binding curve of the sarcolemma of this study, it is presumed that the amount of calcium bound to sarcolemma at the calcium concentration of 25 μM varies parallel with the change of the number of the high-affinity binding sites. It is also presumed that the amount of calcium binding at the calcium concentration of 500 μM roughly reflects the number of low-affinity binding site. Amount of calcium bound to normal sarcolemma at the calcium concentration of 25 μM was 7.13 ± 0.95 nM/mg, while the amount of calcium bound to the sarcolemma from SHR was 4.18 ± 1.24, and that from Goldblatt-hypertensive rats was 3.16 ± 1.92, respectively. The difference between both types of hypertensive rats and normal Wistar rats was significant. The amount of calcium binding of normal Wistar rats, SHR and Goldblatt rats at the calcium concentration of 500 μM was 134 ± 15, 104 ± 31 and 107 ± 28, respectively. There was no significant difference between these values.

Studies from several laboratories have shown that the calcium binding of the plasma membrane was decreased in the erythrocytes (23), adipocytes (7) and vascular smooth muscle (2) of SHR. Transsarcolemmal calcium fluxes are postulated to be facilitated by 1. the receptor complex for muscle agonist, 2. a pore line with fixed negative sites, which has affinity for both sodium and calcium, 3. carrier-mediated sodium calcium exchange, 4. voltage-dependent calcium channel, and 5. ATP-dependent calcium extrusion.

The transport mechanism in which the ATP-independent high-affinity calcium binding site is involved is unknown. However, the first three mechanisms mentioned above are possible candidates, since Langer (21) proposed that the low-affinity calcium binding site of sarcolemma may

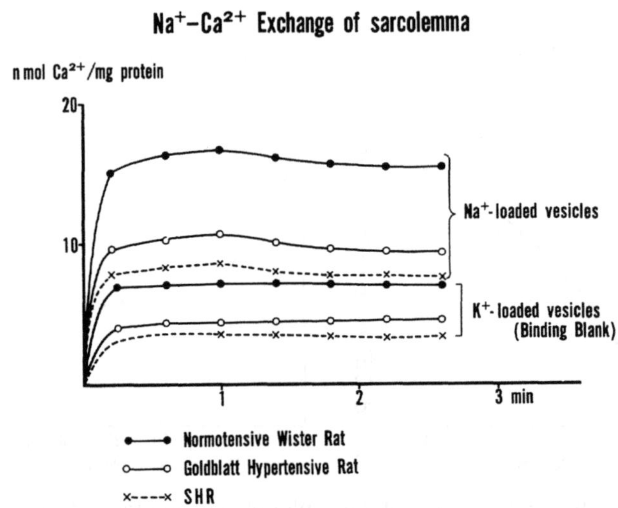

Fig. 3. Na^+-Ca^{++} exchange are estimated by subtracting the Ca^{++} uptake of K^+-preloaded vesicles from the Ca^{++} uptake of Na-preloaded vesicles.

represent the source of contractile-dependent calcium, which is transported through voltage-dependent channels. Bers (22) suggested that the high-affinity calcium binding site is likely to be related to the sodium-calcium exchange system, because the apparent K_m value for this system is similar to the K_m value for calcium uptake by the sodium-calcium exchange.

For this reason, sodium-calcium exchange of myocardial sarcolemma was estimated.

The time course of calcium uptake of sodium-preloaded and potassium-preloaded sarcolemmal vesicles was illustrated in figure 3. To estimate the sodium-calcium exchange, the calcium uptake of potassium-preloaded vesicles was subtracted from the calcium uptake of sodium-preloaded vesicles to correct for passive calcium uptake and for any externally bound calcium. The rate of sodium-calcium exchange of both SHR and Goldblatt-hypertensive rats was lower than normal Wistar rats.

The exact role of sodium-calcium exchange in excitation-contraction coupling has not been defined. Therefore the consequences of alteration in Na^+-Ca^{++} exchange are difficult to predict. Of course, Na^+-Ca^{++} exchange is able to work in both directions, depending on the sodium gradient and membrane potential. However, according to the postulation of Katz (11) as well as Blaustein (10) the Na^+-Ca^{++} exchange will act to pump calcium out of the myocardial cell during the diastole. Therefore inhibition of the rate of sodium-calcium exchange would itself be expected to cause a net increase in cellular calcium if Na^+-Ca^{++} exchange were more important for calcium efflux than influx. In the case of SHR, increase in the intracellular sodium concentration by the diminished sodium-potassium ATPase activity will further decrease the calcium extrusion by a fall of sodium gradient. The increase in the sarcoplasmic calcium concentration may be a cause of the exaggerated aftercontraction or the prolongation of hyper-excitable periods, observed in SHR by Heller (24).

Elevation of the cytoplasmic calcium concentration induces not only functional alteration but also may induce myocardial hypertrophy by accelerating the protein synthesis.

References

1. Limas, C. L., J. N. Cohn: Defective calcium transport by cardiac sarcoplasmic reticulum in spontaneously hypertensive rats. Circulat. Res. **40,** suppl. 1, 62–69 (1979).
2. Wei, J. W., R. A. Janis, E. E. Daniel: Alterations in calcium transport and binding by the plasma membrane of mesenteric arteries from spontaneously hypertensive rats. Blood Vessels **14,** 55–64 (1977).
3. Friedman, S. M., M. Nakashima, R. A. McIndoe: Glass electrode measurement of net Na^+ and K^+ fluxes in erythrocytes of the spontaneously hypertensive rats. Can. J. Physiol. Pharmacol. **55,** 1302–1310 (1977).
4. Kwan, C.-Y., L. Belbeck, E. E. Daniel: Abnormal biochemistry of vascular smooth muscle plasma membrane isolated from hypertensive rats. Mol. Pharmacol. **17,** 137–140 (1979).
5. Mendonca, M. D., M.-L. Grichois, R. P. Garay, J. Sassard, D. Ben-Ishay, P. Meyer: Abnormal net Na^+ and K^+ fluxes in erythrocytes of three varieties of genetically hypertensive rats. Proc. Nat. Acad. Sci. **77,** 4283–4286 (1980).

6. Urry, D. W., T. L. Trapane, S. Andrews, M. M. Long, H. W. Overbeck, S. Oparil: NMR observation of altered interaction with human erythrocyte membranes of essential hypertensives. Biochem. Biophys. Res. Commun. **96,** 514–521 (1980).
7. Postonov, Yu. V., S. N. Orlov, N. I. Pokudin: Alteration of the intracellular calcium pool of adipose tissue in spontaneously hypertensive rats. No effect of peripheral immunosympathectomy. Pflügers Arch. **309,** 256–259 (1980).
8. Devynck, M.-A., M.-G. Pernollet, A.-M. Nunrz, I. Aragon, T. Montenay-Garestier, C. Helene, P. Meyer: Diffuse structural alterations in cell membranes of spontaneously hypertensive rats. Proc. Nat. Acad. Sci. **79,** 5057–5060 (1982).
9. Kawamura, M., S. Watari, E. Nagata, M. Kawanishi, T. Ohkubo, M. Nagano: Study on the Na-K ATPase activity and Ca binding of myocardial sarcolemma of spontaneously hypertensive rats. Proc. 4th International Symposium on rats with spontaneous hypertension and related studies, p. 115–118 (1981).
10. Blaustein, M. P.: Sodium ions, calcium ions, blood pressure regulation, and hypertension: a reassessment and a hypothesis. Amer. J. Physiol. **232,** C 165–C 173 (1977).
11. Katz, A. M.: Physiology of heart. Raven Press (New York 1977).
12. Bers, D. M.: Isolation and characterization of cardiac sarcolemma. Biochim. Biophys. Acta **555,** 131–146 (1979).
13. Mela, L., B. Chance: Spectrophotometric measurements of the kinetics of Ca and Mn accumulation in mitochondria. Biochemistry **7,** 4059–4063 (1968).
14. Jones, A. W.: Altered ion transport in vascular smooth muscle from spontaneously hypertensive rats. Circulat. Res. **33,** 563–572 (1973).
15. Friedman, S. M.: Evidence for enhanced sodium transport in the tail artery of the spontaneously hypertensive rats. Hypertension **1,** 572–582 (1979).
16. Godfraind, T., F. Noel: Sodium activation of heart (Na-K) ATPase from normotensive and spontaneously hypertensive rats. Arch. Int. Pharmacodyn. **245,** 139–144 (1980).
17. Overbeck, H. W., D. E. Grissette: Sodium pump activity in arteries of rats with Goldblatt hypertension. Hypertension **4,** 132–139 (1982).
18. Levin, K.: The stimulating effect of angiotensin and vasopressin on adenosine triphosphatase activity *in vitro*. Acta Physiol. Scand. **79,** 37–49 (1970).
19. Gutman, Y., Y. Shamir, D. Glushevitsky, S. Hochman: Angiotensin increases microsomal (Na-K)-ATPase activity in several tissues. Biochim. Biophys. Acta **273,** 401–405 (1972).
20. Brock, T. A., L. J. Lewis, J. B. Smith: Angiotensin increases Na entry and Na/K pump activity in cultures of smooth muscle from rat aorta. Proc. Nat. Acad. Sci. USA **79,** 1438–1442 (1982).
21. Langer, G. A.: The role of calcium in the control of myocardial contractility: An update. J. Mol. Cell. Cardiol. **12,** 231–239 (1980).
22. Bers, D. M.: Sodium-calcium exchange and sidedness of isolated cardiac sarcolemmal vesicles. Biochim. Biophys. Acta **601,** 358–371 (1980).
23. Postnov, Y. V., S. N. Orlov, N. I. Pokudin: Decrease of calcium binding by the red blood cell membrane in spontaneously hypertensive rats and essential hypertension. Pflügers Arch. **379,** 191–195 (1979).
24. Heller, L. J.: Isovolumetric properties of ventricles of spontaneously hypertensive rats. Amer. J. Physiol. **240,** H927–H933 (1981).

Authors' address:

Dr. M. Kawamura, Dept. Int. Med., Aoto Hospital, Jikei University School of Medicine, Tokyo, Japan

Cardiac Adaptation to Hemodynamic Overload, Training and Stress
Dr. D. Steinkopff Verlag 189–196 (1983)

Cardiac muscle function during the development of hypertrophy in pigs due to pressure overload*)

P. K. Singal**), **K. S. Dhillon, V. Panagia, and N. S. Dhalla**

Experimental Cardiology Section, Department of Physiology,
Faculty of Medicine, University of Manitoba, Winnipeg (Canada)

Summary

Myocardial contractile function was assessed in a chronic, slowly developing hypertrophy in pigs in order to approximate more closely the situation seen in patients with heart hypertrophy due to pressure overload. Presence of heart hypertrophy was confirmed 4 and 8 weeks after the surgery by increased wall thickness and intercapillary distances. Peak developed force at different resting loads as well as +dp/dt and −dP/dt of the trabecular muscle strips did not change at 4 weeks, but these parameters were significantly depressed in the 8-week hypertrophied heart. Positive force-frequency relationship was significantly improved in the 4-week group and depressed or even negative at 8 weeks. It is suggested that a reduction in the contractile performance of the hypertrophied hearts at late stages may be due to combination of factors such as reduced fibre shortening because of increased wall stress and an intrinsic depression of the inotropic state subsequent to changes in subcellular-control mechanisms.

Key words: heart hypertrophy, increased afterload, force-frequency relationship, aortic stenosis

Introduction

The development of ventricular hypertrophy constitutes one of the principal adaptive responses to a chronic increase in work load of the heart. In humans, because of increased wall thickness, the ventricular function is maintained by keeping the wall stress close to control levels (7). Depressed contractile function has been reported in patients where the development of hypertrophy was not enough to counter the increased wall stress (8). Because of these clinical implications, an understanding of changes in the contractile state that accompany increased muscle mass is of considerable interest. Although much has been learnt from studies employing different experimental models, there is still a great controversy in the literature with respect to the contractile performance of hypertrophied cardiac muscle in these models. Accordingly, supernormal (14), normal (5) and subnormal (2, 20) contractile performances of the hypertrophied cardiac muscle have been reported. Varied results may have been due to the model used to induce hypertrophy as well as stage of cardiac

*) Supported by a grant from the Medical Research Council of Canada
**) Canadian Heart Foundation Scholar

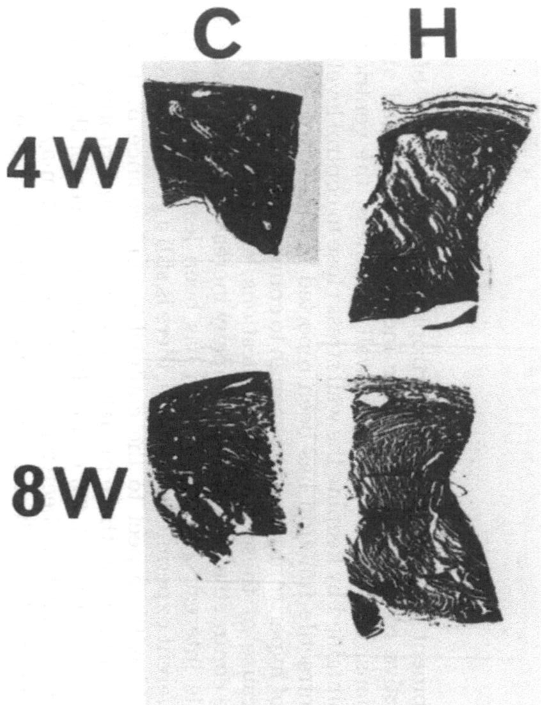

Fig. 1a)

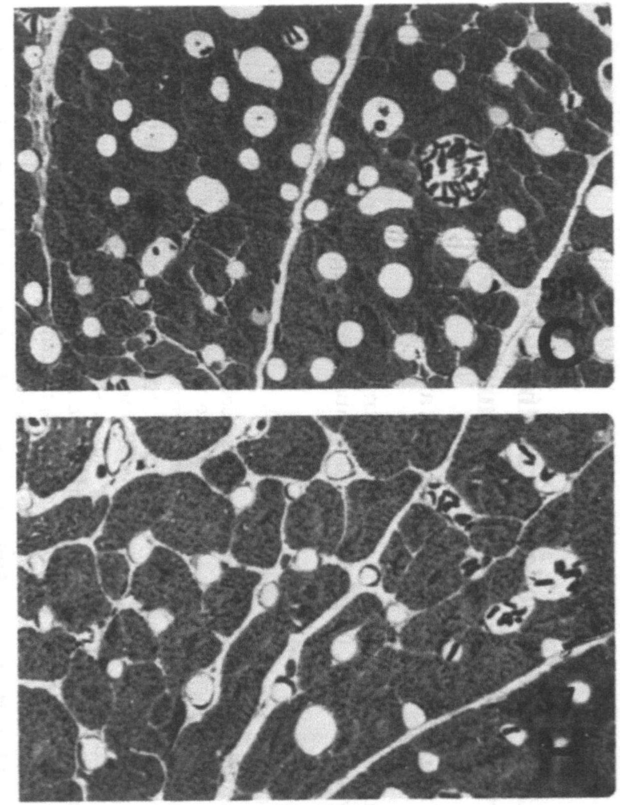

Fig 1b)

Fig. 1. a) Transmural paraffin sections from the mid region of the left ventricle free wall of four (4W) and eight (8W) week sham control (C) and hypertrophied (H) hearts, ×2; b) One-micron-thick sections from control (C) and 8-week hypertrophied (H) myocardium. A significant drop in the number of capillaries per unit area (numbers shown in each figure) in the hypertrophied myocardium is apparent. ×800.

hypertrophy. In animal models where hypertrophy was produced by acutely imposing a pressure overload upon narrowing of the pulmonary artery or aorta, the early changes in cardiac muscle function may not have been strictly due to hypertrophy alone because of the presence of myocardial injury (12, 22) and/or heart failure. It was, therefore, decided to study the contractile function of the cardiac muscle at two stages of hypertrophy in a pig model in which heart hypertrophy was induced by a gradual imposition of pressure overload on the left ventricle.

Methods

Young male pigs employed in this study were maintained on antibiotic-free hog feed and water *ad libitum* for one week prior to the surgery. For producing pressure overload, a snug band was placed around the ascending aorta just above the coronary ostea without constricting the aorta. A graudally increasing aortic stenosis developed as the animals grew in weight. In sham control animals, all surgical procedures were followed except for placing of the band. This experimental model had been employed previously for the assessment of hemodynamic changes during the development of hypertrophy (15). The animals were sacrificed at 4 and 8 weeks after the surgery by a stunning bullet-blow on the forehead and their hearts removed for further studies. Transmural tissue samples from the left ventricular free wall were processed for light microscope studies.

Trabecular muscle strips were quickly dissected out from the apex region of the left ventricular cavity and placed in a beaker filled with oxygenated modified Krebs-Ringer solution. Electrolyte concentrations in this superfusion medium were (mEq): Na, 146.8; K, 5.0; Ca 4.9; HCO_3, 20.14; PO_4, 3.48; Cl, 137.14; and glucose,

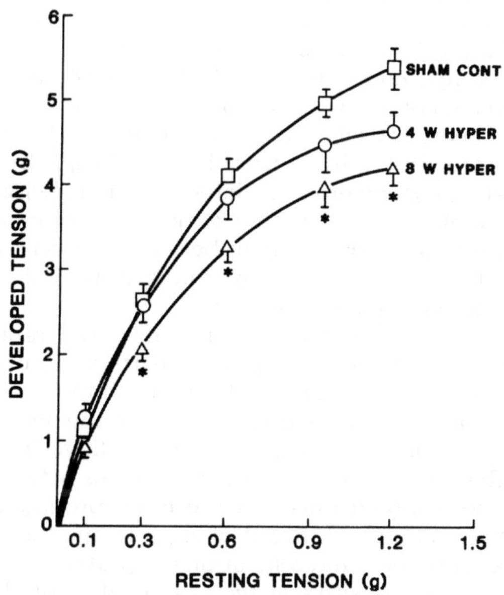

Fig. 2. Effect of different resting loads on the peak developed tension in trabecular muscle strips from control as well as 4- and 8-week hypertrophied myocardium. The muscles were stimulated at 30 beats/min.

Table 1. Maximum rate of cardiac contraction or relaxation of trabecular muscle strips from sham control and hypertrophied pig left ventricle.

Animal group	Cardiac contraction +dp/dt ($g/mm^2/sec$)	Cardiac relaxation −dp/dt ($g/mm^2/sec$)
Sham control (N=7)	14.5 ± 1.0	7.5 ± 0.70
4-week hypertrophy (N=6)	14.6 ± 2.3	8.1 ± 1.86
8-week hypertrophy (N=6)	9.1 ± 0.7*)	4.9 ± 0.46*)

*) Significant ($P < 0.05$). All values shown are at L_{max}. The muscle was stimulated at the rate of 30 beats/min.

45.0 mM (19). A 95 % oxygen/5 % carbon dioxide mixture was continuously bubbled through the solution in the tissue bath, maintaining a pH of 7.3. The bath temperature was 36 °C. The muscle ranged from 5 to 15 mg in weight and from 4 to 6 mm in length with a maximum thickness ranging from 0.8 to 1.2 mm. The muscle and chamber were oriented vertically, one end of the muscle being held firmly by a clamp while the other end tied to a force-displacement (FT 03) transducer.

Results

The development of a concentric hypertrophy of the left ventricle at 4 and 8 weeks was noted in a gross histological examination of the heart. Light microscope studies of the transmural sections of the left ventricular free wall revealed a marked increase in the wall thickness of the hypertrophied hearts as compared to the controls (fig. 1a). Study of one-micron-thick Epon sections, coloured with Mason's trichrome stain, from different regions of the heart revealed a marked decrease in the number of capillaries per unit area in the hypertrophied heart (fig. 1b). These hypertrophic histological changes were associated with narrowing of the aortic lumen at the site of the band. In this experimental model, a gradual increase in the systolic pressure gradient between left ventricle and aorta has been reported to occur without any changes in ejection fraction or clinical signs of pulmonary congestion (15).

The mechanical data for isometric contractions of the trabecular muscle strips from the control and hypertrophied hearts were obtained under different conditions. The active and resting length-tension relationships depicted in figure 2 show a significant reduction in the developed tension during contraction at varied resting loads in the 8-week-hypertrophied muscle but not in the 4-week group. These differences between the control and the 8-week-hypertrophied muscle were more pronounced at higher resting loads. There was no significant change in the maximum rate of tension development (+dp/dt) and relaxation (−dp/dt) at 4 weeks of hypertrophy (table 1). However, positive as well as negative dp/dt values were significantly lower at 8 weeks of hypertrophy. There was a marked improvement in force-frequency relationship at 4 weeks of hypertrophy at all the three frequency increases from 30 to 60, 90 and 120 beats/min (fig. 3).

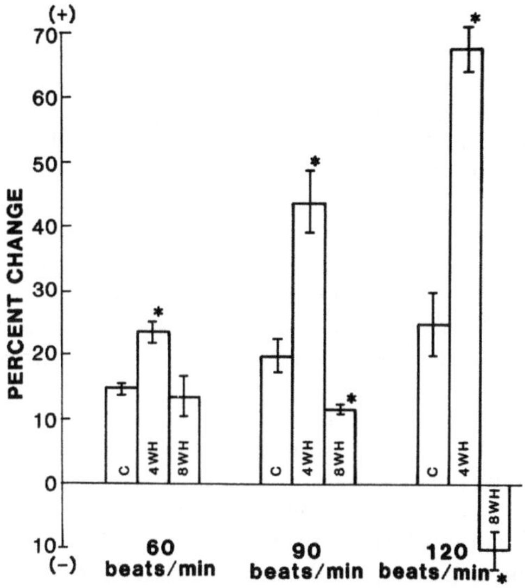

Fig. 3. Effect of increases in the rate of stimulation on the peak developed tension in trabecular muscle strips from control as well as 4- and 8-week hypertrophied myocardium. The muscles were held at L_{max}, and frequency of stimulation was increased from 30 beats/min to 60, 90 and 120 beats/min.

In the 8-week hypertrophy group, the force-frequency relationship was positive when the stimulation rate was increased from 30 to 60 and 90 beats/min, but the percent increase in force was less than the control muscle strips. A negative force-frequency relationship was apparent in the 8-week group when the stimulation rate was increased to 120 from 30 beats/min (fig. 3).

Discussion

It has been reported in literature that changes in the contractile performance of the heart due to experimental hypertrophy vary according to the animal species, duration of the pressure load prior to study and the method used to induce hypertrophy. We feel that the gradual induction of pressure gradient between the left ventricular peak systolic and aortic pressures (15) in the animal model used in this study approximates more closely the situation seen in patients with heart hypertrophy due to chronic pressure overload (1). This approach clearly eliminates changes in the contractile performance because of myocardial injury following acute changes in the cardiac load. In this regard it is pointed out that Spann et al. (20) produced acute right ventricular pressure overload by pulmonary artery constriction in the cat and found a significant decrease in V_{max} after 6 weeks of banding. These findings were confirmed by Williams and Potter (22), however, they also reported a return to normal of V_{max} of hypertrophied right ventricle muscle at 24 weeks of banding, indicating that changes seen after 6 weeks of postbanding may have been due to an acute myocardial injury. Normal or supernormal contractile function have also been observed for the left ventricular muscle following an acute aortic constriction in rats (6, 10). Maintenance of the peak developed force at different resting loads as well as of the rate of contraction and relaxation at L_{max} after 4 weeks of surgery in this study clearly shows that in moderate, gradually developing cardiac hypertrophy, the myocardial contractile performance remains normal. Although it has been shown that ventricular contractile function in concentrically hypertrophied hearts is inversely related to ventricular wall stress (8), the observed increase in left ventricular wall thickness in our study may have normalized wall stress to maintain normal force development at 4 weeks of hypertrophy. However, such a compensatory mechanism may not have been adequate to counter the depressant effect of increased wall stress on the contractile force at 8 weeks of hypertrophy.

In rheumatic heart disease patients, minimally hypertrophied myocardium showed a positive force-frequency relationship, while markedly hypertrophied myocardium showed an oppositive response (3). A similar response was seen in our animal model inasmuch as a markedly improved positive force-frequency relationship was seen at all the frequencies in the 4-week hypertrophied hearts, while a diminished positive response was seen in the 8-week hypertrophied heart only at 60 and 90 beats/min. The negative force-frequency response at 120 beats/min in the 8-week hypertrophied heart probably may have an indication that at this stage of hypertrophy any further stress on these chronic overloaded hearts would result in a failure. Such alterations in force-frequency relationship associated with a progressively developing hypertrophy may be an indication of subcellular changes in the calcium metabolism. In this regard it is pointed out that physiological positive inotropic response of the ventricular muscle has been shown to be due to increased intracellular calcium subsequent to an increase in intracellular sodium due to increased influx (11) as well as sodium pump inhibition (17).

Significant decreases in the peak developed tension at all resting loads as well as in the maximum rates of contraction and relaxation in the 8-week hypertrophied myocardium may have been due to changes at the level of myofibrils and/or subcellular membranes. In this regard, myofibrillar Ca^{2+}-stimulated ATPase activity has been shown to be decreased at 8 weeks in this model (16). Calcium overloads have been reported to be deleterious for heart structure as well as function (4); this may also be a contributing factor in the depressed contractile function. Occurrence of intracellular calcium overload in these 8-week hypertrophied hearts is a real possibility because of the reported decreases in the rate and capacity of calcium uptake by the sarcoplasmic reticulum (9); and a decrease in the sarcolemmal Ca^{2+}-stimulated Mg^{2+}-dependent ATPase activity (18). Some abnormalities in the mitochondrial calcium transport system have also been reported in the 8-week hypertrophied pig hearts (13). Since no apparent symptoms of clinical heart failure were seen in this model (15), depressed contractile function of the cardiac muscle in the 8-week hypertrophied heart observed in this study may represent an important index for the pathological form of hypertrophy (21), whereas normal or supernormal contractile function of the cardiac muscle in the 4-week hypertrophied heart may indicate the presence of physiological hypertrophy.

References

1. Allard, J. R., M. J. O'Neill, Jr., J. I. E. Hoffman: Valvular subcoronary aortic stenosis in dogs. Amer. J. Physiol. **236,** H780–H784 (1979).
2. Alpert, N. R., B. B. Hamrell, W. Halpern: Mechanical and biochemical correlates of cardiac hypertrophy. Circulat. Res. **35,** Suppl. II, 71–82 (1974).
3. Buckley, N. M., Z. J. Penefsky, R. S. Litwak: Comparative force-frequency relationships in human and other mammalian ventricular myocardium. Pflügers Arch. **332,** 259–270 (1972).
4. Dhalla, N. S., G. N. Pierce, V. Panagia, P. K. Singal, R. E. Beamish: Calcium movements in relation to heart function. Basic Res. Cardiol. **77,** 117–139 (1982).
5. Geha, A. S., J. P. Duffy, H. J. C. Swan: Relation of increase muscle mass to performance of hypertrophied right ventricle in the dog. Circulat. Res. **19,** 255–259 (1966).
6. Grimm, A. F., R. Kubota, W. V. Whithborn: Properties of myocardium in cardiomegaly. Circulat. Res. **12,** 118–124 (1963).
7. Grossman, W., D. Jones, L. P. McLaurin: Wall stress and patterns of hypertrophy in the human left ventricle. J. Clin. Invest. **56,** 56–65 (1975).
8. Gunther, S., W. Grossman: Determinants of ventricular function in pressure overload hypertrophy in man. Circulation **59,** 674–688 (1979).
9. Heyliger, C. E., L. E. Alto, G. N. Pierce, V. Panagia, P. K. Singal, N. S. Dhalla: Sarcoplasmic reticular calcium transport changes in hypertrophied pig heart. Proc. Can. Fed. Biol. Soc. **25,** 49 (1982).
10. Kerr, A., jr., A. R. Winterberger, M. Giambatista: Tension developed by papillary muscles from hypertrophied rat hearts. Circulat. Res. **9,** 103–105 (1961).
11. Langer, G. A.: Heart: Excitation contraction coupling. Ann. Rev. Physiol. **35,** 55–86 (1973).
12. Meerson, F. Z.: The myocardium in hyperfunction, hypertrophy and heart failure. Circulat. Res. **25,** Suppl. 2, 1–163 (1969).
13. Pierce, G. N., M. P. Moffat, B. S. Tuana, P. K. Singal, V. Panagia, N. S. Dhalla: Mitochondrial changes in hypertrophied pig heart. Proc. Can. Fed. Biol. Soc. **25,** 3 (1982).
14. Sasayama, S., D. Franklin, J. Ross Jr.: Hyperfunction with normal inotropic state of the hypertrophied left ventricle. Amer. J. Physiol. **232,** H418–H425 (1977).
15. Sharma, G. P., P. K. Singal, N. S. Dhalla: Hemodynamic adaptation of the left ventricle during aortic stenosis in pigs. J. Mol. Cell. Cardiol. **12,** Suppl. 1, 151 (1980).
16. Singal, P. K., K. S. Dhillon, K. S. Dhalla, G. P. Sharma, N. S. Dhalla: Contractility and myofibrillar adenosine triphosphatase activities in hypertrophied pig heart. J. Mol. Cell Cardiol. **12,** Suppl. 1, 155 (1980).
17. Singal, P. K., J. C. Khatter, K. Prasad: Possible mechanism for the frequency-dependent increases in the cardiac contraction in monkey. Can. J. Physiol. Pharmacol. **55,** 734–737 (1977).
18. Singal, P. K., V. Panagia, J. P. Tewari, N. S. Dhalla: Changes in ultrastructure and calcium binding activity of sarcolemma in hypertrophied pig heart. Proc. Can. Fed. Biol. Soc. **25,** 3 (1982).
19. Singal, P. K., K. Prasad: Influence of ouabain on the force-frequency relationship in cardiac muscle. Jap. Heart J. **20,** 341–350 (1979).
20. Spann, J. F., Jr., R. A. Buccino, E. H. Sonnenblick, E. Braunwald: Contractile state of cardiac muscle obtained from cats with experimentally produced right ventricular hypertrophy. Circulat. Res. **21,** 341–354 (1967).
21. Wikman-Coffelt, J., W. W. Parmley, D. T. Mason: The cardiac hypertrophy process: Analyses of factors determining pathological vs. physiological development. Circulat. Res. **45,** 697–707 (1979).

22. Williams, J. F. Jr., R. D. Potter: Normal contractile state of hypertrophied myocardium following pulmonary constriction in the cat. J. Clin. Invest. **54,** 1266–1272 (1974).

Authors' address:

Dr. P. K. Singal, Experimental Cardiology Section, Dep. of Physiology, Faculty of Medicine, Univ. of Manitoba, Winnipeg, Canada, R3E OW3

Cardiac Adaptation to Hemodynamic Overload, Training and Stress
Dr. D. Steinkopff Verlag 197–203 (1983)

Biochemical and mechanical correlates at peak systole in myopathic Syrian Hamster

J. Wikman-Coffelt*, R. Sievers, R. J. Coffelt, and W. W. Parmley

Moffitt Hospital, University of California, San Francisco, California (USA)

Summary

The following studies were carried out to determine the phosphorylation potential of the myopathic Syrian Hamster hearts and whether a decrease in the free energy of ATP hydrolysis and/or shift in isomyosins was responsible for decreased cardiac performance. Hamster hearts were perfused under maximally stressed working conditions, i.e., a workload of 110 mm Hg, high calcium concentrations in the perfusate (3.5 mM) and 10^{-8} M isoproterenol. Mechanical parameters indicated contractility had fallen 50 % in Syrian Hamster hearts under these conditions. Using a specially designed stimulator-triggered freeze-clamp, hearts were terminated at peak systole and tissue content of ATP, ADP, phosphocreatine, creatine, and inorganic phosphate analyzed. Cytosolic concentrations of metabolites were calculated as described by Kammermeier utilizing published data on tissue compartmentation (1, 2). A reduction in contractile performance of the Syrian Hamster hearts not only correlated with a shift in isomyosins but also with a decrease in free energy of ATP hydrolysis from 51.08 kJ/mole in control hearts at peak systole and 45.9 kJ/mole in myopathic hearts at peak systole. These values assume ADP generated from ATP hydrolysis remained free in the cytosol during systole. The low value in myopathic hearts was due to the decrease in ATP and the increase in inorganic phosphate. The reduction in free energy of ATP hydrolysis occurring in Syrian Hamster hearts was sufficient to cause a decrease in contractility: thus a shift in isomyosins, and the cAMP and ATP deficiency appear to be at least partially responsible for a combined coordinate decrease in cardiac performance in the Syrian Hamster.

Key words: Syrian Hamster, contractile performance, phosphorylation potential, ATP hydrolysis, myosin isoenzymes, freeze-clamp

Introduction

The myopathic Syrian Hamster exhibits a decrease in cardiac contractile properties, actin-activated myosin ATPase activity, and is characterized by a calcium overload (3–5). The calcium-blocking agent, verapamil, protects the heart of the myopathic hamster from failure (3). The studies described here were carried out to determine if the decrease in

This work was supported in part by Susan and Don Schleicher

* Career Development Award HL00466

myocardial contractile performance in these animals is due to a shift in isomyosins and/or a drop in the phosphorylation potential of the heart.

Analysis of tissue content of high energy phosphates is important for characterizing myocardial energy metabolism, however acid extraction used in preparation of metabolites results in release of nucleotides from bound and compartmentalized sites, as well as those free in the cytosol. Free cytosol values have been obtained correcting for degree of myocardial compartmentation, degree of binding, and determination of ADP by the creatine kinase equilibrium (1, 2). Such calculations give phosphorylation potential values similar to those obtained with mitochondrial suspensions (2).

Methods

Isolated Hamster heart perfusion. The isolated working rat heart, a modification of that described by Neely, et al. (6), was used in these studies. Media entered the left atrium and was ejected through the aorta. The media was a modified Krebs-Henseleit media (6) with added insulin (0.01 %) and isoproterenol 10^{-8}M); media was flushed with 95 % O_2 and 5 % CO_2; free calcium in the media was 3.5 mM. The afterload chamber was set at 110 mm Hg and the preload chamber at 15 mm Hg. Stimulator leads were placed in the base of the right ventricle. Coronary flow was collected from the right ventricular outflow tract. Arterial oxygen was sampled as described earlier (7). Eighteen hamsters were used for the studies described here, 9 Golden Hamsters and 9 Syrian Hamsters. The Syrian Hamsters were approximately 250 days of age, strain UM-X7-1.

Stimulator-triggered freeze-clamp. The stimulator-triggered freeze-clamp bolts on the face of the perfusion apparatus. Specific details of both systems have been recently described (7, 8), including measurement of temperature in the heart during "smashing". The center of the heart drops from 37 °C to −80 °C in 5 msec with the techniques used here. Measured cooling time is in agreement with calculated cooling time. For the studies described here, the hearts were freeze-clamped at systole.

Tissue extraction. Preparation of acid extracts of the tissue were similar to those described by Morgan et al. (9). The frozen wafer fell from the anvils into liquid

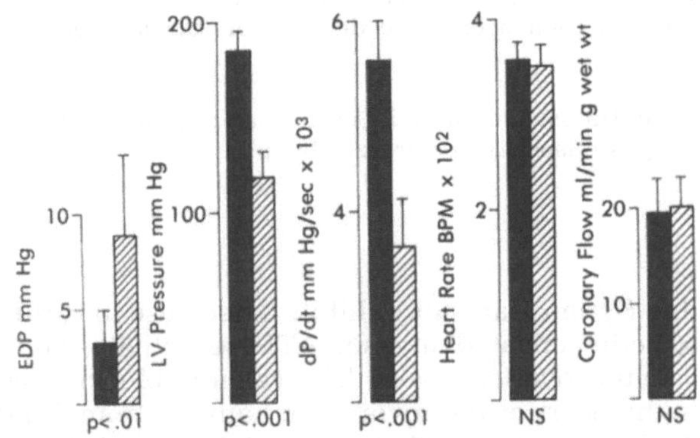

Fig. 1. Differences in cardiac performance between Golden Hamster (solid bars) and Syrian Hamster (stippled bars). Analyses are for: end-diastolic pressure, LV pressure, dP/dt, heart rate, and coronary flow. Standard errors are shown. Statistical evaluation is unpaired t-test. (NS: no significant difference, i.e., p > .05).

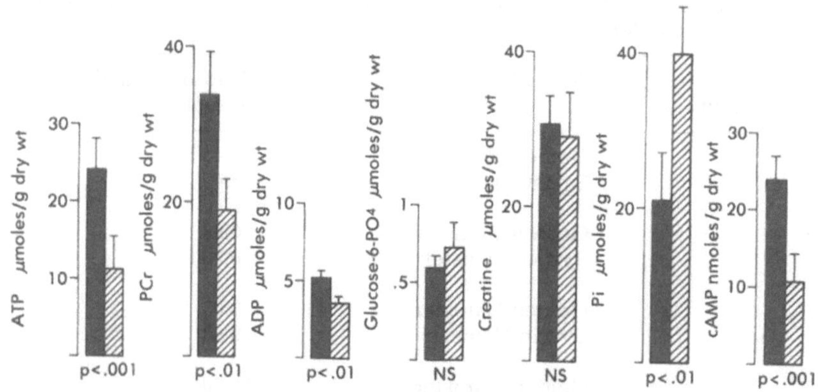

Fig. 2. Differences in metabolites between Golden Hamster (solid bars) and the Syrian Hamster (stippled bars). Analyses are shown for ATP, creatine phosphate, ADP, glucose-6-phosphate, creatine, inorganic phosphate, and cAMP. Standard errors are shown. Statistics the same as in figure 1.

nitrogen when the cylinders were retracted. Tissue was pulverized under liquid nitrogen. A 100 mg sample of the pulverized heart was removed, weighed, dried, and weighed again for assessing wet to dry weight. Acid (−200 °C) (3 ml 10 % PCA) was pulverized separately, then added to the pulverized tissue. Pulverization under liquid nitrogen continued. The frozen mixture was transferred to a Sorvall tube and weighed, then transferred to a mortar. The weight of the cold tube and acid were used as factors in calculating the final tissue weight (wet). The frozen mixture was brought to 0 °C while pulverizing. After centrifugation of the mixture (20,000 × g for 5 min), the extract was weighed, neutralized with 5 N KOH and weighed again for determining volume. The mixture was centrifuged to remove $KClO_4$, and the supernatant stored at −80 °C.

Tissue assays. Using the neutralized extract, standard enzymatic assay methods were carried out to determine concentrations of ATP, ADP, creatine phosphate,

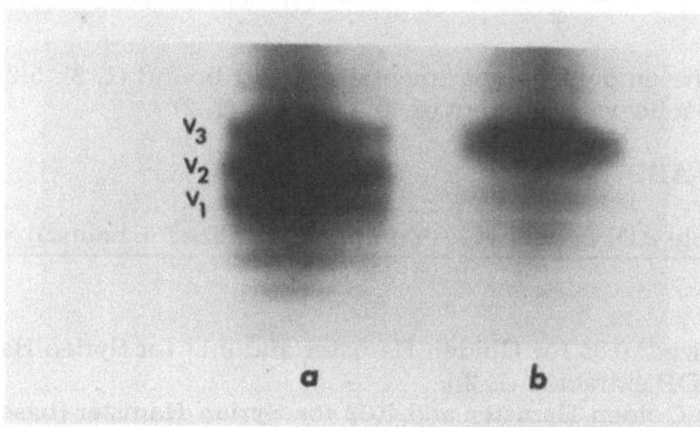

Fig. 3. Gel electrophoresis patterns of myosin isozymes from Golden Hamster (a) and Syrian Hamster (b). Procedures are a modification of that of Hoh (23), except that larger concentrations of chelating and non-complexing agents were included in the dialysis and electrophoresis buffer. Also, the sample was dialyzed extensively in a high concentration of the electrophoresis buffer (sample buffer), and a gradient of 2.5 to 6 % acrylamide was used as the electrophoresis matrix.

Table 1. Metabolites' values during peak systole in the cardiomyopathic Syrian Hamster vs. the Golden Hamster.

Metabolite (μmol/g wet wt.)	Animal	Cytosolic fraction (mmole/l)
ATP	Golden Hamster	8.40
ATP	Syrian Hamster	3.45
ADP	Golden Hamster	0.98
ADP	Syrian Hamster	0.90
Pi	Golden Hamster	3.05
Pi	Syrian Hamster	9.60
PCr	Golden Hamster	12.70
PCr	Syrian Hamster	7.21
Cr	Golden Hamster	12.71
Cr	Syrian Hamster	11.00
$dG/d\varepsilon_{ATP}$	Golden Hamster	51.08 kJ/mole
	Syrian Hamster	45.90 kJ/mole

Calculations for cytosolic fractions are taken from Kammermeier (1, 2) except for corrections made in variance in dry to wet weight and ADP-myosin binding during systole.
Dry weight values are corrected for 15% dry weight fraction. Values are for 9 animals each.

Calculations for cytosolic ATP

$$\frac{\mu\text{mole ATP/g wet wt.} - 0.3 \times 5}{2} = \text{mmole/l cytosolic fraction}$$

0.3 represents the amount compartmentalized and bound (1, 2); 5/2 results from assuming a cytosolic water content of 40% wet wt. (1, 2).

Calculations for ADP

$$\frac{[(\mu\text{mole ADP/g wet wt.}) - (\text{compartmentalized} + \text{bound})] \times 5}{2}$$

Compartmentalized: 0.35 for Golden Hamster and 0.17 for Syrian Hamster [based on percent of ADP extracted (1, 2)].
Bound: 0.03 for Golden Hamster and 0.02 for Syrian Hamster [based on percent myosin-ADP binding. 30% of the dry wt. is myosin giving 0.18 mmole myosin/l; assume a 15% myosin-ADP binding during systole (22)]. 100% myosin ATPase activity in the Golden Hamster and 50% in that of the Syrian (4).

Calculations for cytosolic Pi

$$\frac{(\mu\text{mole/g wet wt.}) - (0.08 \times \text{mole Pi/g wet wt.}) - 1.7 \times 5}{2}$$

0.08 represents 8% bound (1, 2)
1.7 is the value for mitochondrial Pi (1.3 μmol/g) and extracellular Pi (0.4 μmole/g).

Calculations for cytosolic PCr

$$\frac{(\mu\text{mole PCr/g wet wt.}) \times 5}{2}$$

Calculations for cytosolic Cr

$$\frac{(\mu\text{mole Cr/g wet wt.}) \times 5}{2}$$

$$dG/d\varepsilon_{ATP} = \Delta G^{\circ}_{obs\ (ATP)} + RT \ln \frac{(ADP)\ (Pi)}{(ATP)}$$

$\Delta G^{\circ}_{obs\ (ATP)} = -30.5$ kJ/mole (for 37 °C (1 mM Mg^{2+})).

creatine, and glucose-6-phosphate (10–12). Inorganic phosphate was determined as described earlier (13), and cAMP by a radioimmunoassay (14).

Results

Isolated hearts of the Syrian Golden Hamster were perfused under stress conditions, i.e., high calcium (3.5 mM), isoproterenol (10^{-8}M), and a high workload (110 mm Hg). Data indicated that the myopathic hearts could not match the performance of control hearts (fig. 1). The myopathic hearts exhibited a high end-diastolic pressure and a decrease in LV pressure, and dP/dt under stress conditions. There were no significant differences in heart rate and coronary flow between the two groups of animals.

Using a specially designed stimulator-regulated freeze-clamp, metabolic processes were terminated at peak systole and high energy phosphates and other metabolites analyzed. The Syrian Hamsters demonstrated a significant decrease in ATP, PCr, ADP, cAMP, and a significant increase in inorganic phosphate (fig. 2). These values were converted to cytosolic values using the calculations of Kammermeier (1, 2), and the free energy of ATP hydrolysis calculated (table 1). At peak systole under stress conditions, the free energy for ATP hydrolysis was 51.08 kJ/mole for normal hamsters and 45.9 kJ/mole for the Syrian Hamsters. These values would only be obtained if the ADP generated from hydrolysis remained free and was not bound or compartmentalized during systole.

A shift in isomyosins towards V_3 occurs in the Syrian Hamster, whereas all three isomyosins, V_1, V_2, and V_3, are present in the Golden Hamster (fig. 3).

Discussion

The studies described here demonstrate a decrease in high energy phosphates in the myopathic Syrian Hamster at peak systole when maximum work is being performed. They also show a decrease in the free energy of ATP hydrolysis in the heart from 51.08 kJ/mole in the Golden Hamster at systole to 45.9 kJ/mole in the Syrian Hamster. The decrease in free energy is sufficient to cause the observed decrease in contractility (1, 2). The normal values for the free energy of ATP hydrolysis, using a creatine kinase quilibrium value of 10^9, ranges between 58 and 63 kJ/mole (1, 2). The mitochondria are capable of generating values as high as 67 kJ/mol (19). Contractile failure had been shown to occur at 45 kJ/mol (21, 22) and 48 kJ/mol (1, 2). A decrease in cardiac performance has been associated with values between 45 and 50 kJ/mol (1, 2). Since the creatine kinase is not at equilibrium during systole, it is not possible to calculate the free energy of ATP hydrolysis using this method. The present value assumes a rapid binding and compartmentation of nucleotides as described by Kammermeier (1, 2). The decrease in availability of cAMP, ATP and a shift toward isomyosin V_3, the isomyosin associated with low enzymatic activity may, however, cause the decrease in cardiac performance noted in the Syrian Hamster (17–20).

The workload imposed on the ventricles alters both the isomyosin synthesized (19) as well as influences the free cytosolic values of ATP/ADP +Pi (21). The precise control of the type of isozyme synthesized is unknown. It is possible that factors which regulate or are associated with the potential to synthesize ATP may play a role in regulation of isomyosin induction, as a compensatory mechanism (19, 20). Isomyosin V_1, which has an increased rate of ATPase activity, uses ATP less efficiently (17, 18) and may be related to high cytosolic ATP/ADP + Pi ratios, whereas isomyosin V_3, which has a lower ATPase activity but uses ATP more efficiently (17, 18), may be related to lower ATP/ADP + Pi ratios.

Acknowledgement

The authors are grateful to Drs. G. Jasmin and P. Kidd for the Syrian Hamsters used in these studies.

References

1. Giesen, J., H. Kammermeier: Relationship of phosphorylation potential and oxygen consumption in isolated perfused rat hearts. J. Mol. Cell. Cardiol. **12,** 891–907 (1980).
2. Kammermeier, H., P. Schmidt, E. Jungling: Free energy change of ATP-hydrolysis: A causal factor of early hypoxic failure of the myocardium. J. Mol. Cell. Cardiol. **14,** 267–277 (1982).
3. Rouleau, J. L., L. H. S. Chuck, G. Hollosi, P. Kidd, R. Sievers, J. Wikman-Coffelt: Verapamil preserves myocardial contractility in the hereditary cardiomyopathy of the Syrian Hamster. Circulat. Res. **50,** 405–412 (1982).
4. Forman, R., W. W. Parmley, E. H. Sonnenblick: Myocardial contractility in relation to hypertrophy and failure in myopathic Syrian Hamsters, J. Mol. Cell. Cardiol. **4,** 203–211 (1972).
5. Pang, D. C., W. B. Weglicki: Alterations of myofibrillar ATPase activities in hearts of cardiomyopathic hamsters. J. Mol. Cell. Cardiol. **12,** 445–456 (1980).
6. Neely, J. R., H. Liebermeister, E. J. Battersby, H. E. Morgan: Effect of pressure development on oxygen consumption by isolated rat heart. Amer. J. Physiol. **212,** 804–814 (1967).

7. Wikman-Coffelt, J., R. J. Coffelt, M. Rapscak, R. Sievers, J. L. Rouleau, W. W. Parmley: A new apex-ejecting perfused rat heart preparation: relation between coronary flow and loading conditions. Cardiovasc. Res. (in press).
8. Wikman-Coffelt, J., R. J. Coffelt: A stimulator-regulated rapid freeze-clamp for terminating metabolic processes of the heart during normal physiological working conditions. IEEE Transactions on Biomedical Engineering **29,** 448–453 (1982).
9. Morgan, H. E., B. H. L. Chua, E. O. Fuller, D. Siehl: Regulation of protein synthesis and degradation during in vitro cardiac work. Amer. J. Physiol. **238,** E431–442 (1980).
10. Lowry, O. H., J. V. Passoneau: In: Methods of Enzymatic Analysis (Bergmeyer, H. U., ed.) Vol. 2, pp. 276–279. Academic Press (New York 1972).
11. Lamprecht, W. I., I. Trautschold: Determination with hexokinase and glucose-6-phosphate dehydrogenase. In: Methods of Enzymatic Analysis (Bergmeyer, H. U., ed.). Vol. 1, pp. 543–551, Academic Press (New York 1965).
12. Bergmeyer, H. U., E. Bernt, F. Schmidt, H. Stork: In: Methods of Enzymatic Analysis (Bergmeyer, H. U., and Gawehn, K., eds.) vol. 3, pp. 1196–1201, Academic Press (New York 1974).
13. Srivastava, S., R. Cooke, J. Wikman-Coffelt: Studies on the role of myosin light chain LC_2 in tension generation. Biochem. Biophys. Res. Commun. **92,** 1–7 (1980).
14. Stewart, D., T. Kamiyama, D. T. Mason, R. Miller, J. Wikman-Coffelt: Alteration in canine cardiac basal levels of cAMP and cGMP and elevated tissue pCO_2 levels, induced by coronary ligation. J. Mol. Cell. Cardiol. **10,** 125–136 (1978).
15. Wikman-Coffelt, J., R. Sievers, R. J. Coffelt, W. W. Parmley: The Cardiac Cycle: Regulation and energy oscillations. Amer. J. Physiol. (submitted).
16. Lawson, J. W., R. L. Veech: Effects of pH and free Mg^{2+} on the K_{eq} of the creatine kinase reaction and other phosphate hydrolyses and phosphate transfer reactions. J. Biol. Chem. **254,** 6528–6537 (1979).
17. Alpert, N. R., L. A. Muliere, R. Z. Litten: Functional significance of altered myosin adenosine triphosphatase activity in enlarged hearts. Amer. J. Cardiol. **44,** 947–953 (1979).
18. Alpert, N. R., L. A. Mulieri: The functional significance of altered tension-dependent heat and thyrotoxic myocardial hypertrophy. Basic Res. Cardiol. **75,** 179–184 (1980).
19. Wikman-Coffelt, J., W. W. Parmley, D. T. Mason: The cardiac hypertrophy process: Analyses of factors determining pathological vs physiological development. Circ. Res. **45,** 697–707 (1979).
20. Wikman-Coffelt, J., W. W. Parmley: Relation of myosin isozymes to the heart as a pump. Amer. Heart J., **103,** 934–940 (1982).
21. Hearse, D. J.: Oxygen deprivation and early myocardial contractile failure: A reassessment of the possible role of adenosine triphosphate. Amer. J. Cardiol. **44,** 1115–1151 (1979).
22. Nishiki, K., M. Erecinka, D. F. Wilson: Energy relationships between cytosolic metabolism and mitochondrial respiration in rat heart. Amer. J. Physiol. (Cell Physiol.) **3(2),** C73–C81 (1978).
23. Hoh, J. F. Y.: Developmental changes in chicken skeletal myosin isoenzymes. FEBS Lett. **98,** 267–270 (1979).

Authors' address:

Joan Wikman-Coffelt, Ph.D., Moffitt Hospital Rm M1186, University of California, San Francisco, San Francisco, California 94143, USA

Cardiac Adaptation to Hemodynamic Overload, Training and Stress
Dr. D. Steinkopff Verlag 204–210 (1983)

Buffer capacity of the myocardium after swimming training*)

G. Kissling and A. Beyer

Physiologisches Institut II der Universität Tübingen (FRG)

Summary

The effect of enhanced myocardial activity on myocardial buffer capacity was investigated in swimming-trained rats and age-matched controls. Conclusions about myocardial buffer capacity were drawn from the response of cardiac mechanics to changes in arterial pH induced by hypercapnia and hypocapnia. The observed changes of left ventricular mechanics were found to be less pronounced in the swimming-trained animals than in the controls. Assuming the existence of active transport of bicarbonate and/or hydrogen ions across the cell membrane by specific pump mechanisms, the present results could be interpreted such that swimming training causes an increase in activity of such ionic pumps.

Key words: swimming training of rats, left ventricular mechanics, myocardial buffer capacity, hypercapnia, hypocapnia

Introduction

In vivo the buffer capacity of myocardium is substantially higher than that of skeletal muscle (2). In the rat heart even higher myocardial buffer capacity was found in the early stage of chronic pressure overload (1, 3, 4, 7). It seems that the intracellular buffer capacity of the heart correlates well with the state of myocardial activity (1). Therefore myocardial buffer capacity should also be improved by physical training.

We have investigated the effects of hypercapnia and hypocapnia on cardiac mechanics of swimming-trained rats and age-matched controls since intracellular pH is much more influenced by changes in extracellular pH due to CO_2 than by changes of extracellular pH due to noncarbonic acids. Although myocardial buffer capacity was not measured directly, conclusions about myocardial buffer capacity may be drawn from the response of the cardiac mechanics to changes in arterial P_{CO_2} since H^+ ions are known to influence the effects of Ca^{++} ions.

Materials and methods

Young male Sprague-Dawley rats were subjected to swimming training of 2 hours per day. After 13 weeks, experiments were performed on the trained animals and age-matched controls.

*) Supported by the Deutsche Forschungsgemeinschaft.

Table 1. Mean values and standard error ($\bar{x} \pm s_{\bar{x}}$) of body weight, heart weight, left ventricular weight, heart weight/100 g body weight, and left ventricular weight/ 100 g body weight in swimming-trained rats and age-matched controls.

	Body weight (g)	Heart weight (mg)	Left ventricular weight (mg)	Heart weight / 100 g body weight (mg)	Left ventricular weight / 100 g body weight (mg)
Controls (n=21) (age-matched)	538 ± 29	1324 ± 102	884 ± 68	246 ± 17	164 ± 12
Swimming-trained rats (n=23)	434 ± 29	1269 ± 108	861 ± 87	293 ± 24	198 ± 18
Δ (percent of control value)	−19 %	−4 %	−3 %	+19 %	+21 %
p <	0.0005	n.s.	n.s.	0.0005	0.0005

The experimental set-up has been described in detail elsewhere (5), and therefore only a brief description is provided below. After opening the chest under urethane anesthesia (1.2–1.5 g/kg b.w.), the pericardium was removed, and the left ventricle was pierced with a cannula at the apex for pressure measurement and withdrawal of arterial blood samples. The superior and inferior venae cavae as well as the ascending aorta were ligated. The ligatures cut off the entire systemic circulation with the exception of coronary circulation, whereas pulmonary circulation remains intact.

Hypercapnia as well as hypocapnia were produced by ventilating the animals with gas mixtures of oxygen and variable concentrations of carbon dioxide (0–10 Vol% CO_2). Steady-state values of arterial P_{CO_2} and p_H were attained within 2 minutes after the change of the ventilation gas mixture. P_{CO_2} and p_H were measured in arterial blood samples with a p_H blood gas analyzer (I L 213/329, Instrumentation Laboratory Inc.).

Results and discussion

Body weight, heart weight, and left ventricular weight of the swimming-trained rats and the age-matched controls are summarized in table 1. Differences in heart weight and left ventricular weight can be shown only when heart weight and left ventricular weight are related to body weight, whereas the absolute values of heart weight and left ventricular weight are almost identical in both groups.

In the early phase of hypercapnia (2 min), heart rate, left ventricular peak pressure, and maximum rate of pressure development are significantly decreased. In the early phase of hypocapnia (2 min), heart rate, left ventricular peak pressure, and maximum rate of pressure rise are significantly increased. Since left ventricular enddiastolic pressure remains constant, the observed changes in left ventricular mechanics cannot be attributed to the Frank-Starling mechanism. However, the changes in left ventricular mechanics are less pronounced in the swimming-trained animals than in the controls.

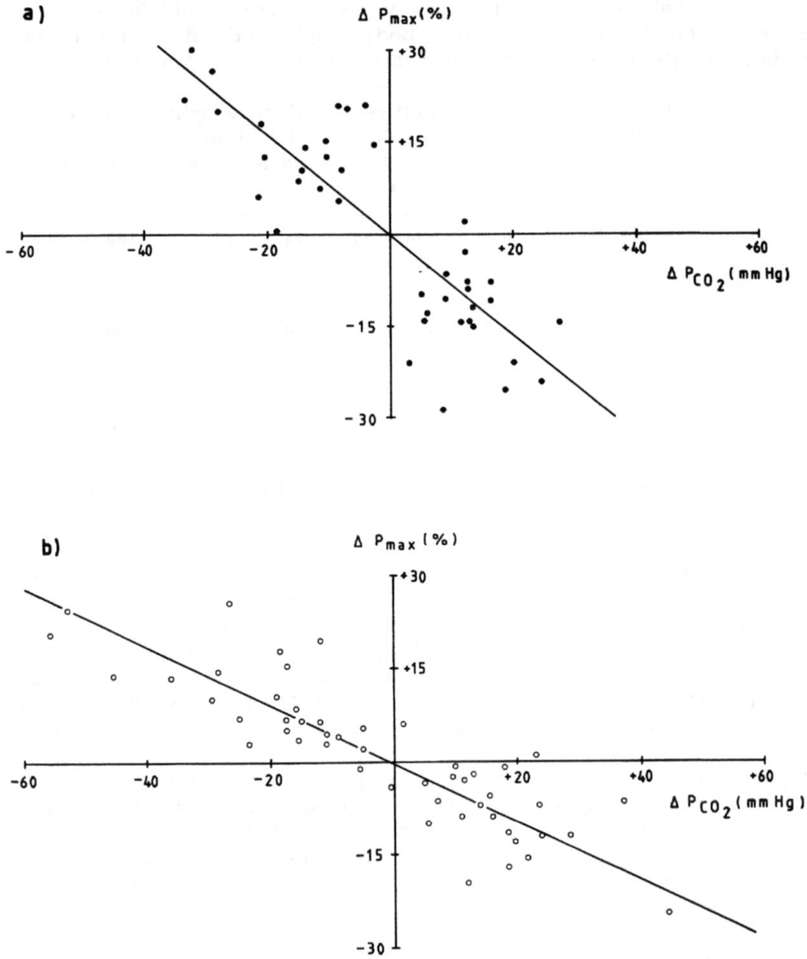

Fig. 1. Dependence of the percentage change of left ventricular peak pressure in the early phase of hypercapnia and hypocapnia on the absolute change of P_{CO_2}. Respiratory acidosis results in a decrease in left ventricular peak pressure, respiratory alkalosis in an increase. In controls (a) the change in left ventricular peak pressure due to hypercapnia and hypocapnia is significantly greater than in swimming-trained rats (b). a) ● controls: $\Delta P_{max} = -0.82\ \Delta P_{CO_2} - 0.04$ ($r = 0.85$); b) ○ swimming-trained rats: $\Delta P_{max} = -\ 0.47\ \Delta P_{CO_2} - 0.4$ ($r = 0.88$). Difference in slope: $p < 0.0005$.

Figure 1 shows the dependence of the relative change in left ventricular peak pressure on the absolute change of P_{CO_2}. For a given change of P_{CO_2} the relative change in left ventricular peak pressure is significantly smaller in swimming-trained rats (fig. 1b) than in the controls (Fig. 1a).

However, this phenomenon could be explained by an improved buffer capacity in the blood of the swimming-trained animals. In fact, the correlation between p_H and P_{CO_2} shows a change to higher p_H-values in the swimming-trained rats (fig. 2a). At a given ΔP_{CO_2} the change in concentration of hydrogen ions is significantly smaller in the blood of the swimming-trained rats, which suggests an improved buffer capacity in the blood of these animals (fig. 2b and fig. 2c).

However, the less pronounced hemodynamic reactions of the swimming-trained animals to hypercapnia or hypocapnia are not solely due to

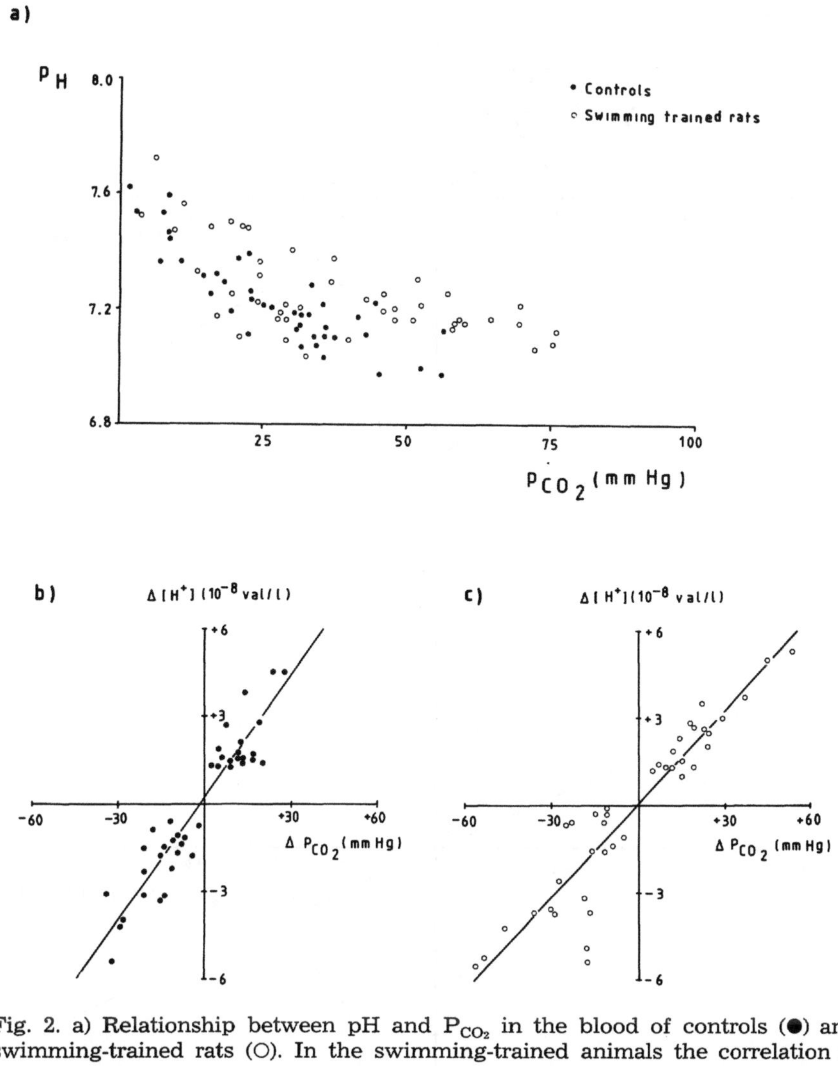

Fig. 2. a) Relationship between pH and P_{CO_2} in the blood of controls (●) and swimming-trained rats (○). In the swimming-trained animals the correlation is shifted to higher pH values. b) and c): Dependence of the change in concentration of hydrogen ions on the change in P_{CO_2} in controls (b) and swimming-trained rats (c). At a given ΔP_{CO_2} the change in concentration of hydrogen ions is significantly smaller in the blood of swimming-trained animals. ● Controls: $10^{-8}\ \Delta(H^+) = 0.1401\ \Delta P_{CO_2} + 0.1415 \cdot 10^{-8}$ ($r = 0.938$). ○ Swimming-trained rats: $10^{-8}\ \Delta(H^+) = 0.1065\ \Delta P_{CO_2} + 0.0345 \cdot 10^{-8}$ ($r = 0.930$). Difference in slope: $p < 0.05$.

improved buffer capacity of the blood, but also to improved myocardial buffer capacity. This is shown in the plots of ΔP_{max} against the concentration of hydrogen ions (fig. 3). At a certain change of the H^+ concentration, the absolute change of P_{max} and dP/dt_{max}, as well as the percentage change

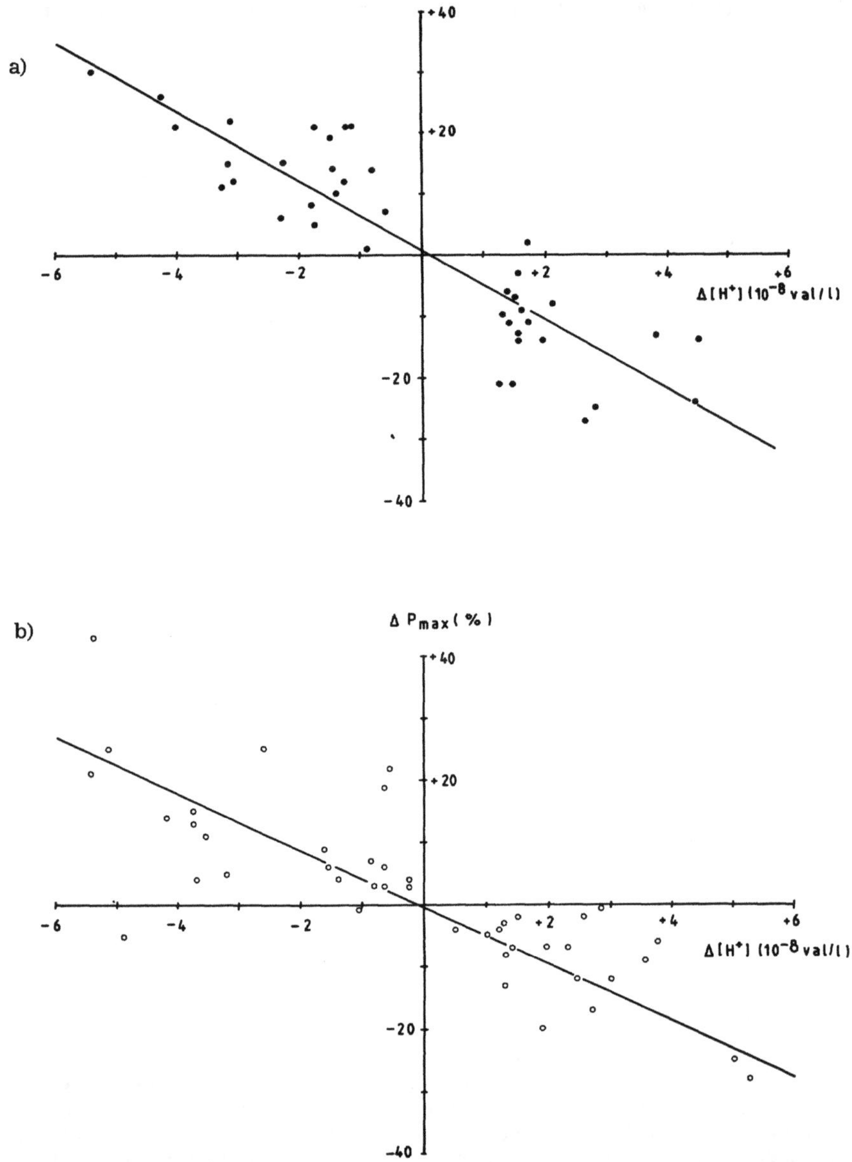

Fig. 3. Dependence of the percentage change of left ventricular peak pressure on the absolute change of the concentration of hydrogen ions. a) ● controls: $\Delta P_{max} = -5.6618 \cdot 10^{-8}\ \Delta(H^+) + 0.8830$ ($r = 0.876$); b) ○ swimming-trained rats: $\Delta P_{max} = -4.0563 \cdot 10^{-8}\ \Delta(H^+) - 0.0292$ ($r = 0.822$). Difference in slope: $p < 0.0125$.

of these parameters is significantly smaller in swimming-trained rats than in the controls.

In the present preparation, the blood values of P_{CO_2} and p_H attain a new steady state within 2 minutes after the start of hypercapnia or hypocapnia and show no change within the following 10 minutes, due to the fact that renal compensation cannot take place. Hemodynamic parameters, however, show still considerable changes, which are an indication of further myocardial buffering processes. Longer duration of hypercapnia is tolerated by all animals; controls can even compensate for the initial decrease of P_{max} and dP/dt_{max}. Longer duration of hypocapnia, however, is only tolerated by the swimming-trained animals, whereas in controls it inevitably leads to heart failure.

The observed reactions of left ventricular mechanics to hypercapnia and hypocapnia may be related to the effect of the competition between H^+ and Ca^{++} on cardiac contractile function (9). The enhanced myocardial buffer capacity of the swimming-trained animals may be due to several factors: 1. The content of noncarbonic buffers may be higher in the myocardium of the swimming-trained rats. However, this explanation seems to be unlikely since no difference in noncarbonic buffers was found in the rat heart after aortic constriction (3). 2. The change in intracellular p_H due to hypercapnia and hypocapnia remains the same, but its effect on electromechanical coupling is less pronounced in the myocardium of the swimming-trained animals. This possibility also seems to be unlikely since the intracellular p_H in hypertrophied myocardium was found to be increased and to change less than in controls (3, 7). 3. Finally, exchange of bicarbonate and/or hydrogen ions between the intracellular and extracellular space may be enhanced (1, 3, 6, 7, 8).

Assuming the existence of ionic pumps, our results could be interpreted such that swimming training results in an increase in activity of these pumps. Due to the increase in pump activity, hypercapnia and hypocapnia result in smaller changes of intracellular p_H and therefore in smaller changes of mechanical activity.

References

1. Albers, C.: The intracellular p_H and the buffer capacity of the heart. Basic Res. Cardiol. **72,** 274–278 (1977).
2. Clancy, R. L., R. B. Brown: In vivo CO_2 buffer curves of skeletal and cardiac muscle. Amer. J. Physiol. **211,** 1309–1312 (1966).
3. Gonzales, N. C., H.-G. Wemken, N. Heisler: Intracellular pH regulation of normal and hypertrophied rat myocardium. J. Appl. Physiol. **47,** 651–656 (1979).
4. Herten, W., C. Albers: Das intrazelluläre pH des Rattenherzens bei chronischer Hypertrophie. Verh. Dtsch. Ges. Kreislaufforschg. **41,** 298–301 (1975).
5. Kissling, G., L. Malloy, H. Rupp: Energetics of the rat heart in chronic pressure overload. This issue, p. 166–172.
6. Lai, Y. L., B. A. Attebery, E. B. Brown: Mechanism of cardiac muscle adjustment to hypercapnia. Respiration Physiology **19,** 123–129 (1973).
7. Saborowski, F., Ch. Scholand, D. Lang, C. Albers: Intracellular pH and CO_2 combining curve of hypertrophic cardiac muscle in rats. Respiration Physiology **18,** 171–177 (1973).

8. Strome, D. R., R. L. Clancy, N. C. Gonzales: Myocardial CO_2 buffering: role of transmembrane transport of H^+ or HCO_3^- ions. Amer. J. Physiol. **230,** 1037–1041 (1976).
9. Williamson, J. R., B. Safer, T. Rich, S. Schaffer, K. Kobayaski: Effects of acidosis on myocardial contractility and metabolism. Acta med. Scand. Suppl. **587,** 95–111 (1975).

Authors' address:

Prof. Dr. G. Kissling, Physiol. Institut II d. Univ. Tübingen, Gmelinstraße 5, 7400 Tübingen, FRG

Coronary circulation, ischemia, adenine nucleotide content in cardiac overload

Cardiac Adaptation to Hemodynamic Overload, Training and Stress
Dr. D. Steinkopff Verlag 213–219 (1983)

Coronary reserve in spontaneously hypertensive rats: the effect of blood pressure, hypertrophy and long-term vasodilator therapy

M. Klepzig and B. E. Strauer

Department of Medicine, University of Munich (FRG)

Summary

Coronary reserve in man is reduced in concentric hypertensive hypertrophy. In 65-week-old spontaneously hypertensive rats (SHR) we found similar changes; in perfusion studies on isolated hearts the vasodilating capacity was restricted in comparison to Wistar Kyoto rats (WKY). Minimal coronary vascular resistance was 0.12 mmHg · min · 100 g/ml versus 0.05 units in WKY ($p < 0.0001$). 60 weeks of antihypertensive therapy with hydralazine reduced coronary vascular resistance to 0.07 units ($p < 0.0001$). Under this treatment, blood pressure and heart weight/body weight ratios were also significantly reduced. Metoprolol, even when applied in high doses, reduced coronary vascular resistance only to 0.09 units ($p < 0.0001$); despite a modest reduction in blood pressure, the degree of myocardial hypertrophy remained constant. It may be concluded that an increase in coronary vascular resistance in SHR can be prevented by antihypertensive treatment with hydralazine; metoprolol treatment is less effective.

Key words: coronary reserve, coronary resistance, SHR – long-term antihypertensive therapy, hydralazine, metoprolol, essential hypertension, cardiac hypertrophy

Introduction

Patients with essential hypertension have a higher risk of vascular complications such as rhythm disturbances, coronary insufficiency, cardiac failure and myocardial infarctions. In studies on coronary hemodynamics in man, coronary reserve has been found to be significantly reduced in concentric hypertensive hypertrophy (14). The spontaneously hypertensive rats (SHR) are still the best experimental model for comparison with essential hypertension in humans, so they are expected to show similar changes of the coronary vascular bed. The purpose of this study was to quantify both the coronary reserve and the coronary vascular resistance in SHR in order to evaluate how they are effected by long-term antihypertensive treatment and whether therapeutical consequences can be derived from these long-term studies.

Methods

The experiments were conducted on 56 rats at the age of 65 weeks. Antihypertensive treatment of the SHR started at the age of 5 weeks and lasted for 60 weeks.

12 SHR (group 0) and 12 WKY rats served as control animals and had no antihypertensive treatment. The remaining 32 SHR were divided into 4 groups receiving the following therapy: group H: 15 mg/kg · day hydralazine (Ciba-Geigy); group M_1: 50 mg/kg · day metoprolol (Astra), group M_2: 175 mg/kg · day metoprolol; group M_1 + H: 50 mg/kg · day metoprolol and 15 mg/kg · day hydralazine. The drugs were applied with drinking water. Blood pressures and heart rates were measured under light ether anesthesia using the tail cuff method (11). After iv. heparinisation with 500 IU, the hearts were immediately removed, put into iced saline solution and cannulated via the aorta according to the Langendorff method (7). During preparation, the isolated hearts were perfused with a modified Krebs-Ringer solution.

Composition of the solutions (mM): Krebs-Ringer solution: NaCl 127.2, KCl 4.7, $CaCl_2$ 2.5, KH_2PO_4 1.2, $NaHCO_2$ 10.46, glucose 5.5, Na-pyruvate 2. Vasoconstricting solution: NaCl 91.9, KCl 40, $CaCl_2$ 2.5, KH_2PO_4 1.2, $NaHCO_2$ 10.46, glucose 5.5, Na-pyruvate 2. Vasodilating solution: NaCl 127.2, KCl 4.7, KH_2PO_4 1.2, $NaHCO_3$ 10.46, glucose 5.5, Na-pyruvate 2, EGTA 5, adenosine 0.1.

All chemicals were obtained from Merck except adenosine (Boehringer Mannheim) and EGTA (Serva, Heidelberg). The solutions were gassed with 95 % O_2/5 % CO_2 and kept at 0 °C.

After preparation, the hearts were perfused with the solutions at 300, 600 and 900 ml/h, 10 min at each level. Perfusion pressure was recorded continuously (Statham P 23 Gb, Kipp Zonen Micrograph BD 6). Moreover, left and right ventricular heart wet weights and body weights were determined. Statistical analysis was made with the unpaired Student's t-test.

Results

As one should expect, heart rates were increased by hydralazine treatment and decreased dose-dependently by metroprolol. Heart rate remained constant in the group receiving the combined treatment (table 1). Systolic pressures were significantly lower in all groups receiving antihypertensive therapy for 60 weeks. The decrease produced by hydralazine (group H, M_1 + H) was more pronounced than in the metoprolol groups. Similarly, heart weights were effected by our antihypertensive treatment. In the hydralazine-treated group, the reduction in heart weight again was more pronounced. The reduction in heart weight was mainly caused by the prevention of left ventricular hypertrophy, whereas the right ventricular weights remained constant (table 1). The heart weight/body weight ratios expressing the degree of myocardial hypertrophy were decreased in the hydralazine-treated groups; the reduction did not reach statistical significance in the metoprolol groups, because the body weights were reduced at the same time. Even in group M_2, the rats receiving high-dose metoprolol, the prevention of myocardial hypertrophy was not significant.

Figure 1 shows the pressure-flow relations for SHR after 60 weeks of antihypertensive therapy; figure 2 shows the calculated coronary vascular resistance including the statistical analysis. In untreated SHR, coronary vascular resistance was 150 % higher than in the WKY rats. At vasoconstriction, the difference was 162 %. This increase in coronary vascular resistance could be prevented by antihypertensive therapy; in the untreated SHR, it was at vasodilatation 0.12 mm Hg · min · 100 g/ml; after 60 weeks of antihypertensive therapy with hydralazine, it was only 0.07 units; in the metoprolol groups, the values were about 0.09 units. The

Table 1. The effect of 60 weeks of antihypertensive treatment on SHR. Group 0: no treatment; group H: 15 mg/kg · day hydralazine; group M_1: 50 mg/kg · day metoprolol; group M_2: 175 mg/kg · day metoprolol; group M_1+H: 50 mg/kg · day metoprolol and 15 mg/kg · day hydralazine. Mean values ± standard deviation. Significances versus group 0: *: $p < 0.05$; **: $p < 0.01$; ***: $p < 0.0001$. Note the reduction of coronary vascular resistance by antihypertensive treatment.

Group	0	H	M_1	M_2	M_1+H
Blood pressure (mm Hg)	220 ± 30	123 ± 14**	156 ± 16**	164 ± 11**	112 ± 26**
Heart rate (l/min)	401 ± 15	428 ± 16*	367 ± 21*	298 ± 43*	377 ± 47
Left ventricular weight (mg)	1499 ± 197	1068 ± 132**	1259 ± 137**	1159 ± 66**	1085 ± 166***
Right ventricular weight (mg)	273 ± 73	244 ± 44	255 ± 58	242 ± 24	288 ± 130
Heart weight (g)	1.77 ± 0.26	1.30 ± 0.17**	1.51 ± 0.17**	1.27 ± 0.38**	1.28 ± 0.16**
Heart weight/body weight (mg/g)	4.88 ± 0.5	4.04 ± 0.5*	4.47 ± 0.5	4.48 ± 0.7	4.09 ± 0.5*
R cor vasodilation (mm Hg · min · 100 g/ml)	0.12 ± 0.013	0.07 ± 0.014***	0.09 ± 0.012***	0.09 ± 0.005***	0.07 ± 0.05***
R cor vasoconstriction (mm Hg · min · 100 g/ml)	0.35 ± 0.06	0.25 ± 0.07*	0.33 ± 0.06	0.34 ± 0.05	0.25 ± 0.05*

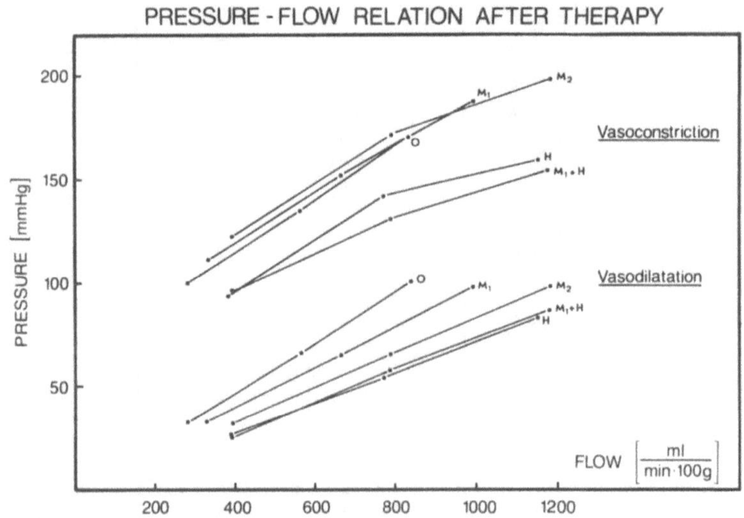

Fig. 1. Pressure-flow relationship after 60 weeks of antihypertensive therapy. The control SHR have a higher minimal perfusion pressure at any given flow in comparison with the hydralazine-treated animals. The steepness of the curves representing the vascular resistance is reduced by hydralazine treatment.

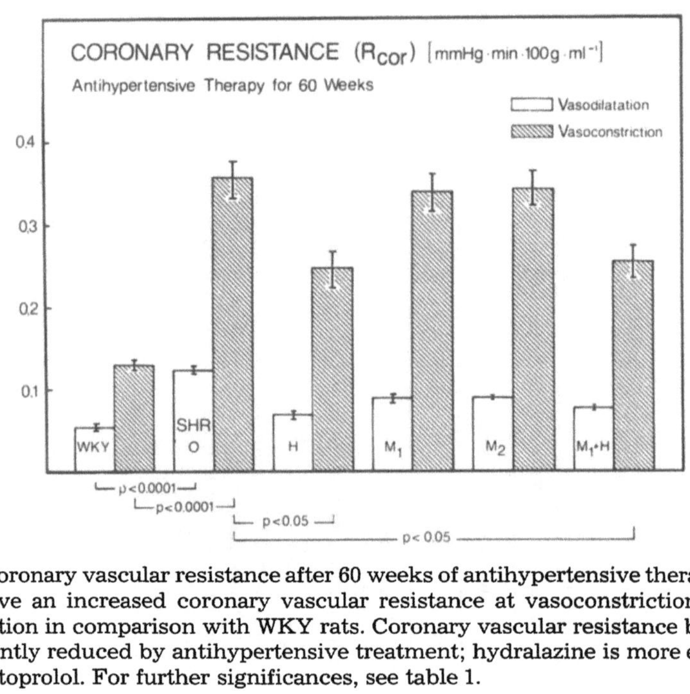

Fig. 2. Coronary vascular resistance after 60 weeks of antihypertensive therapy. The SHR have an increased coronary vascular resistance at vasoconstriction and at vasodilation in comparison with WKY rats. Coronary vascular resistance becomes significantly reduced by antihypertensive treatment; hydralazine is more effective than metoprolol. For further significances, see table 1.

higher dose of metoprolol did not show any further effect. The WKY control values of 0.05 units were not reached in any group. The results at vasoconstriction gave basically the same information.

Discussion

The fact that antihypertensive therapy was quite efficient is mainly due to two reasons:
1. we used very high doses of hydralazine and metoprolol,
2. we treated the rats for a very long period of time.

That is probably why Weiss (19), Sen (12), Pfeffer (10), and our group achieved prevention or regression of myocardial hypertrophy parallel with blood pressure reduction, in contrast to Pegram and Frohlich (8), Boström (2) and earlier studies of Pfeffer (9), who only treated for quite shorter periods.

The better response to hydralazine treatment in comparison to metoprolol therapy is not a question of the applied doses; probably it is caused by the different sites of action. Hydralazine is a peripheral vasodilator (1, 4). Therefore it can reduce blood pressure very effectively by lowering the increased peripheral resistance in SHR. The prevention of myocardial hypertrophy can be explained with the good control of blood pressure. The increased coronary vascular resistance in SHR at vasodilatation corresponds to the reduced vasodilating capacity in patients with essential hypertension, expressed as a reduced coronary reserve (14). The increased minimal coronary resistance in SHR is the result of at least 3 factors:
1. Media hypertrophy of the small coronary vessels. Media hypertrophy in coronary arteries has been described by Yamory (20). According to Folkow's theories, an encroachment of the media upon the lumen would result in an increased minimal vascular resistance (13, 18).
2. Increased proliferation of connective tissue. Such a proliferation has been shown by Sen and Tarazi (12). They found out that an increased hydroxyproline production in SHR can be reduced by antihypertensive treatment.
3. Hypertrophy of myocardium with inadequate growth of the coronary vascular bed. This has been described by Wearn (17). Henrich (3) found a rarefication of mesenteric vessels in SHR.

In vivo some more factors might play a role, such as differences in blood viscosity and cellular water content (15).

It is difficult to decide which of these factors is the most important explanation for the increased coronary vascular resistance in SHR and for its prevention by antihypertensive therapy. The role of the media hypertrophy has to be investigated in further experiments on isolated coronary arteries. The myocardial hypertrophy with inadequate vascular growth is certainly not the only explanation. Coronary resistance is enhanced in SHR and can be prevented by antihypertensive therapy even if the values are not normalised to heart weights.

Marcus produced two kinds of myocardial hypertrophy in dogs: by volume-overloading (A) and by pressure-overloading (B). Coronary vascular resistance is decreased in group (A) and increased in group (B). That means the coronary vascular bed can adapt adequately to myocardial hypertrophy, but this is not the case in hypertension. So there must be some coronary-vascular alteration in hypertension (6).

This is in good correlation with our clinical finding that patients with essential hypertension already have a reduced coronary reserve in early stages of the development. The significance of this study is that we have been able to achieve prevention of the pathophysiological changes in coronary hemodynamics in an appropriate model.

References

1. Ablad, B.: Hemodynamic effects of hydralazine. Arch. Pharmacol. Toxicol. (Suppl.) **20,** 5–53 (1963).
2. Boström, S. L., J. Fryklund: Protein synthesis and composition of cardiac and vascular tissue in spontaneously hypertensive rats and the effects of beta-adrenergic antagonist treatment. Clinical science **57,** 39–41 (1979).
3. Henrich, H., R. Hertel, R. Assmann: Structural differences in the mesentery microcirculation between normotensive and spontaneously hypertensive rats. Pflügers Arch. **375,** 153–159 (1978).
4. Kment, A., M. Klepzig, U. Büll, B. E. Strauer: Koronare Hämodynamik und myokardialer Sauerstoffverbrauch unter Dihydralazininfusion. Verh. dtsch. Ges. inn. Med. **86,** 633–636 (1980).
5. Koch-Weser, J.: Hydralazine. N. Engl. J. Med. **295,** 320–323 (1976).
6. Marcus, M., M. Müller, C. L. Eastham: Effect of short-term ventricular hypertrophy on coronary circulation. Amer. J. Physiol. **241,** H 358–362 (1981).
7. Neely, J. R., H. Liebermeiser, E. J. Battersby, H. E. Morgan: Effect of pressure development on oxygen consumption by isolated rat heart. Amer. J. Physiol. **212** (4), 804–814 (1967).
8. Pegram, B., S. Ishise, E. D. Frohlich: Effect of methyldopa, clonidine and hydralazine on cardiac mass and hemodynamics in WKY and SHR. Cardiovasc. Res. **16,** 40–46 (1982).
9. Pfeffer, M., J. Pfeffer, K. Weiss, E. Frohlich: Development of hypertension and cardiac hypertrophy during prolonged beta blockade. Amer. J. Physiol. **232** (6), H 639–H 644 (1977).
10. Pfeffer, J., M. Pfeffer, P. Fletcher, M. Fishbein, E. Braunwald: Favorable effects of therapy on cardiac performance in SHR. Amer. J. Physiol. **242,** H 776–H 784 (1982).
11. Pfeffer, J., M. Pfeffer, E. Frohlich: Validity of an indirect tail cuff method for determining systolic arterial pressure in unanesthesized normotensive and spontaneously hypertensive rats. J. Lab. Clin. Med. 957–961 (1971).
12. Sen, S., F. M. Bumpus: Collagen synthesis in development and reversal of cardiac hypertrophy in SHR. Amer. J. Cardiol. **44,** 954–958 (1979).
13. Sivertson, R.: The hemodynamic importance of structural vascular changes in essential hypertension. Acta Physiol. Scand., Suppl. **343,** 1–56 (1970).
14. Strauer, B. E.: Hypertensive heart disease. Springer (Berlin–Heidelberg–New York 1980).
15. Strauer, B. E.: Koronare Mikrozirkulationsstörungen. Klin. Wschr. **59,** 1125–1137 (1981).
16. Wangler, R. D., K. Peters, M. Marcus, R. Tomanek: Effect of duration of arterial hypertension and cardiac hypertrophy on coronary vasodilatator reserve. Circulat. Res. **51,** 10–18 (1982).
17. Wearn, J. T.: Alterations in heart accompanying growth and hypertrophy. Bull. Johns Hopk. Hosp. **68,** 363–374 (1941).

18. Weiss, L.: Aspects of the relation between functional and structural cardiovascular factors in primary hypertension. Acta Physiol. Scand., Suppl. 409 (1974).
19. Weiss, L., Y. Lundgren: Left ventricular hypertrophy and its reversibility in young spontaneously hypertensive rats. Cardiovasc. Res. **12,** 635–638 (1978).
20. Yamori, Y., et al.: Cardiac hypertrophy in early hypertension. Amer. J. Cardiol. **44,** 964–969 (1979).

Authors' address:

Dr. med. M. Klepzig, Medizinische Klinik I, Klinikum Großhadern, Marchioninistraße 15, 8000 München 70, FRG

Cardiac Adaptation to Hemodynamic Overload, Training and Stress
Dr. D. Steinkopff Verlag 220–227 (1983)

Effect of aortic constriction on rat heart function and mortality*)

H.-G. Zimmer

Physiologisches Institut der Universität München (FRG)

Summary

The maximal rate of rise of left ventricular pressure (LV dP/dt_{max}) measured in closed-chest rats by means of an ultraminiature catheter pressure transducer served as an indicator of cardiac contractility (6). It was slightly increased subsequent to constriction of the abdominal aorta and markedly enhanced after administration of isoproterenol and triiodothyronine. In all three models of cardiac hypertrophy, the enhancement of contractility occurred prior to the maximal stimulation of myocardial adenine nucleotide and protein synthesis. Combination of severe aortic constriction with simultaneous administration of isoproterenol induced an impairment of rat heart function. 24 hours after this intervention, heart rate, left ventricular systolic pressure, and LV dP/dt_{max} were all depressed by more than 20 %, and the content of cardiac ATP was also diminished to about the same extent. The mortality of rats with severe aortic constriction, which was 46 % when physiologic saline was applied as continuous i.v. infusion for 48 hours, was reduced to 18 % by ribose.

Key words: adenine nucleotide biosynthesis, afterload, cardiac ATP content, cardiac contractility, cardioprotection, isoproterenol, triiodothyronine

Introduction

The metabolic changes occurring in the myocardium during the development of experimentally induced cardiac hypertrophy have been well characterized (8, 10, 12, 15, 18). However, there are only few reports on the hemodynamics in intact small laboratory animals in vivo after aortic constriction (2, 3). In particular, information on left ventricular function is lacking due to methodological difficulties in obtaining hemodynamic parameters. These have recently been overcome by the availability of an ultraminiature catheter pressure transducer with dimensions suitable for catheterization of the left heart via the carotid artery in small animals (19, 20). It was one of the aims of the present study to measure changes in basic parameters of heart function in rats after aortic constriction and to correlate them with some characteristic metabolic alterations. For comparison, similar studies have been performed in two other types of cardiac hypertrophy, which were induced chemically by administration of isoproterenol and triiodothyronine, respectively.

---

*) This study was supported by the Deutsche Forschungsgemeinschaft (Zi 199/4-3)

Another purpose of the present investigations was to examine whether impairment of heart function can be induced in rats by combination of two interventions both of which leading to cardiac hypertrophy when applied alone. Such a combination which elicits a reduction in cardiac hemodynamic parameters turned out to be severe aortic constriction and simultaneous administration of isoproterenol. This model of a reduced rat heart function in vivo has been characterized both in functional and metabolic terms.

The final aim of the study concerns the effect of ribose. This pentose has been shown previously to have pronounced effects on myocardial adenine nucleotide metabolism (16) and on the function (19) as well as on the morphology of the isoproterenol-stimulated heart (17). In view of these beneficial effects of ribose, the question remained as to whether this pentose may also influence the mortality of rats with severe aortic constriction.

Methods

All experiments were done on female Sprague-Dawley rats (200–240 g body weight) fed a diet of Altromin® with free access to water. DL-Isoproterenol-HCl and 3,3',5-triiodo-L-thyronine-sodium salt were purchased from Sigma Chemie München. Pressure-induced cardiac hypertrophy was elicited by constriction of the abdominal aorta to a final diameter of 0.65 mm using the method described previously (12). The other two types of myocardial hypertrophy were induced chemically. Isoproterenol which has been shown to produce hypertrophy of both ventricles (11) was given as a single s.c. injection in a dose of 25 mg/kg. Triiodothyronine was administered daily as a single s.c. dose of 0.2 mg/kg (15).

To measure the function of the heart in closed-chest rats anesthetized with thiobutabarbital-sodium (Inactin® Buyk, 80 mg/kg, i.p.), an ultraminiature catheter pressure transducer (model PR-249, Millar Instruments, Inc., Houston, Texas) was inserted into the right carotid artery and then quickly advanced into the left ventricle. Heart rate, left ventricular pressure (LVP), and the maximal rate of rise of left ventricular pressure (LV dP/dt_{max}) were continuously recorded on a multichannel Beckman RM type dynograph or a Gould Brush 2600 recorder. Measurements were taken 15 min after catheterization of the left ventricle when a steady state had been reached. Details of the procedure have been described recently (19, 20). For continuous i.v. infusion of ribose, a steriflex catheter (Vygon Company, Aachen) with an outside diameter of 1 mm was placed in the right jugular vein of rats in ether anesthesia, fixed thoroughly and connected to a 20-ml syringe filled with physiologic saline or ribose (200 mg/kg/h). The syringe was placed in an infusion pump (type 5003, Infors AG, Hofstetten). The infusion rate was 5 ml/kg body weight/h and maintained for up to 48 hours during which time the animals could move around freely in their individual cages.

Rates of cardiac adenine nucleotide biosynthesis were determined after an in-vivo exposure time of 60 min to 1-^{14}C-glycine (specific activity: 54.2 mCi/mmole, obtained from Amersham International, Inc., Braunschweig, 250 µCi/kg body weight, injected into the tail vein) by relating the total radioactivity of myocardial adenine nucleotides due to the incorporation of 1-^{14}C-glycine to the mean specific activity of the tissue glycine precursor pool (13). Relative rates of cardiac protein synthesis were also obtained by means of 1-^{14}C-glycine taking into account the radioactivity of total cardiac proteins and the mean specific activity of glycine in the tissue (12). The cardiac ATP content was determined using the method of Gerlach et al. (5). Statistical analysis of the data was done by means of the unpaired Student's t-test or the χ^2 test.

Results

1 Changes in cardiac contractility after aortic constriction in relation to metabolic alterations. Comparison with other hypertrophy models

After constriction of the abdominal aorta, heart rate decreased slightly, and left ventricular systolic pressure increased to a maximum of 178 ± 8 mm Hg (n = 11) after 48 hours (data not shown). Contractility measured as the maximal rate of rise of left ventricular pressure development (LV dP/dt_{max}) did not change within the first 5 hours after the intervention, at a time when both adenine nucleotide and protein synthesis were depressed (fig. 1). Thereafter, LV dP/dt_{max} increased reaching the level of significance after 24 hours. At that time, adenine nucleotide biosynthesis was also enhanced, but protein synthesis had not yet changed. Thus the increase in contractility in this model of cardiac hypertrophy occurred prior to the maximal stimulation of adenine nucleotide and protein synthesis.

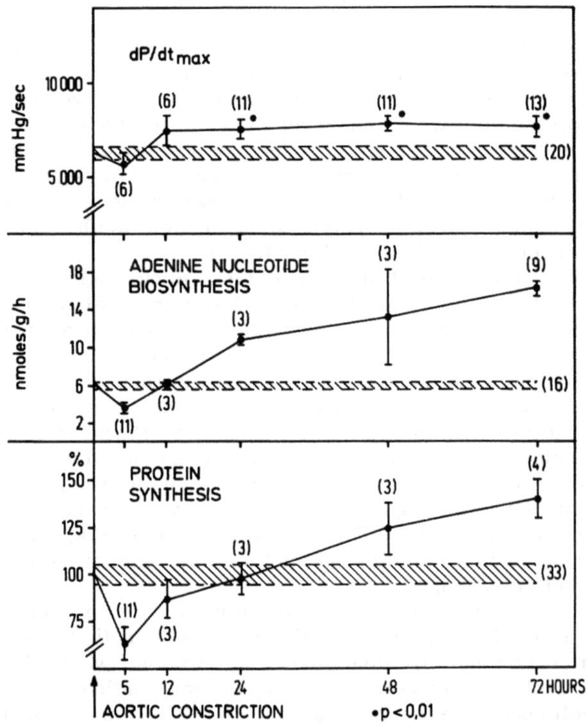

Fig. 1. Changes in the maximal rate of rise of left ventricular pressure (dP/dt_{max}), in myocardial adenine nucleotide biosynthesis, and in protein synthesis in rats subsequent to aortic constriction. Measurements of dP/dt_{max} were taken at the time points indicated 15 min after placement of the ultraminiature catheter pressure transducer in the left ventricle. Mean values ± SEM, number of experiments in parentheses.

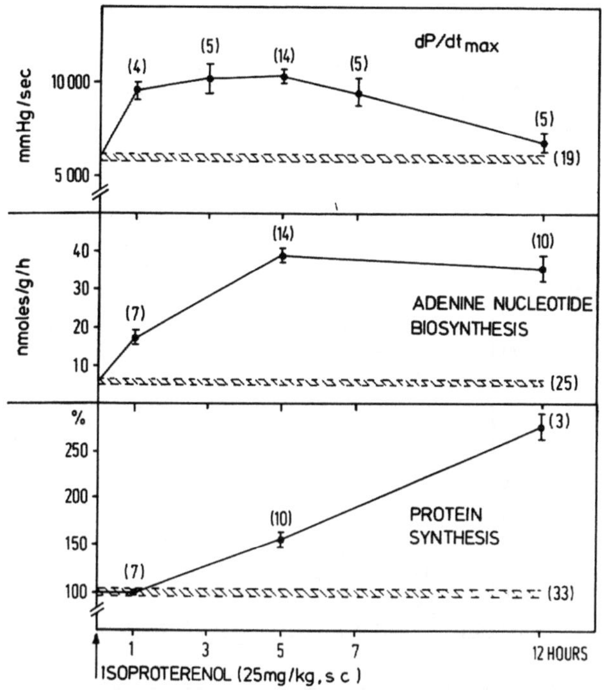

Fig. 2. Effect of a single s.c. injection of isoproterenol on left ventricular dP/dt_{max} and on myocardial adenine nucleotide as well as protein synthesis. The increase of the functional and metabolic parameters was statistically significant at any time as calculated by means of the unpaired Student's t-test. Mean values ± SEM, number of experiments in parentheses.

A similar relationship between changes in contractility and in metabolic parameters was observed in the other two models. Subsequent to administration of isoproterenol, heart rate increased (14) and left ventricular systolic pressure decreased slightly within the first 12 hours (data not shown). There was a pronounced elevation in LV dP/dt_{max} (fig. 2), which occurred before adenine nucleotide and protein synthesis attained their respective maxima. When triiodothyronine was administered, there was also an immediate and marked increase in contractility, which occurred before the maximal rise in adenine nucleotide and protein synthesis occurred (fig. 3).

2 Reduction of heart function by aortic constriction in combination with simultaneous administration of isoproterenol

All types of experimentally induced cardiac hypertrophy were characterized by an enhancement of contractility, though to different extents. It was therefore of interest to examine whether it may be possible to induce a reduction in heart function by combination of two of the methods applied. It turned out that increased afterload due to constriction of the abdominal

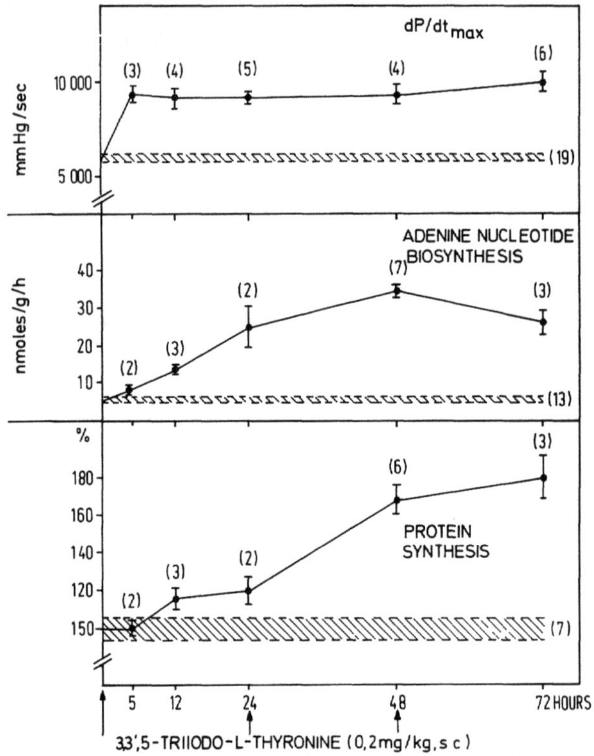

Fig. 3. Successive increases in LV dP/dt_{max}, in myocardial adenine nucleotide as well as in protein synthesis under the influence of multiple doses of triiodothyronine. Mean values ± SEM, number of experiments in parentheses.

aorta and simultaneous administration of isoproterenol is a combination that leads to impairment of left ventricular hemodynamic parameters. 24 hours after this intervention, heart rate was diminished, left ventricular systolic pressure was reduced and LV dP/dt_{max} was also depressed, the

Table 1. Effect of constriction of the abdominal aorta (final diameter: 0.65 mm) in combination with simultaneous administration of isoproterenol (25 mg/kg, s.c.) on heart rate, left ventricular systolic pressure (LVSP) and the maximal rate of rise in left ventricular pressure (LV dP/dt_{max}) as well as on the content of cardiac ATP in rats. Measurements were made 24 hours after the intervention. Mean values ± SEM, number of experiments in parentheses.

	Control	Aortic constriction + isoproterenol
Heart rate (beats/min)	409 ± 7 (19)	304 ± 32 (11)*
LVSP (mm Hg)	142 ± 4 (19)	111 ± 5 (11)*
LV dP/dt_{max} (mm Hg/sec)	6073 ± 187 (19)	4699 ± 338 (11)*
ATP (μmoles/g)	4.4 ± 0.1 (38)	3.4 ± 0.1 (14)*

* $p < 0.0005$

Table 2. Effect of ribose on the mortality of rats with severe constriction of the abdominal aorta (final diameter: 0.65 mm). The unanesthetized and unrestrained rats received continuous i.v. infusion of either 0.9% NaCl or ribose (200 mg/kg/h) for 48 hours.

Treatment	Number of rats with aortic constriction	Deaths within 48 hours	Mortality
NaCl-infusion	28	13	46%
Ribose infusion	28	5	18%

decline of all parameters being of about the same extent (table 1). Also the ATP content turned out to be diminished after this experimental procedure.

3 Improvement of survival of rats with aortic constriction by ribose

After severe constriction of the abdominal aorta, the mortality of rats which had received continuous i.v. infusion of physiologic saline was 46 %. When the rats were infused with ribose for 48 hours, however, the mortality was considerably reduced (table 2). This difference was statistically significant as calculated with the χ^2 test.

Discussion

This study shows that contractility measured as the maximal rate of rise in left ventricular pressure (LV dP/dt_{max}) is enhanced, though to different extents, in all three models of cardiac hypertrophy. The increase in LV dP/dt_{max} after aortic constriction occurs late and is quite moderate compared to that observed after administration of isoproterenol or triiodothyronine (figs. 1–3). After a single injection of isoproterenol, LV dP/dt_{max} is elevated very early, but this positive inotropic effect subsides so that contractility is almost in the normal range after 12 hours. In the triiodothyronine model, there is also an immediate increase in LV dP/dt_{max}, which persists when the hormone is administered every 24 hours. A feature common to all hypertrophy models is that the enhancement of contractility occurs before the maximal rise in adenine nucleotide and protein synthesis is attained.

Given these changes in contractility, it may be asked whether the control LV dP/dt_{max} value determined by means of the ultraminiature catheter pressure transducer is representative for the normal in-vivo situation in the rat. A comparison with data in the literature reveals that the value obtained in the present study (6,073 ± 187 mm Hg/sec, n = 19) is much lower than that measured with a fluid-filled catheter (17,647 ± 1,045 mm Hg/sec, n = 17) (9) or by direct puncture of the left heart after thoracotomy (10,000 to 12,000 mm Hg/sec) (4). These differences in dP/dt_{max} may be due to the well-known problems associated with fluidfilled catheter pressure measurement systems. In contrast, its low mass makes the ultraminiature catheter pressure transducer used in this study insensitive to acceleration forces and the "catheter whip" phenomenon. On the other hand, subsequent to thoracotomy, catecholamines may have been released and may be responsible for the higher dP/dt_{max} (4). Thus the obvious discrepancies in the magnitude of the dP/dt_{max} values are most likely due to methodological differences.

Since the increase in cardiac contractility subsequent to aortic constriction is only moderate, it appeared possible to induce a reduction in heart function by additional administration of a catecholamine. Catecholamines have recently been shown to ultimately impair left ventricular function when carefully studied in open-chest rabbits (7). The combination of increased afterload due to aortic constriction with simultaneous administration of isoproterenol in fact elicited a marked reduction of all hemodynamic parameters determined as well as of the myocardial ATP content (table 1). Since it is quite difficult to induce an impairment of heart function in rats in vivo, this appears to be a suitable model to test the effect of metabolic interventions in an attempt to restore myocardial contractility.

The final aspect of this study concerns the effect of ribose on the mortality of rats with severe aortic constriction. Continuous i.v. infusion of ribose for 48 hours improved significantly the survival (table 2). Thus aortic constriction appears to be an appropriate experimental condition for survival studies in contrast to myocardial infarction due to ligation of the descending branch of the left coronary artery, which is also characterized by a reduction in contractility. In this situation, however, early arrhythmias and ventricular fibrillations occur early and frequently (1) so that there is only a minimal chance for ribose to exerts its beneficial effects (unpublished observations).

In order to explain the pronounced effect on mortality, one has to take into consideration that ribose has been shown to enhance adenine nucleotide biosynthesis in various pathophysiologic situations such as recovery from asphyxia (16) and stimulation with isoproterenol (17). In the latter situation, the ribose-induced further enhancement of cardiac adenine nucleotide biosynthesis was of such a magnitude that the decline in the ATP level was prevented. This normalization of cardiac ATP has already been demonstrated to be associated with an improvement of the isoproterenol-elicited positive inotropic effect (19) and with a significant reduction of the focal myocardial cell lesions that regularly occur when isoproterenol is administered in rats (17). Accordingly, the improvement of the survival of rats subsequent to aortic constriction may also be regarded to be due to the pronounced effect of ribose on myocardial adenine nucleotide metabolism.

References

1. Bergey, J. L., K. Nocella, J. D. McCallum: Acute coronary artery occlusion-reperfusion-induced arrhythmias in rats, dogs and pigs: Antiarrhythmic evaluation of quinidine, procainamide and lidocaine. Eur. J. Pharmacol. **81,** 205–216 (1982).
2. Beznák, M.: The effect of the pituitary and growth hormone on the blood pressure and on the ability of the heart to hypertrophy. J. Physiol. **116,** 74–83 (1952).

3. Bezňák, M.: The effect of different degrees of subdiaphragmatic aortic constriction on heart weight and blood pressure of normal and hypophysectomized rats. Can. J. Biochem. Physiol. **33,** 985–994 (1955).
4. Dowell, R. T., A. F. Cutilletta, P. C. Sodt: Functional evaluation of the rat heart in situ. J. Appl. Physiol. **39,** 1043–1047 (1975).
5. Gerlach, E., B. Deuticke, R. H. Dreisbach: Zum Verhalten von Nucleotiden und ihren dephosphorylierten Abbauprodukten in der Niere bei Ischämie und kurzzeitiger post-ischämischer Wiederdurchblutung. Pflügers Arch. **278,** 296–315 (1963).
6. Gleason, W. L., E. Braunwald: Studies on the first derivative of the ventricular pressure pulse in man. J. Clin. Invest. **41,** 80–91 (1962).
7. Lee, J. C., S. E. Downing: Ventricular function in norepinephrine-induced cardiomyopathic rabbits. Amer. J. Physiol. **242,** H191–H196 (1982).
8. Meerson, F. Z.: Compensatory hyperfunction of the heart and cardiac insufficiency. Circulat. Res. **10,** 250–258 (1962).
9. Pfeffer, J. M., M. A. Pfeffer, P. Fletcher, M. C. Fishbein, E. Braunwald: Favorable effects of therapy on cardiac performance in spontaneously hypertensive rats. Amer. J. Physiol. **242,** H776–H784 (1982).
10. Rabinowitz, M., R. Zak: Biochemical and cellular changes in cardiac hypertrophy. Ann. Rev. Med. **23,** 245–262 (1972).
11. Stanton, H. C., G. Brenner, E. D. Mayfield: Studies on isoproterenol-induced cardiomegaly in rats. Amer. Heart J. **177,** 72–80 (1969).
12. Zimmer, H.-G., G. Steinkopff, E. Gerlach: Changes of protein synthesis in the hypertrophying rat heart. Pflügers Arch. **336,** 311–325 (1972).
13. Zimmer, H.-G., C. Trendelenburg, H. Kammermeier, E. Gerlach: De novo synthesis of myocardial adenine nucleotides in the rat. Acceleration during recovery from oxygen deficiency. Circulat. Res. **32,** 635–642 (1973).
14. Zimmer, H.-G., E. Gerlach: Effect of beta-adrenergic stimulation on myocardial adenine nucleotide metabolism. Circulat. Res. **35,** 536–543 (1974).
15. Zimmer, H.-G., E. Gerlach: Early metabolic alterations during the development of experimentally induced cardiac hypertrophy. Arzneim.-Forsch./Drug Res. **30** (II), 11a, 2001–2007 (1980).
16. Zimmer, H.-G.: Restitution of myocardial adenine nucleotides: acceleration by administration of ribose. J. Physiol., Paris **76,** 769–775 (1980).
17. Zimmer, H.-G., H. Ibel, G. Steinkopff, G. Korb: Reduction of the isoproterenol-induced alterations in cardiac adenine nucleotides and morphology by ribose. Science **207,** 319–321 (1980).
18. Zimmer, H.-G., E. Gerlach: Some metabolic features of the development of experimentally induced cardiac hypertrophy. Europ. Heart J. **3** (Suppl. A), 83–92 (1982).
19. Zimmer, H.-G.: Ribose enhances the isoproterenol-elicited positive inotropic effect in rats in vivo. J. Mol. Cell. Cardiol. **14,** 479–482 (1982).
20. Zimmer, H.-G.: Measurement of left ventricular hemodynamic parameters in closed-chest rats under control and various pathophysiologic conditions. Basic Res. Cardiol. (in press).

Author's address:

Prof. Dr. H.-G. Zimmer, Physiologisches Institut der Universität, Pettenkoferstraße 12, D-8000 München 2, FRG

Cardiac Adaptation to Hemodynamic Overload, Training and Stress
Dr. D. Steinkopff Verlag 228–234 (1983)

Metabolic effects of low-flow ischemia on the perfused hypertrophied rat heart: a phosphorus (^{31}P) nuclear magnetic resonance (NMR) study

N. Lavanchy, J. Martin, J. Aussedat, A. Ray, and A. Rossi

Laboratoire de Physiologie animale de l'Université Scientifique et Médicale de Grenoble (France)

Summary

Phosphorus nuclear magnetic resonance (^{31}P NMR) spectroscopy was used to ascertain whether the metabolic response of hypertrophying hearts to ischemia differs from that of control hearts. Cardiac hypertrophy was induced in rats either by abdominal aortic stenosis or by chronic beta-receptor stimulation (7 daily injections of isoproterenol 5 $mg \cdot kg^{-1}{}_{bw}$). Ten days after placing the clip or two days following the last isoproterenol injection, hearts were perfused in a Langendorff mode and submitted to a 24-min global low-flow ischemia (0.2 $ml \cdot min^{-1}$) followed by reperfusion for 30 min. When compared to the changes occurring in control hearts during the sequence ischemia-reperfusion, the perfused hypertrophying hearts exhibit a lower relative ATP depletion, a smaller rate and extent of intracellular acidosis, and a better restoration of the ratio phosphocreatine/inorganic phosphate on reperfusion. All these observations seem to indicate that the extent of metabolic cellular injury due to ischemia is reduced during the stage of developing cardiac hypertrophy. The assumption is made that this may be related to a reduction in the effect of endogenous catecholamines during ischemia; such a reduction may reduce the activation of anaerobic metabolism, which in turn results in a reduction in the acidification of the intracellular medium.

Key words: cardiac hypertrophy, ischemia, phosphorus nuclear magnetic resonance spectroscopy, ATP depletion, intracellular pH

Introduction

Cardiac hypertrophy develops when a sustained cardiac workload creates chronic conditions of desequilibrium between energy production and demand. In ischemia, acute reduction in oxygen and substrate delivery to the heart also induces disturbances in energy balance. Thus, development of cardiomegaly and impairment of cardiac function and tissue damage due to ischemia present similar changes in "energy metabolism". It is therefore of interest to investigate whether (and how) the early metabolic changes due to ischemia and reperfusion are different from normal hearts during the phase of developing hypertrophy. Among the various biochemical indices available, changes in the level of ATP, creatine phosphate (CP) and inorganic phosphate (Pi) are the more sensitive indicators of tissue injury; however, owing to the very short half-life of these compounds, the usual biochemical methods of measurement give no information about the continuing changes in energy metabolism. A non-invasive technique such as phosphorus-31 nuclear magnetic resonance (^{31}P-NMR) allows measurement of the highly dynamic process of energy metabolism in the isolated heart (1, 2). With this method it is possible to continuously monitor the tissue level of phosphate compounds in the isolated perfused heart. In addition, this technique gives an indirect but fairly precise measurement of intracellular pH, another parameter that can play an important role in the pathogenesis of ischemic injury. This technique was therefore used to describe the metabolic changes occurring in the hypertrophying rat heart submitted to temporary ischemia. Cardiac hypertrophy was induced in rats either by producing an aortic stenosis or by administering isoproterenol. The hearts were perfused in a Langendorff mode and submitted to a 24-min global low-flow ischemia followed by reperfusion. Level of high energy phosphate compounds and intracellular pH were measured every 3 min by NMR.

Methods

Animals

The experiments were carried out on rats weighing 200 to 250 g. Two models were used for experimental cardiac hypertrophy, 1) left ventricular hypertrophy due to abdominal aortic constriction, 2) symmetrical cardiomegaly induced by seven daily subcutaneous injections of 5 $mg \cdot kg^{-1}{}_{b.w.}$ of isoproterenol. Hearts were perfused on the 10th day after placing the clip or two days following the last isoproterenol injection.

Perfusion

The hearts were perfused in a Langendorff mode with a phosphate-free Krebs-Henseleit bicarbonate buffer. The medium was bubbled with a mixture of 95 % oxygen, 5 % carbon dioxide, the pH at the level of the heart being adjusted to 7.4 by adding sodium bicarbonate. The perfusion pressure was 100 cm water and the temperature 37 °C. Temperature and gas content of the perfusion fluid were maintained by using thermostatically controlled glass tubing. The hearts were placed into a 15-mm diameter teflon-stoppered tube and immersed in a little volume of perfusate, the excess of effluent being evacuated via a peristaltic pump. The NMR tube was then placed in the bore of the superconducting magnet. Following a 30-min perfusion, the hearts were submitted to 24 minutes of global low-flow ischemia, the coronary flow being adjusted to 0.2 $ml \cdot min^{-1}$ by means of a peristaltic pump. The hearts were then again perfused for 30 minutes under constant aortic pressure. At the end of perfusion, the ventricles were freeze-clamped to allow biochemical determinations and measurement of ventricular weight.

NMR conditions

^{31}P-NMR experiments were performed in a Bruker WM 250 spectrometer operating at 101.3 MHz. Fourier-transform 3 min spectra (132 transients) were obtained intermittently by applying 45° RF pulses. PC, ATP and Pi concentrations were calculated by integrating the areas under the respective peaks. The data were normalized by expressing the results as percentages of their own control value taken from the last pre-ischemic spectrum (27–30-min perfusion). Intramyocardial pH (pHi) was calculated from the chemical shift of the peak of Pi (pH dependant) relative to the PC peak (pH independant). A calibration curve was plotted from the experimental values obtained in a cardiac perchloric extract buffered by phosphate. Results were analyzed for significance by the Student's t test taking P = 0.05 as the limit of significance. Ten hearts were used in each condition, the results were compared to those obtained in 16 control hearts.

Biochemical measurements

Biochemical determinations of adenine nucleotide content of the tissue were performed on the ventricles freeze-clamped at the end of NMR experiments, and on hearts taken "in situ". Nucleotides were extracted by 0.6 N perchloric acid (7 vol: w.weight) and after neutralization by potassium carbonate, 20 microlitres of the extract were analyzed by high performance liquid chromatography. The column (partisil-10 ODS, 0.4 × 18 cm, Wathman) was eluted with a pyrophosphate buffer (25 mM, pH 5.75) at a flow rate of 1.7 ml·min^{-1}.

Results

The degree of cardiomegaly reached in the two experimental models was different. Isoproterenol-treated rats exhibit an increase in heart weight (ventricles) of 43 %, while in those with aortic stenosis the extent of cardiac hypertrophy was about 16 %.

Figure 1 shows the time-course of changes in pHi. In control hearts the pH decreased from 7.08 ± 0.01 to 6.04 ± 0.26 (means ± S.E.) after 24 min of ischemia. In hypertrophying hearts, in both groups, the pHi corresponding to the main peak of Pi did not fall below 6.50. In the isoproterenol group, but not in hearts from rats with aortic stenosis, tissue areas with a pH of 5.80 were revealed by secondary peaks of Pi. On reflow the intracellular pH returned rapidly to near neutrality except in the isoproterenol group where it remained slightly below the pre-ischemic value.

Figure 2 shows that, during ischemia, the degradation of PC was similar in the various groups, but that a greater rephosphorylation of creatine occurred in hypertrophying hearts. In these groups PC levels exceeded pre-ischemic values after 10-min reperfusion before decreasing to about

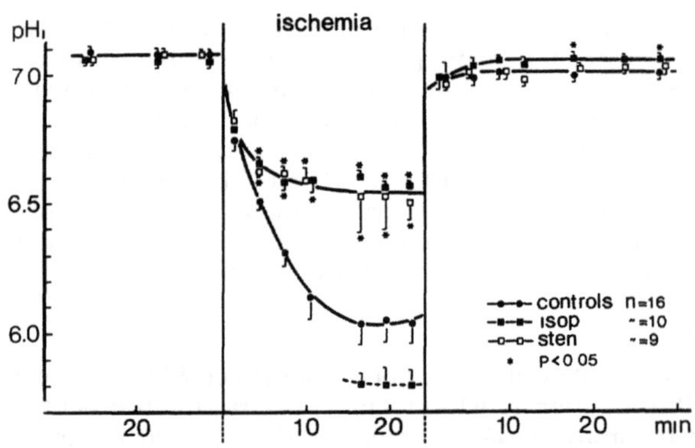

Fig. 1. Changes in intracellular pH of perfused rat hearts during and after ischemia. Low-flow ischemia (0.2 ml·min^{-1}) lasting 24 min was followed by a 30-min reperfusion. Means ± SEM. Values of hearts from isoproterenol-treated rats (isop.) and from rats with aortic stenosis (sten.) were compared with control values. For the isop. group a secondary area with more acidotic pH is indicated by dotted lines.

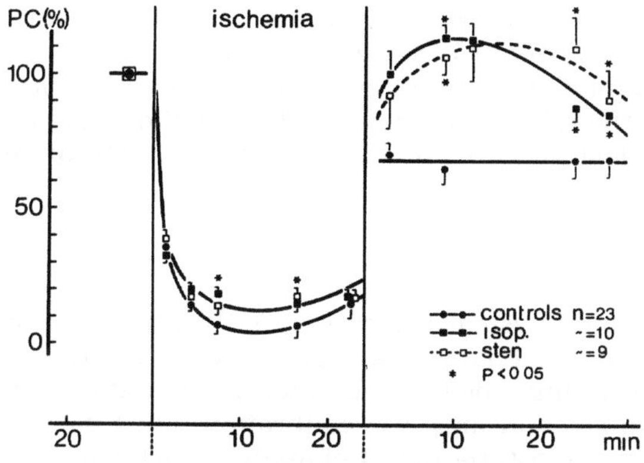

Fig. 2. Percentage changes in phosphocreatine of perfused rat hearts on ischemia and reperfusion. A low-flow ischemia (0.2 ml·min^{-1}) lasting 24 min was followed by a 30-min reperfusion. Means ± SEM. Isop: hearts from isoproterenol-treated rats. Sten: hearts from rats with aortic stenosis. Values for hypertrophying hearts were compared to values from control rats.

90 % of the initial value by the end of reperfusion. These final values differ significantly from the value of 70 % found in control hearts.

Inorganic phosphate level changed in the opposite direction. In control hearts, Pi concentration was increased by about 5 times at the end of the ischemic period; although decreasing on reperfusion, Pi levels remained near 200 % of control values after 30 min. In the isoproterenol-treated group the increase of Pi during ischemia was significantly lower than in controls and pre-ischemic values of Pi were rapidly restored on reperfusion. In hearts from rats with aortic stenosis, the changes of Pi were not significantly different from controls.

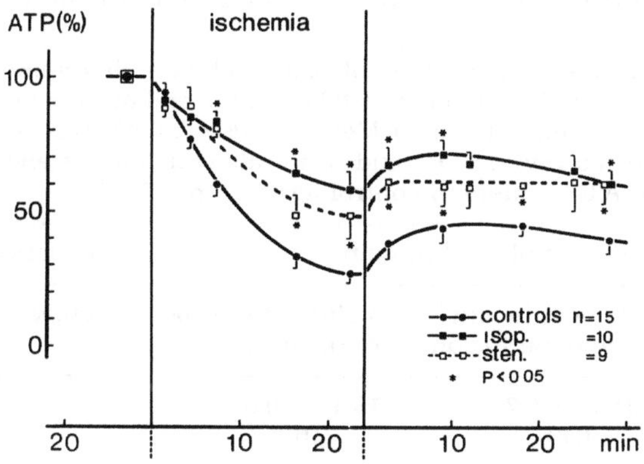

Fig. 3. Percentage changes in ATP of perfused rat hearts on ischemia and reperfusion. A low-flow ischemia (0.2 ml·min^{-1}) lasting 24 min was followed by a 30-min reperfusion. Means ± SEM. Isop: hearts from isoproterenol-treated rats. Sten: hearts from rats with aortic stenosis. Values for hypertrophying hearts were compared to values from control rats.

Figure 3 shows the changes in tissue ATP levels. In control hearts ATP fell progressively by about 70 % during ischemia and was restored to 40 % of the initial value at the end of reperfusion. In both groups of hypertrophying hearts, the relative decrease of ATP due to ischemia was less than in controls and at the end of the experiment 60 % of the initial level remained.

Discussion

Although the biophysical technique of ^{31}P-NMR is a useful probe to follow the metabolic changes associated with global ischemia in the isolated heart, care must be taken in interpreting data. Values for pHi may be subjected to error in absolute calibration, but this should have only small effects on the estimation of changes in pH. Our results show that there is a reduction of the ischemia-induced intracellular acidosis in the hypertrophying hearts suggesting that the metabolic response of the tissue is altered.

The possibility that the myocardium responds heterogeneously to ischemia is suggested by the existence of several peaks of Pi in hearts from isoproterenol-treated rats. It is probable that localized tissue necrosis (due to the chronic isoproterenol treatment) are thus revealed by ischemia. Of interest is the observation that on reperfusion, only one Pi peak remains, whereas, when hearts fail, multiple peaks of Pi are still present (7). Concerning the measurement of myocardial contents of ATP, PC and Pi, the technique has the advantage that it allows serial data to be obtained on the same heart. In practice it is difficult to calibrate signal areas in terms of absolute tissue concentration, and so the values are usually – as in this work – expressed as percentages of the initial value. Since this pre-ischemic value may be different from that of control hearts, the technique does not give similar information to that obtained by biochemical methods. In fact, when the myocardial content of ATP is determined chromatographically on a perchloric acid extract of the tissue no differ-

Table 1. Changes in ATP of perfused rat hearts. ATP was determined biochemically in hearts taken "in situ" and in hearts taken at the end of the sequence perfusion-ischemia-reperfusion (see Methods). Means ± SEM (n). ATP content of hearts from isoproterenol-treated rats (ISOP.) and from rats with aortic-stenosis (STEN.) was compared to the ATP content of control hearts. *($p < 0.05$)

	ATP μmol · g^{-1} protein		Variation	
	Values "in situ" before perfusion	Values at the end of reperfusion	μmole · g^{-1}	% change
CONTROLS	31.4 ± 0.7 (28)	18.4 ± 0.5 (16)	13	41.4
ISOP.	31.9 ± 0.1 (7)	18.7 ± 0.4 (8)	13.2	41.3
STEN.	26.4 ± 1.1* (5)	14.9 ± 0.9* (7)	11.5	43.5

ences appear in the ischemia-induced ATP degradation between control hearts and hypertrophied hearts (table 1).

Probably the pool of ATP, which is subjected to magnetic resonance, is not identical to the pool of ATP estimated by conventional destructive methods. We have no information about the nature and localization of such pools. However, considering the relative changes in phosphocreatine and inorganic phosphate levels, the results show that in the hypertrophying myocardium there is a better rephosphorylation of creatine on reflow than in control hearts. This demonstrates that mitochondria are still capable of resynthesizing ATP, and it could well be that phosphocreatine is a better indicator than ATP of the ATP/ADP cytoplasmic ratio.

A reasonable explanation of these observations could be that the activation of metabolic processes by catecholamines, which normally occurs at the onset of ischemia, is considerably reduced in hypertrophying rat hearts. A reduction of the effect of catecholamines would indeed lower the rate of glycogenolysis and the extent of acidosis, which is probably correlated with the hydrolysis of glycolytically produced ATP (4, 5). Moreover, the transmembrane influx of Ca^{++} that produces myofilament overstimulation and excessive breakdown of ATP is also reduced in these conditions. Several data both from this work and that of others argues in favour of this hypothesis. Wollenberger et al. (6) showed that heart hypertrophy resulting from aortic constriction was associated with severe depletion of cardiac catecholamines and that ischemia failed to induce a rise in cyclic AMP and activation of phosphorylase. On the other hand, as demonstrated by Hein and coll. (7), the responsiveness to beta-adrenergic stimulation was greatly depressed in hypertrophied hearts of chronically isoproterenol-treated rats. In all models of hypertrophy, such a reduction of the efficiency of beta-adrenergic stimulation occurs as the result of long-term overstimulation of the sympathetic nervous system (8, 9). Finally, our hypothesis is supported by the work of Pieper et al. (10) who have shown a similar reduction in the degree of acidosis and a better preservation of high-energy phosphate compounds in the presence of a beta-blocker.

Heart contractility was not measured in these experiments, and the consequences of the metabolic resistance of the hypertrophying heart on heart function remain unclear. The relationship between functional recovery, necrosis, pHi, and cellular energetics are incompletely understood, although recent NMR experiments have shown that on reflow a rapid decline in inorganic phosphate and a rapid increase in phosphocreatine is associated with stable recovery of mechanical function (3).

Acknowledgement

The help of Dr. D. Harding for preparing the text and of Mrs. A Dubourdeaux for typing the manuscript is gratefully acknowledged. Supported by grants of INSERM. PRC n° 130068.

References

1. Hoult, D. I., S. J. W. Busby, D. G. Gadian, G. K. Radda, R. E. Richards, P. J. Seeley: Observation of tissue metabolites using ^{31}P nuclear magnetic resonance. Nature **252**, 285–287 (1974).

2. Gadian, D. G., D. I. Hoult, G. K. Radda, P. J. Seeley, B. Chance, C. Barlow: Phosphorus nuclear magnetic resonance studies on normoxic and ischemic cardiac tissue. Proc. Nat. Acad. Sci. USA **73,** 4446–4448 (1976).
3. Bailey, J. A., A. M. L. Seymour, G. K. Radda: A ^{31}P-NMR study of the effects of reflow on the ischaemic rat heart. Biochim. Biophys. Acta **637,** 1–7 (1981).
4. Gevers, W.: Generation of protons by metabolic processes in heart cells. J. Mol. Cell. Cardiol. **9,** 867–873 (1977).
5. Seelye, R. N.: Proton generation and control during anaerobic glycolysis in heart cells. J. Mol. Cell. Cardiol. **12,** 1483–1486 (1980).
6. Wollenberger, A., L. Will Shahab, E. G. Krause, S. Genz, W. Warbanow, S. Nitschkoff: Effect of acute ischemia on myocardial cyclic AMP, phosphorylase a and lactate levels in various forms of cardiac hypertrophy, 551–559. Recent Advances in Studies on Cardiac Structure and Metabolism. Vol. 3, ed. N. S. Dhalla, University Park Press (Baltimore, London, Tokyo 1972).
7. Hein, B., R. Hein, J. Janke: Restriction of beta-adrenergic responsiveness in hypertrophied hearts of chronically isoproterenol-treated rats, 359–367. Recent Advances in Studies on Cardiac Structure and Metabolism. Vol. 7, ed. P. Harris, R. J. Bing, A. Fleckenstein, University Park Press (Baltimore 1976).
8. Hoffman, B. B., R. J. Lefkowitz: Adrenergic receptors in the heart. Ann. Rev. Physiol. **44,** 475–484 (1982).
9. Poupa, O., Z. Turek, V. Pelouch, J. Prochazka, K. Krofta: Increased resistance of the myocardium to anoxia in vitro after repeated application of isoprenaline. Physiol. Bohemoslov. **14,** 536–540 (1965).
10. Pieper, G. M., G. L. Todd, S. T. Wu, J. M. Salhany, F. C. Clayton, R. S. Eliot: Attenuation of myocardial acidosis by propranolol during ischaemic arrest and reperfusion: evidence with ^{31}P nuclear magnetic resonance. Cardiovasc. Res. **14,** 646–653 (1980).

Authors' address:

N. Lavanchy, Laboratoire de Physiologie animale, BP n° 68, 38402 Saint Martin d'Hères, Cedex, France

Cardiac Adaptation to Hemodynamic Overload, Training and Stress
Dr. D. Steinkopff Verlag 235–244 (1983)

Myocardial mechanics of infarcted and hypertrophied non-infarcted myocardium following experimental coronary artery occlusion

O. H. L. Bing, W. W. Brooks, C. H. Conrad, K. B. Weinstein, J. Spadaro, and P. Radvany

Thorndike Laboratory and Department of Medicine, Harvard Medical School; and Beth Israel Hospital, Boston, Massachusetts; and Department of Medicine, Boston VA Medical Center, Boston, Massachusetts (USA)

Summary

The physiology of the intact heart with myocardial infarction is complex, in part, because it is comprised of a heterogenous population of infarcted, fibrotic and noninfarcted tissue. To further define the mechanical performance of these differing elements, we have examined isolated muscle mechanics of infarcted and noninfarcted myocardium from the same heart.

We have found that: (1) Hypertrophy is present in noninfarcted myocardium of hearts sustaining a myocardial infarction; (2) Infarcted tissue which appears to be grossly fibrotic by eye contains visible myocardium on microscopy, and significant contractile activity persists; (3) Functional changes in the hypertrophied posterior papillary muscle from hearts with infarction include prolonged electro-mechanical delay time and time-to-peak force, with no change in active force, or force-velocity relations. Resting force measured at the apex of the length-force curve is increased; (4) In the infarcted anterior papillary muscle, active force and force-velocity relations are depressed, electro-mechanical delay time is prolonged, and passive stiffness, determined from the passive length-force relation, is increased.

Key words: myocardial infarction, ventricular hypertrophy, myocardial mechanics, isolated muscle preparation

Introduction

While cardiac hypertrophy is uniformly acknowledged to be an adaptive response of the myocardium to chronic loading, its presence in regional myocardial disease is less well recognized. Nonetheless, compensatory growth of noninfarcted myocardium was described by Busch (5). He observed that in massive infarctions of the left ventricle, there was hypertrophy of the non-infarcted left ventricular free wall. Friedberg (10) esti-

---

Supported, in part, by Grants HL-20552 and HL-18338 from the National Heart, Lung, and Blood Institute; and Grant RR-01032 from the General Clinical Research Centers Program of the Division of Research Resources, National Institutes of Health; and funds from the Medical Research Service of the Veterans Administration. O. H. L. Bing is a recipient of a Career Development Award (HL-00072) from the National Institutes of Health.

mates that at least two-thirds of patients who survive myocardial infarction due to coronary occlusion demonstrate cardiac hypertrophy. While it is not clear in the clinical setting whether hypertrophy precedes or follows infarction, experimental studies in rats (18) demonstrate a significant increase in heart weight 6 and 12 weeks after ligation of the left anterior descending coronary artery. In dogs, Gudbjarnason and co-workers (11) noted an increase in protein synthesis in the noninfarcted regions of the left ventricle.

In a number of experimental studies of pressure overload hypertrophy, the intrinsic contractile function of isolated papillary muscles has been shown to be altered (1, 3, 6, 14, 16, 19). However, the mechanical properties of papillary muscles which have undergone hypertrophy in a ventricle with myocardial infarction have not been previously reported.

In the present investigation, a ligation of the left anterior descending coronary artery resulted in infarction of the left ventricle. Animals were sacrified three weeks later. The contractile behavior of the noninfarcted posterior and infarcted anterior papillary muscles was studied. Comparable studies were done with muscles from sham-operated animals. Myocardial infarct size was quantified, and infarcted and noninfarcted papillary muscle preparations were fixed for histological comparison to those obtained from sham-operated animals.

Methods

Charles River CD rats weighing between 180 and 200 grams were studied. Myocardial infarction was produced by ligation of the left anterior coronary artery utilizing a method similar to that described by Johns and Olson (13). Three weeks later, sham-operated and infarcted animals were sacrificed. Only hearts in which the anterior papillary muscle was obviously infarcted, while the posterior papillary muscle appeared uninvolved, were studied. The anterior and posterior papillary muscles of the left ventricle were dissected free and mounted vertically in chambers containing Krebs-Henseleit solution (17) at 28 °C and oxygenated with 95 % O_2 and 5 % CO_2. Muscles were stimulated at a rate of 12/minute by parallel platinum electrodes delivering 5-msec pulses at voltages 10 % greater than the minimum necessary to produce a maximum mechanical response. The spring clip on the tendon-end of the muscle was connected to the lever arm of a low-inertia DC motor (General Scanning G100PD); the lower clip was attached to a semiconductor strain gauge transducer (Kistler-Morse DSC-3) immersed in the bath.

Either the length or tension of the preparation could be controlled by means of an electronic servosystem controlled by a digital computer (Data General Nova 2). Muscle contractions were recorded by sampling length and force at a rate of 2 kHz. Quantitation error was less than 5 µm for length and 20 mg for force. All contractions were examined on a CRT display screen and, if acceptable, recorded on LINC tape or disk for future analysis.

After a 60-minute equilibration period, muscles were gradually lengthened to the peak of the length-tension curve (L_{max}) by means of an automatic computer routine. The L_{max} routine was repeated five times, and after a consistent length at L_{max} was determined, muscles contracted isometrically at that length for 5 minutes; five isometric contractions were then recorded for later analysis. The length of the muscle was measured using a Gaertner cathetometer and telescope. Muscle cross-sectional areas were calculated by assuming cylindrical uniformity and a density of 1.0 g/cm^3. All force data were normalized by the cross-sectional area of the muscle, and all length data by the muscle length. Force velocity curves were obtained by the quick release method at 50 % time to peak tension (isometric contractions). Loads ranged from 0.5 grams to the maximum developed force for each muscle.

For microscopic studies, the muscles (after weighing) were quickly resuspended in the muscle chamber and stretched again to L_{max}. All muscles were fixed at L_{max} by the addition of 10 % formalin to the bath for 1 hour. Fixation was then continued for an additional 8 hours. Tissues were then sectioned, stained with trichrome, and slides prepared. Myofibril diameters were measured in longitudinal section under light microscopy.

To determine myocardial infarct size, the left ventricles were cut from apex to base into four transverse slices, which were processed in a routine manner for histological study. Sections 10 μm thick were cut, stained with Masson's trichrome stain, and mounted (8). The histological sections of the all left ventricular slices were projected onto a screen, and infarct size was calculated from planimetered data as described previously (9). Data were evaluated statistically using the unpaired t test, analysis of variance and the Newman-Keuls multiple sample comparison test.

Results

Rat heart and body weights

In table 1, data are presented on cardiac chamber weight, total heart weight, animal weight, LV to body weight and RV to body weight ratios. Animals with infarction demonstrated a significantly larger heart weight than sham-operated controls. The increase in heart weight was primarily due to an enlarged right ventricle. No differences in LV weight and body weight between groups were present. Myocardial infarct size measured by planimetry was 43 ± 2 % (mean ± SEM) of left ventricular mass in the hearts with myocardial infarction.

Length-tension data

Muscle preparations were stretched in 1 % increments to L_{max} (fig. 1). Active tension was depressed in infarcted anterior papillary muscle preparations in comparison to all other groups. Resting tension values were uniformly higher in posterior papillary muscle preparations from hearts with infarction in comparison to the posterior papillary muscles from the sham-operated group. Stiffness was determined from passive length-ten-

Table 1. Rat heart and body weights.

	LV wt. (g)	RV wt. (g)	Heart wt. (g)	Body wt. (g)	LV/BW ratio	RV/BW ratio
Infarct (n = 7)	0.632±0.050	0.376±0.029	1.264±0.065	312±18	2.02±0.07	1.24±0.12
	NS	p < 0.01	p < 0.01	NS	NS	p < 0.01
Sham (n = 6)	0.588±0.039	0.183±0.014	0.878±0.057	308±26	1.92±0.05	0.65±0.07

Values are means ± SEM

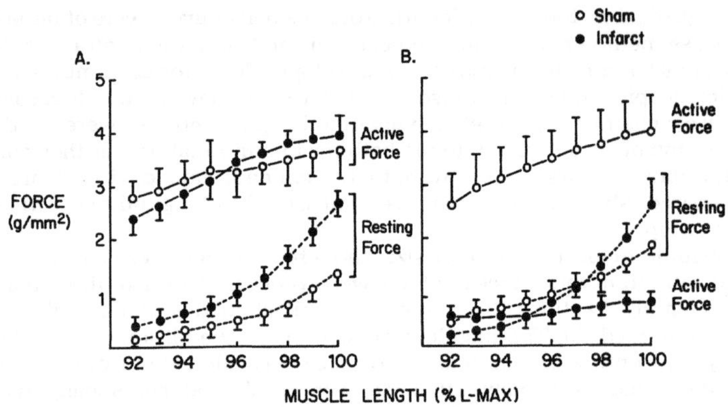

Fig. 1. Active and passive (resting) length-force relationships for muscle preparations from rats three weeks after myocardial infarction and sham operation. In A, data are shown from posterior papillary muscle preparations, while in B, data are from anterior papillary muscle preparations. In hearts with infarction, the anterior papillary muscle appears grossly fibrotic, while the posterior papillary muscle appears largely uninvolved.

sion relationships in each group by an exponential curve fit to the formula

$$\text{Force} = A + B\, e^{C(L-90)}$$

where L = muscle length (% L_{max}) and C is the exponential stiffness constant. A significant increase in C was found in infarcted anterior papillary muscles (table 2). No significant increase in C was seen in hypertrophied posterior papillary muscles from hearts with infarction.

Isometric performance

Resting force was found to be significantly increased in hypertrophied posterior papillary muscles from hearts with infarction in comparison to preparations from sham-operated control animals (table 2). The electromechanical delay time and time-to-peak force were also significantly prolonged in posterior papillary muscle preparations from infarcted hearts in comparison to controls.

The active tension and maximum rate of tension development of anterior (infarcted) preparations was significantly depressed in comparison to sham-operated animals. The electromechanical delay time was markedly prolonged in comparison to values from sham-operated animals. Because of the slow onset of contraction and the low total amplitude of tension present in infarcted muscles, our computer algorithm may have had difficulty in detecting the precise time of onset of mechanical activity. Examination of raw data from contractions obtained in hypertrophied posterior and infarcted anterior papillary muscles (fig. 2) indicate that electromechanical delay time and time-to-peak tension were prolonged following myocardial infarction.

Force-velocity data

Force-velocity data were not significantly different in hypertrophied posterior papillary muscle preparations from hearts with infarction than

Table 2. Papillary muscle mechanics: isometric force parameters at L_{max} and passive stiffness.

	Cross-sect. area	EM delay	Time-to-peak force	Relaxation time (50 %)	Resting force	Active force	Total force	+dF/dt	−dF/dt	Passive stiffness (C)
	(mm^2)	(msec)	(msec)	(msec)	(g/mm^2)	(g/mm^2)	(g/mm^2)	(g/mm^2/sec)	(g/mm^2/sec)	
PPM infarct (n = 9)	1.62±0.15	33.0±1.1	139±4	170±6	2.10±0.20	3.88±0.28	5.98±0.32	42.5±5.1	17.6±1.9	0.214±0.021
	NS	$p < 0.001$	$p<0.01$	NS	$p<0.001$	NS	NS	NS	NS	NS
PPM sham (n = 8)	1.50±0.18	25.0±0.9	120±3	178±14	1.00±0.18	3.72±0.53	4.71±0.67	42.0±5.6	16.3±1.6	0.223±0.013
APM infarct (n = 9)	1.47±0.21	74.2±10.4	120±9	128±5	2.12±0.24	0.78±0.26	2.90±0.32	9.0±2.7	6.3±1.3	0.301±0.023
	$p < 0.05$	$p < 0.001$	NS	$p < 0.05$	NS	$p < 0.001$	$p < 0.001$	$p < 0.001$	$p < 0.001$	$p < 0.01$
APM sham (n = 8)	0.94±0.10	28.9±2.4	116±5	162±16	1.52±0.20	4.47±1.72	5.99±0.68	53.4±7.1	21.8±2.6	0.166±0.012

PPM = posterior papillary muscle
APM = anterior papillary muscle
Values are means ± SEM

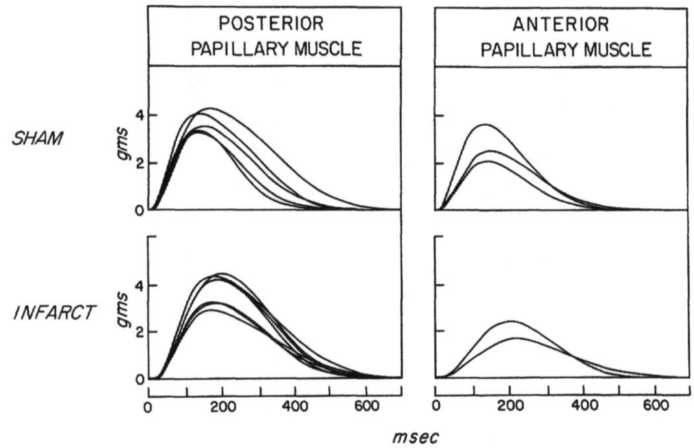

Fig. 2. Isometric contractions from posterior and anterior papillary muscle preparations redrawn from original tracings. As in figure 1, in hearts with coronary occlusion, it is the anterior papillary muscle which is infarcted. Note the relatively slow onset of mechanical activity in both posterior and anterior papillary muscle preparations from hearts with myocardial infarction.

those from sham-operated animals. The force-velocity relations of infarcted anterior papillary muscles were found to be significantly depressed at all loads examined. No differences in force-velocity relationships between anterior and posterior papillary muscles from sham-operated animals were present.

Microscopic data

Sham-operated control preparations demonstrated less than 5 % fibrosis. Fiber diameters from anterior and posterior papillary muscle preparations averaged 12.8 ± 0.99 and 12.9 ± 1.03 μm, respectively. In the

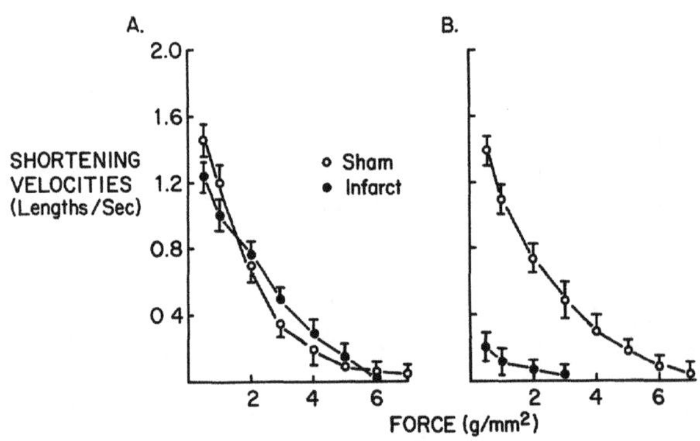

Fig. 3. Quick-release force-velocity relationships. Releases were performed at 50 percent time-to-peak tension (isometric contractions). Velocities were measured at increasing loads 17 msec after release. As in figure 1, A and B indicate data from posterior and anterior papillary muscle preparations, respectively.

infarcted group, between 50 and 75 % fibrosis of the anterior papillary muscles was found, while less than 25 % fibrosis was observed in posterior non-infarcted papillary muscles. The fiber diameters of these preparations were 14.4 ± 1.37 and 17.5 ± 1.28 μm, respectively. Fiber diameters of posterior papillary muscles of the infarcted group were increased compared to posterior papillary muscles from sham-operated control hearts ($p < 0.001$).

Discussion

Although the LV/body weight ratio was not elevated in hearts with infarction in the present study, the noninfarcted papillary muscle was hypertrophied as evidenced by the increase in muscle fiber diameter. This observation is consistent with previous findings by Turek et al. (22) who noted that rats with an old left ventricular infarction demonstrated an increase in muscle fiber diameter of the non-infarcted papillary muscle. In that study, regional hypertrophy was also not accompanied by an increase in total left ventricular mass. Since the LV/BW ratio in animals with a large left ventricular infarction was not different from sham-operated animals, it is likely that hypertrophy was responsible for normalizing this ratio. That is to say, had hypertrophy not developed, myocardial mass lost in the infarcted region would likely have resulted in a decrease in the LV/BW ratio. Turek and co-workers (22) found a similar degree of right ventricular hypertrophy in rats with 4½-week-old myocardial infarctions to that observed in the present study.

Passive stiffness was evaluated in the present study, both by examination of the slope (C) of the resting length-force relationship, and by measuring resting force at L_{max}. A significant increase in C was found only in infarcted muscles, which were found to have over 50 % fibrosis by point counting. Resting force values were found to be elevated only in the non-infarcted hypertrophied papillary muscle. Resting force values at L_{max} are uncertain in the infarcted papillary muscles as it is difficult to define a clear peak in the length-active tension curve (see fig. 1). The resting tension curve is rising steeply, and a small underestimation of L_{max} would have resulted in considerably larger resting tension values at L_{max}.

It is interesting that resting tension values at L_{max} are elevated in the hypertrophied, non-infarcted papillary muscle without an increase in the slope of the stiffness-stress relationships. These studies point out that increased stiffness as measured by C may not necessarily be associated with resting tension elevations. Likewise, preparations with an elevated resting tension at L_{max} may not have an increased C value. The reason for the apparent diversity in findings with respect to indices of stiffness is not clear but may be related to difficulties in defining L_{max}, as pointed out, as well as the quantity, location or properties of collagenous structures within the myocardium. An increase in resting tension of hypertrophied left ventricular papillary muscles measured at L_{max} has been observed previously in cardiac hypertrophy which follows acute aortic banding (2, 3). Stiffness has been reported to be increased in other models of pressure overload hypertrophy as well (1, 12, 16).

Infarcted anterior papillary muscles exhibit considerable depression of both maximum force development and velocity of shortening at all loads. It was of interest that seemingly totally fibrotic myocardium exhibited significant contractile activity. By eye, these muscles were white and frequently adherent to the ventricular wall. Nevertheless, microscopic examination of these preparations revealed approximately 25–50 % persisting myocardium. Thus it is important to consider that apparent scar may contain residual myocardium with the capacity for significant contractile activity.

As has been previously observed, left ventricular hypertrophy in rats due to pressure overload is associated with a variable depression of maximum shortening velocity and a prolonged time-to-peak tension, whereas developed tension and maximum rate of tension development are largely unchanged (2–4, 6, 14, 16). Similar findings are noted in the present study. In addition, the onset of mechanical activity appears to be delayed in both the infarcted anterior and the hypertrophied posterior papillary muscle.

While noninfarcted hypertrophied papillary muscles from hearts with coronary ligation studied 21 days postinfarction do not demonstrate significantly altered force-velocity relationships when compared with muscles from sham-operated animals, there was a tendency for velocity at light loads to be depressed although not to the $p < 0.05$ level of significance. We have also determined force-velocity relations from physiological sequenced contractions (20). It is interesting that a greater depression of shortening velocity at light loads is seen in physiologically sequenced contractions in comparison to quick-release data. Velocities of shortening measured in physiologically sequenced contractions, as in afterloaded isotonic contractions, are measured at progressively later times in the contraction. Velocities at light loads, measured very early, may be relatively depressed if the onset of mechanical activity is slowed as may be the case in models of pressure overload hypertrophy where it has been shown that time-to-peak tension is prolonged (2, 6, 14, 16).

Similar to the situation with acute aortic banding, non-infarcted left ventricular myocardium is suddenly subjected to an acute load after coronary artery occlusion. Findings from hypertrophied myocardium of the rat with myocardial infarction are in large part similar to those in animals subjected to acute banding but appear to differ from studies of chronic, slowly developing hypertrophy (15, 23) or volume overload hypertrophy (7, 21). It further remains to be determined whether the responses to an abruptly imposed load represent an adaptation of the myocardium and/or whether these changes are in part responsible for hemodynamic impairment.

Acknowledgements

The authors wish to thank Susan Pierce for her assistance in the preparation of this manuscript. Data organization and analysis were performed on the Prophet system, a national computer resource sponsored by the Division of Research Resources, National Institutes of Health.

References

1. Alpert, N. R., B. B. Hamrell, W. Halpern: Mechanical and biochemical correlates of cardiac hypertrophy. Circulat. Res. **35** II, 71–82 (1974).
2. Bing, O. H. L., S. Matsushita, B. L. Fanburg, H. J. Levine: Mechanical properties of rat cardiac muscle during experimental hypertrophy. Circulat. Res. **28**, 234–245 (1971).
3. Bing, O. H. L., B. L. Fanburg, W. W. Brooks, S. Matsushita: The effect of the lathyrogen beta-amino proprionitrile on the mechanical properties of experimentally hypertrophied rat cardiac muscle. Circulat. Res. **43**, 632–637 (1978).
4. Bing, O. H. L., A. W. Wiegner: Myocardial mechanics in the spontaneously hypertensive rat: Changes with age (in press).
5. Busch, W.: Die vikarierende Hypertrophie in der linken Herzkammer. Cardiologia (Basel) **22**, 366–371 (1953).
6. Capasso, J. M., J. E. Strobeck, E. H. Sonnenblick: Myocardial mechanical alterations during gradual onset long-term hypertension in rats. Amer. J. Physiol. **241**, H435–H441 (1981).
7. Cooper, G., F. J. Puga, K. J. Zujko, C. E. Harrison, H. N. Coleman: Normal myocardial function and energetics in volume-overloaded hypertrophy in cat. Circulat. Res. **32**, 140–148 (1973).
8. Fishbein, M. C., D. MacLean, P. R. Maroko: Experimental myocardial infarction in the rat. Amer. J. Pathol. **90**, 57–70 (1978).
9. Fishbein, M. C., D. MacLean, P. R. Maroko: The histopathologic evaluation of myocardial infarction. Chest **73**, 843–849 (1978).
10. Friedberg, C. K.: Diseases of the Heart, ed. 3, p. 790, W. B. Saunders (Philadelphia 1966).
11. Gudbjarnason, S., W. Braasch, R. J. Bing: Protein synthesis in cardiac hypertrophy and heart failure. *In:* Heart Failure, Pathophysiological and Clinical Aspects, edited by H. Reindell, G. Stuttgart, Thieme Verlag, p. 184–196 (1968).
12. Jacob, R., B. Brenner, G. Ebrecht, C. Holubarsch, I. Medugorac: Elastic and contractile properties of the myocardium in experimental cardiac hypertrophy of the rat. Methodological and pathological considerations. Basic Res. Cardiol. **75**, 253–261 (1980).
13. Johns, T. P. N., B. J. Olson: Experimental myocardial infarction. I. A method of coronary occlusion in small animals. Ann. Surg. **140**, 675–682 (1954).
14. Jouannot, P., P. Y. Hatt: Rat myocardial mechanics during pressure-induced hypertrophy development and reversal. Amer. J. Physiol. **229**, 355–364 (1974).
15. Julian, F. J., D. L. Morgan, R. L. Moss, M. Gonzalez, P. Dwivedi: Myocyte growth without physiologic impairment in gradually induced rat cardiac hypertrophy. Circulat. Res. **49**, 1300–1310 (1981).
16. Kämmereit, A., R. Jacob: Alterations in rat myocardial mechanics under Goldblatt hypertension and experimental aortic stenosis. Basic Res. Cardiol. **74**, 389–405 (1979).
17. Krebs, H. A., K. Henseleit: Untersuchungen über die Harnstoffbildung im Tierkörper. Z. Physiol. Chem. **210**, 33–66 (1932).
18. Norman, T. D., C. R. Coers: Cardiac hypertrophy after coronary artery ligation in rats. Arch. Path. **69**, 181–184 (1960).
19. Spann, J. F., R. A. Buccino, E. H. Sonnenblick, E. Braunwald: Contractile state of cardiac muscle obtained from cats with experimentally produced ventricular hypertrophy and heart failure. Circulat. Res. **21**, 341–354 (1967).
20. Sulman, D. L., O. H. L. Bing, R. G. Mark, S. K. Burns: Physiologic loading of isolated heart muscle. Biochem. Biophys. Res. Commun. **56**, 947–951 (1974).
21. Taylor, R. R., J. W. Covell, J. Ross: Left ventricular function in experimental aorto-caval fistulae with circulatory congestion and fluid retention. J. Clin. Invest. **47**, 1333–1342 (1968).

22. Turek, Z., M. Grandtner, K. Kubat, B. E. M. Ringnalda, F. Kreuzer: Arterial blood gases, muscle fiber diameter and intercapillary distance in cardiac hypertrophy of rats with an old myocardial infarction. Pflügers Arch. **376,** 209–215 (1978).
23. Williams, J. F. Jr., R. D. Potter: Normal contractile state of hypertrophied myocardium after pulmonary artery constriction in cat. J. Clin. Invest. **54,** 1266–1272 (1974).

Authors' address:

Oscar H. L. Bing, M.D. ACOS/R & D (151), Boston VA Medical Center, 150 S. Huntington Avenue, Boston, Massachusetts 02130, (617) 739–3457, USA

Cardiac Adaptation to Hemodynamic Overload, Training and Stress
Dr. D. Steinkopff Verlag 245–250 (1983)

The interference of respiratory chain function with lipid metabolism in the left ventricular myocardium of rats with compensated chronical volume overload

J. Moravec and J. Nzonzi, with technical assistance of A. Corsin, A. Courtalon, and P. Pocholle

I.N.S.E.R.M. U2, Hôpital Léon Bernard, Limeil-Brévannes (France)

Summary

Isolated atrially perfused hearts from rats with chronical volume overload (3-month-old aorto-caval fistula) were exposed to a 15 min lasting ischemia using the one-way valve developed by Neely. Biochemical consequences of decreated coronary perfusion (50 % of its initial values) were studied and compared to those observed in control hearts. In both groups of hearts, the diffuse ischemia leads to a significant reduction of total pyridine nucleotide and to a significant decrease of adenine nucleotide phosphate potential. In control hearts, a 100 % increase of succinate and of long chain acyl CoA regularly occurs. These latter modifications are considerably attenuated in the hearts from rats with chronical volume overload. This may underlie the improved utilization of the intracellular oxygen previously described in volume-overloaded hearts recovering from transient anoxia (Moravec, 1980).

Key words: chronical volume overload, aorto-caval fistula, isolated perfused rat heart, ischemia, long chain acyl-CoA, succinate

Introduction

In our recent work we showed that, in hearts of rats with one-month-old aorto-caval fistula, both cytochrome aa_3 and pyridine nucleotides can remain fully oxidized at significantly lower intracellular $[O_2]$'s than those required by control hearts (Moravec et al., 1981; Moravec et al., 1982). This apparent decrease of critical pO_2 was followed by an acceleration of reduced pyridine nucleotide reoxidation occurring during the recovery of the overloaded hearts from a short anoxia (Moravec, 1980). In addition, the mechanically overloaded hearts did not accumulate any long chain-acyl esters of CoA which, under similar conditions, were increasing by about 100 % in hearts of control rats (Moravec, 1980). In this work, metabolic changes related to a diffuse ischemia (50 % reduction of coronary flow rate by means of a one-way valve, Neely et al., 1975) were studied. The prospective relationship between respiratory chain function and lipid metabolism was thus re-examined under conditions of a partial inhibition of the electron transport.

Methods

An aorto-caval communication was surgically created in two-month-old female rats. Sham-operated animals were used as controls. The animals were sacrificed three months after the surgery and their hearts were atrially perfused with a bicarbonate buffer containing 10 mM glucose. The perfusate (200 ml) was recirculated. All hearts were preperfused for 15 min. Then, in some of them, a 50 % reduction of coronary flow was induced by the insertion of a one-way valve into the aortic outflow tract (Neely et al., 1973). Left ventricular function was assessed by monitoring of the aortic pressure and of the heart rate. The aortic and coronary flow were measured by means of the appropriate rotameters (Manostat 36-541-12 and 36-541-07). At the end of the perfusion (30 min), the hearts were deep-frozen in liquid nitrogen and the ventricular fragments processed for CP, ATP, ADP and inorganic phosphate. An aliquot of frozen tissue was used for CoA and long-chain acyl CoA (Garland et al., 1965) determinations. Tissue levels of citrate, succinate and that of pyridine nucleotides (NAD and NADH) were determined fluorimetrically (Williamson, 1963).

Results

Under normoxic conditions, the hemodynamic performance of the overloaded heart was comparable to that of controls. The insertion of the one-way valve into the aortic outflow tract was followed in both groups studied by a 50 % decrease of the coronary flow rate and by a 40 % reduction of the aortic ejection. The left ventricular pressure development was less

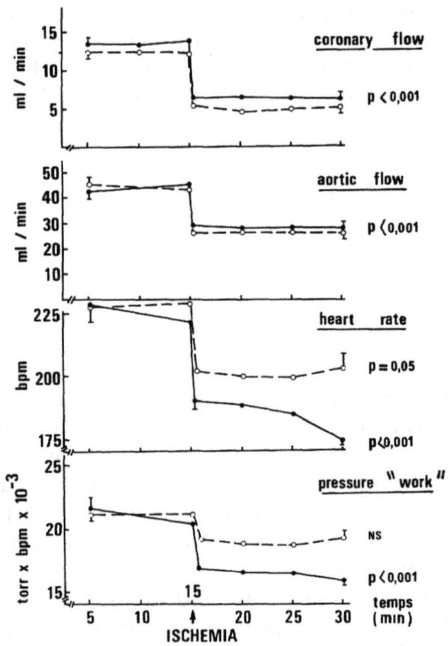

Fig. 1. Hemodynamic effects of reduced coronary flow rate (50 % reduction, 15 min) as observed in control and mechanically overloaded hearts. Note better preservation of the heart rate and of resulting isometric work (HR × peak AoP) in hearts from animals with the aorto-caval fistula (●——● controls, ○ - - - - ○ fistulas).

Table 1. Effect of diffuse ischemia on tissue levels of adenine nucleotides and those of lipid intermediates in isolated hearts from control and overloaded hearts.

		CP	ATP	ADP	Pi	ATP/ ADP · Pi	Long-chain acyl-CoA	Succinate
		(µmoles/gdw)					(nmoles/gdw)	
Control	Normoxic	31.20 ± 2.5	19.00 ± 0.38	3.30 ± 0.10	24.75 ± 1.40	0.24 ± 0.02	133 ± 7	1,375 ± 200
	Ischemic	20.15* ± 1.5	16.80 ± 0.50	4.90 ± 0.10	38.45* ± 3.17	0.08* ± 0.01	256* ± 10	2,695* ± 260
Fistulae	Normoxic	28.81 ± 4.11	18.50 ± 0.98	3.50 ± 0.44	25.40 ± 4.14	0.23 ± 0.03	128 ± 13	1,525 ± 360
	Ischemic	19.9 * ± 2.55	15.75 ± 0.41	3.78 ± 0.28	31.40* ± 2.02	0.14* ± 0.02	153 ± 16	2,202 ± 320

m ± SEM; n = 6–10; * = $p < 0.05$.

affected during the ischemic period. The heart rate was only slightly depressed in the hearts from rats with the aorto-caval fistula. In the control hearts, the acute ischemia was followed by a more pronounced bradycardia and by frequent ectopic beats (fig. 1). Biochemically, the normoxic overloaded hearts resembled their normoxic controls, except for higher steady-state reduction of total tissue pyridine nucleotides. After 15 min of ischemia, the redox states of total pyridine nucleotides decreased considerably in both groups of hearts, the resulting NAD/NADH ratio being not significantly different any longer. On the other hand, following differences between the control and the overloaded hearts have occurred (table 1). The ATP/ADP · Pi ratio fell to 30 % of its normoxic value in the control hearts, it equalled to 60 % in the overloaded one. In addition, the control hearts accumulated a large amount of long-chain acyl esters of CoA during the ischemic period. This accumulation of lipid intermediates was considerably attenuated in the hearts from rats with aorto-caval fistula (table 1). In this respect, our data concerning the succinate concentrations are of interest. In the control hearts exposed to ischemia, the succinate increased by about 100 per cent. Only 40 per cent increase of succinate concentrations occurred in the mechanically overloaded hearts exposed to the same conditions. In both of the ischemic groups, a non-significant increase of citrate concentrations could also be detected.

Discussion

The metabolic effects of acute ischemia on the heart have been extensively studied in the past (Rovetto, 1973; Neely, 1979; Shug et al., 1975). These studies have established that a decrease of oxygen supply to tissue immediately leads to intracellular reduction and rapid loss of left ventricular contractility (Williamson, 1979). The intracellular phosphate potential decreases rapidly (Garfinkel, 1979), which explains the initial activation of the anaerobic glycolysis. Later on, the glycolytic flux becomes limited because of the intracellular acidification (Neely et al., 1975). The utilization of exogenous fatty acids is impaired under ischemic conditions (Neely et al., 1979) and, in the intracellular space, an accumulation of long-chain acyl intermediates of lipid metabolism (acyl carnitine, acyl CoA) has been detected (Shug et al., 1975; Neely et al., 1979). This accumulation of long-chain acyl esters persists even in absence of any exogenous fatty acids. It occurs, perhaps to a smaller extent, in hearts perfused with glucose only (Neely et al., 1979; Moravec, 1980). This suggests that at least one part of long-chain acyl radicals could be generated by the mitochondrial fatty-acid-synthetizing pathway described by Hülsmann (1962). This author demonstrated that the reduction of pyridine nucleotides resulting from an incomplete oxidation of different intermediates of citric acid cycle favors the conversion of labeled acetate into the long-chain acyl moities by isolated cardiac mitochondria. The rate of this acetate incorporation into the mitochondrial lipids is further accelerated under conditions leading to a partial inhibition of the respiratory chain (Hull and Whereat, 1967). In contrast, this process is virtually inexistent when the electron transport and thus the NADH oxidation via respiratory chain is maintained elevated by means of an uncoupler or by exogenous ADP (Whereat, 1967). In vitro,

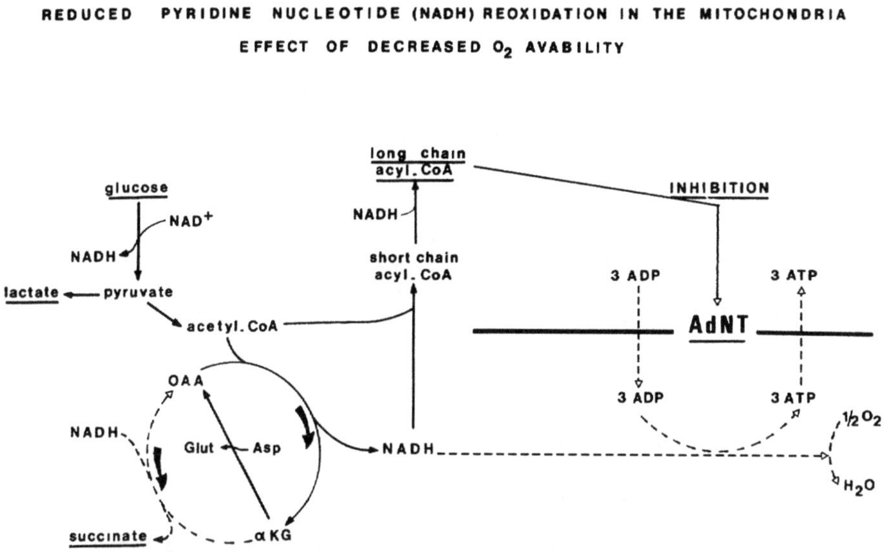

Fig. 2. Schematic representation of the interference between the respiratory chain and lipid metabolism at the level of reduced pyridine nucleotide reoxidation. Under normal condition, most of the NAD^+ necessary for the maintenance of metabolic activity is regenerated by the respiratory chain. Under conditions of decreased oxygenation, the respiratory chain function becomes O_2-limited. Small amounts of NAD^+ can then be regenerated by enhanced transaminations and by the intramitochondrial synthesis of free fatty acids (Whereat, 1967; Hochachka, 1980). During the development of cardiac hypertrophy, the oxygen requirements of the respiratory chain function are decreased. The accumulation of long-chain acyl intermediates of lipid metabolism can thus be attenuated.

the intramitochondrial neo-synthesis of FFA was found stimulated by the succinate (Whereat et al., 1967) which, by the reversal of the first span of the respiratory chain (Klingenberg et al., 1961), can directly generate a large amount of the intramitochondrial NADH. In this respect, it should be noted that succinate has been identified as one of the end products of the hypoxic myocardium (Hochachka, 1977; 1980).

In our work, we found succinate accumulation in the control hearts exposed to 50 % reduction of the coronary flow rate. This succinate accumulation was considerably attenuated in the hearts from rats with the chronical aorto-caval fistula. In the light of this finding, as well as of our previous data concerning the decreased oxygen requirements for respiratory chain oxidation (Moravec, 1980; Moravec et al., 1981), the absence of FFA accumulation in the overloaded hearts exposed to diffuse ischemia can be related to the following factors: (1) improved ability of the respiratory chain to utilize intracellular oxygen, which maintains a residual electron transport and thus the NADH oxidation under conditions of decreased O_2 availability; (2) absence of the excessive succinate accumulation necessary for the initiation of the NADH removal via the reversal of β-oxidation (fig. 2).

References

1. Garfinkel, D., M. J. Achs: Metabolism of the acutely ischemic dog heart. II. Interpretation of a model. Amer. J. Physiol. **5,** R31–R39 (1979).
2. Hochachka, P., J. R. Neely, W. R. Driedric: Integration of lipid metabolism with Krebs cycle activity in muscle. Fed. Proc. **36,** 2009–2014 (1977).
3. Hochachka, P.: Living Without Oxygen. Hochachka, P. (ed.), Harvard University Press (Cambridge, Mass. 1980).
4. Hull, F. E., A. F. Whereat: The effect of rotenone on the regulation of fatty acid synthesis in heart mitochondria. J. Biol. Chem. **242,** 4023–4028 (1967).
5. Hülsmann, W. C.: Citrate-induced synthesis of free fatty acids in rabbit heart mitochondria. Biochim. Biophys. Acta **58,** 417–425 (1962).
6. Moravec, J.: Possible relationships between tissue level of long-chain acyl-CoA and the ability of the overloaded heart to reoxidize an excess of reduced pyridine nucleotide. FEBS Lett. **113,** 134–136 (1980).
7. Moravec, J., M. Moravec, P. Y. Hatt: Rate of pyridine nucleotide oxidation and cytochrome oxidase interaction with intracellular oxygen in hearts from rats with chronical volume overload. Pflügers Arch. **392,** 106–114 (1981).
8. Neely, J. R., M. J. Rovetto, J. T. Whitmar, M. E. Morgan: Effects of ischemia on ventricular function and metabolism in isolated working heart. Amer. J. Physiol. **225,** 651–658 (1973).
9. Neely, J. R., J. T. Whitmar, M. J. Rovetto. – Effect of coronary blood flow on glycolytic flux and intracellular pH in isolated rat hearts. Circulat. Res. **37,** 733–751 (1975).
10. Neely, J. R., D. Garber, K. McDonough, J. Iddel-Wenger: Relationship between ventricular function and intermediates of fatty acid metabolism during myocardial ischemia. In: Ischemic Myocardium and Antianginal Drugs. Winburg, M. M., Abiko, Y (Eds), pp. 225–234 (New York 1979).
11. Shug, A. L., E. Shrago, H. Bittar, J. D. Folts, J. R. Koke: Acyl-CoA inhibition of adenine nucleotide translocation in ischemic myocardium. Amer. J. Physiol. **228,** 689–692 (1975).
12. Whereat, A. F., E. Hull, M. W. Orishimo: The role of succinate in the regulation of fatty acid synthesis by heart mitochondria. J. Biol. Chem. **242,** 4013–4022 (1967).
13. Williamson, J. R., B. E. Corkey: Assay of intermediates of the citric acid cycle and related compounds by fluorimetric methods. In: Methods in Enzymology, vol. 13. Lowenstein, J. M. (ed.), pp. 434–446, Academic Press (New York 1963).
14. Williamson, J. R.: Mitochondrial function in the heart. Ann. Rev. Physiol. **41,** 485–506 (1979).

Authors' address:

Dr. J. Moravec, I.N.S.E.R.M. U2, Hôpital Léon Bernard, Limeil-Brévannes, France

Neuroendocrine, cardiac and vascular alterations in hypertension and stress
– Pathogenesis and effects of interventions –

Cardiac Adaptation to Hemodynamic Overload, Training and Stress
Dr. D. Steinkopff Verlag 253–257 (1983)

Cardiovascular abnormalities in spontaneously hypertensive rats. Causes or consequences of the increased blood pressure?

M. J. Mulvany, E. Mikkelsen, O. Lederballe Pedersen, N. Nyborg, and L. T. Jespersen

Biophysics and Pharmacology Institutes, Aarhus University, Aarhus C (Denmark)

Summary

Three cardiovascular parameters have been investigated in 14-week-old adult spontaneously hypertensive (SHR) and control Wistar-Kyoto (WKY) rats, which had been treated with hydralazine, and in SHR/WKY hybrids (F_2-generation). The three parameters were heart mass/body mass, resistance vessel media thickness/lumen diameter and resistance vessel calcium sensitivity, all of which are increased in adult SHRs. None of these parameters was affected by the anti-hypertensive treatment, although the treatment normalized the blood pressure of the SHRs. In the SHR/WKY hybrids, the only parameter which correlated significantly with blood pressure was resistance vessel calcium sensitivity. The results suggest that none of the parameters investigated is a consequence of hypertension. Furthermore, they suggest that of the parameters only the increased calcium sensitivity of the SHR resistance vessels could be closely associated with the cause of hypertension in 14-week SHRs.

Key words: spontaneously hypertensive rat, cardiac hypertrophy, resistance vessel abnormalities, anti-hypertensive therapy, SHR/WKY hybrids, hypertension, calcium, hydralazine, noradrenaline, tunica media, vascular smooth muscle

Introduction

The increased blood pressure of the spontaneously hypertensive rat is associated with cardiac hypertrophy (Sen et al., 1974) as well as both structural (Folkow et al., 1973) and sensitivity (Lais and Brody, 1978) abnormalities in the resistance vessels. However, it has not been clear whether these abnormalities are causes of the hypertension, as opposed to being consequences of or just incidental to the hypertension. Three strategies have been used to try and clarify this question (for review see Mulvany, 1983). First, investigators have made use of the fact that young SHRs are almost normotensive, so that any abnormalities seen there are not consequences of hypertension. Second, anti-hypertensive therapy has been used to determine whether blood pressure normalization is accompanied by regression of the abnormality: again, the absence of regression would indicate that the abnormality was not a consequence of the hypertension. Finally, cross-breeding experiments have been used to determine whether there is any correlation between blood pressure and the abnormality in the hybrid offspring: such a correlation would indicate that the abnormality was at least not incidental to the hypertension.

In previous investigations of adult SHRs we have also found cardiac hypertrophy (increased heart mass/body mass), as well as evidence for both structural and sensitivity abnormalities in resistance vessels, in that isolated 150-μm resistance vessels had an increased media thickness/lumen diameter and an increased noradrenaline activated calcium sensitivity (Mulvany et al., 1978, 1980a, 1980b). These studies also indicated that heart mass/body mass and resistance vessel calcium sensitivity were increased in young pre-hypertensive SHRs, whereas resistance vessel media thickness/lumen diameter was normal in these young SHRs.

To elucidate further whether these abnormalities are involved in the etiology of hypertension in the SHR, we have here conducted anti-hypertensive experiments as well as a pilot cross-breeding study.

Methods

Spontaneously hypertensive rats (SHRs) and control Wistar-Kyoto rats (WKYs) were supplied at age 4 weeks from Møllegaards Avlslaboratorium, Denmark. In the therapy study, the anti-hypertensive treatment consisted of adding 159 mg/l hydralazine (CIBA) to the drinking water from age 4 weeks. Treatment was stopped 3 days before experiments. For the pilot cross-breeding study, one SHR and one WKY were crossed; the offspring of these (F_1-generation) were then crossed, and the male offspring of these (F_2-generation) were reared. Blood pressures were measured regularly using the tail cuff method.

Rats were sacrificed at age 14 weeks, heart (ventricle) and body masses were determined, and segments of mesenteric resistance vessels were isolated and mounted on an isometric myograph (Mulvany and Halpern, 1976). Vessels were set to internal circumference $L_o = 0.9\ L_{100}$, where L_{100} is an estimate of the internal circumference the vessel would have had in situ under a transmural pressure of 100 mm Hg (Mulvany and Halpern, 1977).

Vessels were normally held in physiological salt solution (PSS) of the following composition (mmol/l): NaCl, 119; $NaHCO_3$, 25; KCl, 4.7; KH_2PO_4, 1.18; $MgSO_4$, 1.17; $CaCl_2$, 2.5; ethylene-diaminetetraacetic acid (EDTA), 0.026; glucose, 5.5, bubbled with 5 % CO_2 in O_2, adjusted to pH 7.4 and held at 37 °C. After 30 min equilibration in PSS, media thickness, m_o, of vessels when held at L_o was determined by light microscopy (Mulvany et al., 1978). Calcium dose response curves were performed as described previously (Mulvany and Nyborg, 1980b) to determine the calcium concentration giving half maximal response when the vessel was activated with 10 μmol/l noradrenaline (Ca-ED_{50}). The negative logarithm of the Ca-ED_{50} (mol/l) was taken as a measure of the resistance vessel calcium sensitivity.

Results

The results of the therapy study are shown in table 1. Although hydralazine treatment prevented the SHRs becoming hypertensive, the treatment had no effect on heart mass/body mass, resistance vessel media thickness/lumen diameter or resistance vessel calcium sensitivity in either SHRs or WKYs. Hydralazine treatment did not affect the blood pressure of the WKYs.

Table 1. Effect of hydralazine treatment on the cardiovascular parameters investigated in spontaneously hypertensive (SHR) and control Wistar-Kyoto (WKY) rats.

		Hydralazine-treated	Control	P
Mean				
Blood pressure	SHR	93 ± 5 (6)	126 ± 9 (6)	P < 0.01
(mm Hg)	WKY	97 ± 5 (6)	98 ± 6 (6)	n. s.
Heart mass / Body mass (mg/g)	SHR	3.54 ± 0.25 (6)	3.47 ± 0.10 (6)	n. s.
	WKY	2.94 ± 0.06 (6)	3.09 ± 0.06 (6)	n. s.
Media thickness / Lumen diameter	SHR	0.070 ± 0.003 (6)	0.077 ± 0.007 (12)	n. s.
	WKY	0.042 ± 0.003 (6)	0.049 ± 0.006 (12)	n. s.
$-\log$ (Ca– ED_{50})	SHR	4.11 ± 0.08 (6)	4.11 ± 0.04 (12)	n. s.
	WKY	3.83 ± 0.01 (6)	3.77 ± 0.03 (12)	n. s.

Six rats per group, 1 or 2 vessels per rat. Values show mean ± SE (number of determinations). P-values show significance of effect of treatment (2-tail t-test). n.s. = not significant ($P > 0.05$). For further details see text.

The results of the pilot cross-breeding experiments were shown in figure 1. In the SHR/WKY hybrids there was no correlation between heart mass/ body mass and blood pressure or between resistance vessel media thickness/lumen diameter and blood pressure. However, there was a significant ($P < 0.05$) correlation between resistance vessel calcium sensitivity and blood pressure.

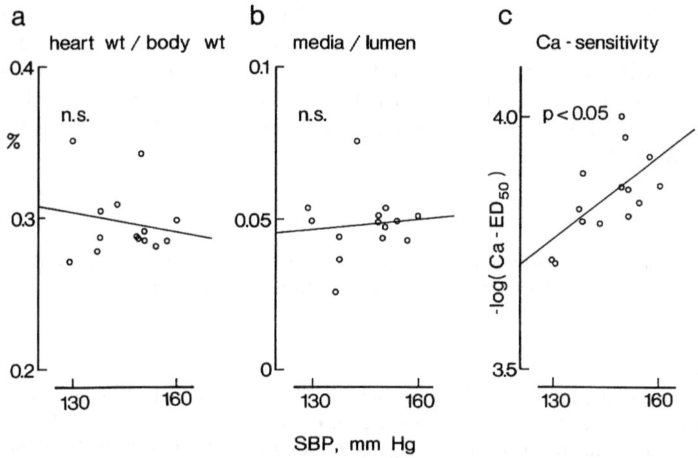

Fig. 1. (a) Heart mass/body mass, (b) resistance vessel media thickness/lumen diameter, (c) resistance vessel calcium sensitivity (negative logarithm of calcium concentration to give half maximal response when activated with 10 µmol/l noradrenaline) as a function of systolic blood pressure (SBP) in hybrid SHR/WKYs (F_2-generation). The lines show the correlation of the parameters on SBP. In (a), (b) the significance of the correlation was not significant (n.s.); in (c) the correlation was significant ($P < 0.05$). For further details see text.

Discussion

The aim of the present study was to investigate whether 3 cardiovascular abnormalities seen in adult (14 wk) SHRs (increased heart mass/body mass; increased resistance vessel media thickness/lumen diameter; increased resistance vessel calcium sensitivity) were causes or effects of the increased blood pressure of these animals.

Heart mass/body mass. This parameter was previously found to be increased in young pre-hypertensive SHRs. Here, the parameter was found to be unaffected by anti-hypertensive treatment. Furthermore the parameter did not correlate with blood pressure in the hybrid SHR/WKYs. It therefore seems that increased heart mass/body mass is not a consequence of increased blood pressure. Thus it appears that this abnormality is a genetic difference between SHRs and WKYs, a difference which is not in itself sufficient to cause hypertension.

Resistance vessel media thickness/lumen diameter. This parameter was previously found to be normal in young pre-hypertensive SHRs (Mulvany et al., 1980a, 1980b), only being increased in SHRs at age 12 weeks or older. The parameter did not, however, normalize as a result of anti-hypertensive treatment, nor did it correlate with blood pressure in the hybrid SHR/WKYs. Therefore, again it seems that the increase which occurs up to age 12 weeks is not a consequence of the increasing blood pressure. Therefore the abnormality may be a genetic difference between SHRs and WKYs, a difference which again is not in itself sufficient to cause high blood pressure.

Resistance vessel calcium sensitivity. This parameter was previously found to be increased in young pre-hypertensive SHRs (Mulvany and Nyborg, 1980). Here we found that the parameter was unaffected by anti-hypertensive treatment, but that it did correlate positively with blood pressure in the hybrid SHR/WKYs. It therefore seems, on the basis of the strategy outlined in the Introduction, that this abnormality is neither a consequence of, nor incidental to, high blood pressure. Indeed, it seems that the abnormality may be closely associated with the cause of hypertension in the SHR.

Acknowledgements

We thank Jørgen Andresen and Lone Larsen for excellent technical assistance. The work was supported by the Danish Medical Research Council.

References

1. Folkow, B., M. Hallbäck, Y. Lundgreen, R. Sivertsson, L. Weiss: Importance of adaptive changes in vascular design for establishment of primary hypertension, studied in man in spontaneously hypertensive rats. Circulat. Res. Suppl. I **32** and **33**, 2–13 (1973).
2. Lais, L. T., M. J. Brody: Vasoconstrictor hyperresponsiveness: an early pathogenic mechanism in the spontaneously hypertensive rat. Europ. J. Pharmacol. **17**, 177–189 (1978).
3. Mulvany, M. J.: Do resistance vessel abnormalities contribute to the elevated blood pressure of spontaneously hypertensive rats? A review of some of the evidence. Blood Vessels **20**, 1–22 (1983).

4. Mulvany, M. J., C. Aalkjær, J. Christensen: Changes in noradrenaline sensitivity and morphology of arterial resistance vessels during development of high blood pressure in spontaneously hypertensive rats. Hypertension **2,** 664–671 (1980a).
5. Mulvany, M. J., W. Halpern: Mechanical properties of vascular smooth muscle cells in situ. Nature **260,** 617–619 (1976).
6. Mulvany, M. J., W. Halpern: Contractile properties of small arterial resistance vessels in spontaneously hypertensive and normotensive rats. Circulat. Res. **41,** 19–26 (1977).
7. Mulvany, M. J., P. K. Hansen, C. Aalkjær: Direct evidence that the greater contractility of resistance vessels in spontaneously hypertensive rats is associated with a narrower lumen, a thicker media and a greater number of smooth muscle cell layers. Circulat. Res. **43,** 854–864 (1978).
8. Mulvany, M. J., N. Nyborg: An increased calcium sensitivity of mesenteric resistance vessels in young and adult spontaneously hypertensive rats. Brit. J. Pharmacol. **71,** 585–596 (1980b).
9. Sen, S., R. C. Tarazi, P. A. Khairallah, F. M. Bumpus: Cardiac hypertrophy in spontaneously hypertensive rats. Circulat. Res. **35,** 775–781 (1974).

Authors' address:

M. J. Mulvany, Biophysics Institute, Universitetsparken 185, DK-8000 Aarhus C, Denmark

Cardiac Adaptation to Hemodynamic Overload, Training and Stress
Dr. D. Steinkopff Verlag 258–264 (1983)

Mechanisms of heart sarcoplasmic reticulum damage under stress

Yu. V. Arkhipenko, V. E. Kagan, and F. Z. Meerson

Institute of General Pathology and Pathological Physiology, U.S.S.R. Academy of Medical Sciences and School of Biology, Moscow State University, Moscow, U.S.S.R.

Summary

It has been demonstrated that emotional painful stress paralleled with activation of lipid peroxidation (LPO) causes functional damage of the Ca^{2+} pump of heart sarcoplasmic reticulum (SR) membranes. Preliminary injection to rats of a free radical scavenger, 4-methyl-2,6-di(tert-butyl)phenol prevents this damage. The observed effects were studied in a model system *"in vitro"* during LPO induction by the Fe^{2+} + ascorbate system in isolated SR membranes. Investigation of mechanisms responsible for Ca^{2+} pump damage induced by LPO showed that the Ca^{2+}-accumulating properties of SR vesicles are decreased due to increased membrane permeability in the lipid bilayer region in which "peroxide clusters" are formed, as well as in the region of protein-lipid interactions. The decrease of Ca-ATPase activity in late steps of LPO is due to the deficiency of polyenoic lipids in the enzmye molecule microenvironment and to formation of intermolecular cross-links.

Key words: sarcoplasmic reticulum, stress, emotional painful, lipid peroxidation, calcium accumulation, calcium transport ATPase, membrane fluidity

Introduction

It is general knowledge that emotional painful stress (EPS) impairs the contractile function of the heart. This is manifested in the hypersensitivity of the myocardium to exogenous Ca^{2+} and in the appearance of local contractures (1, 2). Earlier it was demonstrated that the functional damage of cardiac myocytes is paralleled with an increase in the number of lipid peroxidation (LPO) products (2). The accumulation of these products and the changes in the functional parameters of the heart can be prevented by injection of free radical scavengers prior to EPS. It was therefore assumed that LPO is one of the most essential pathogenetic mechanisms causing heart damage in stress situations.

However, the exact molecular mechanisms of damage of the Ca transport system of sarcoplasmic reticulum (SR) in EPS and the role of LPO in this damage still remain obscure. The present paper sums up the results of an experimental analysis of the role of LPO in SR damage of skeletal and cardiac muscles and postulates possible use of free radical scavengers for prevention or restriction of the damaging effect of LPO on the Ca transport system.

Methods

EPS was induced in Wistar rats as described by Desiderato (3). 4-methyl-2,6-di(tert-butyl-)phenol (butylated hydroxytoluene, BHT) in a dose of 20 mg/kg was injected to rats daily for 3 days as a 5 % suspension in Tween prior to EPS exposure.

The microsomal fractions from rat hearts or from rabbit white skeletal muscles were isolated by the method of Martonosi (4) with slight modifications. Protein was determined by a biuret reaction.

The rate of Ca^{2+} transport and the Ca-ATPase activity of microsomal membranes were measured pH-metrically and by $^{45}CaCl_2$ accumulation. The rate of Ca^{2+} efflux from calcium oxalate-loaded SR vesicles was determined using a Ca^{2+}-selective electrode. The model system of contracting myofibrils was prepared as described in (5). *"In vitro"* activation of LPO in membrane suspension was performed using Fe^{2+} (10 nmole/mg of protein) + ascorbate (2 mM). BHT dissolved in ethanol solution was added to the membrane suspension to a concentration of 5.10^{-5} M. Membrane lipids were extracted in a chloroform-methanol (2:1) system. The amount of phospholipid hydroperoxides in the extracts was determined polarographically with a mercury-dropping electrode (6) or spectrophotometrically ($\lambda = 232$ nm) (7). The end products of LPO, i.e., Schiff bases, were determined from the fluorescence at 350–420 nm (8). The concentration of carbonyl products of LPO in membrane suspension was measured in a reaction with 2-thiobarbituric acid (9). The phospholipid content was determined by thin-layer chromatography on Kieselgel-coated plates ('Merck', No. 5721); the fatty acid composition of phospholipid was established using a 'Perkin-Elmer F22' gas chromatograph unit. Protein composition of the membranes was determined by SDS polyacrylamide gel electrophoresis. The polarity, fluidity, and cluster formation of SR membrane lipids were investigated using TEMPO and TEMPO-palmitate spin labels.

Results

The main structural components of the myocytes that control the level of Ca^{2+} in the sarcoplasm are the SR membranes and sarcolemma. Damage of these structures will inevitably result in the appearance of Ca^{2+} excess in the sarcoplasm. Indeed, table 1 demonstrates that the microsomal fraction from the hearts of control rats, which predominantly consists of SR and sarcolemma, has a far more efficient Ca^{2+} pump than the same fraction of the animals subjected to EPS. When injected prior to EPS exposure, the free radical scavenger, BHT, prevents the damage of the Ca^{2+}-accumulating properties of the microsomal fraction. Thus the damage of the enzymatic system of Ca^{2+} transport induced by LPO activation

Table 1. Parameters of Ca-transport system in heart SR under EPS.

Activity, nmole · min^{-1} · mg of $protein^{-1}$	Control	EPS	BHT	BHT + EPS
Ca-ATPase	502 ± 48	359 ± 77 $P<0.05$	488 ± 71	469 ± 68
Mg-ATPase	694 ± 113	642 ± 103	688 ± 93	640 ± 87
Accumulation of Ca^{2+}	37.2 ± 4.0	23.1 ± 4.2 $P<0.05$	36.2 ± 3.2	29.0 ± 3.8

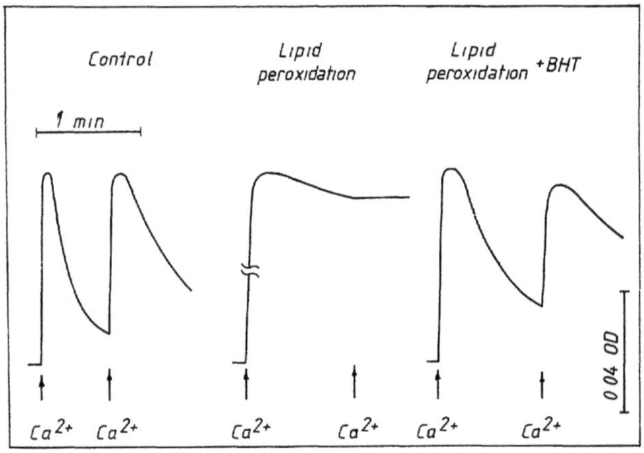

Fig. 1. Myofibrillar contraction-relaxation cycles in the presence of SR vesicles recorded by light-scattering at 540 nm.

under EPS may be a key link in the pathogenetic chain of the stressory damage of the heart.

This assumption can be confirmed by the following data from model experiments. The curves showing the changes in the light-scattering pattern of a suspension containing isolated myofibrils and SR membranes are shown in figure 1. It can be seen that an addition of Ca^{2+} to the incubation medium rapidly increases the turbidity of the membrane suspension due to myofibrillar contraction. However, shortly thereafter the myofibrils are relaxed again, since the SR present in the medium traps practically all the Ca^{2+} inside the vesicles.

Further additions of exogenous Ca^{2+} to this system simulate the contraction-relaxation cycles of the myocardium up to the moment when the medium contains ATP. However, when the LPO process is induced in such a system, no myofibrillar contraction occurs. As under "in vivo" conditions, BHT protects the SR vesicles against the LPO-induced damage. This suggests that LPO activation in SR membrane results in a loss of the Ca^{2+}-accumulating capacity and is associated with myofibrillar contractility impairment.

In order to study the molecular mechanisms causing Ca^{2+} pump damage induced by LPO, we used preparations of skeletal muscle SR possessing more stable functional characteristics than the corresponding fraction from the heart.

The main components of the Ca^{2+}-accumulating system of SR are i) Ca-ATPase (a transmembrane protein responsible for Ca^{2+} transport inside the cisterns), and ii) lipid bilayer possessing low passive permeability for Ca^{2+}

LPO induction in SR membranes by the Fe^{2+} + ascorbate system is accompanied by accumulation of some specific products. Figure 2 shows the kinetics of an increase in the number of primary (phospholipid hydroperoxides and conjugated dienes), secondary (carbonyl compounds of the malonyl dialdehyde type) and end products of LPO (fluorescent Schiff

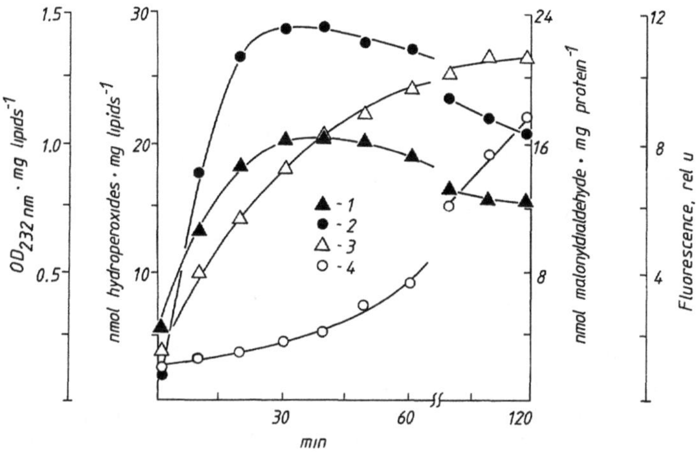

Fig. 2. Accumulation of LPO products in SR membranes induced *"in vitro"* by the Fe^{2+} + ascorbate system. 1 – phospholipid hydroperoxides; 2 – conjugation dienes; 3 – malonyl dialdehyde; 4 – fluorescent products.

bases). Parallel to the accumulation of the above-mentioned products in the SR membranes, the amount of polyunsaturated fatty acyls in the lipids and the amount of the most unsaturated phospholipid, phosphatidyl ethanolamine, are decreased. These alterations in the membrane lipid composition are associated with an emergence of intermolecular protein cross-links and a simultaneous decrease of the protein with a molecular weight of about 10^5 corresponding to Ca-ATPase.

Figure 3 shows the experimental data on the functional parameters of the Ca^{2+} pump. In the course of LPO induction, the Ca/ATP ratio demon-

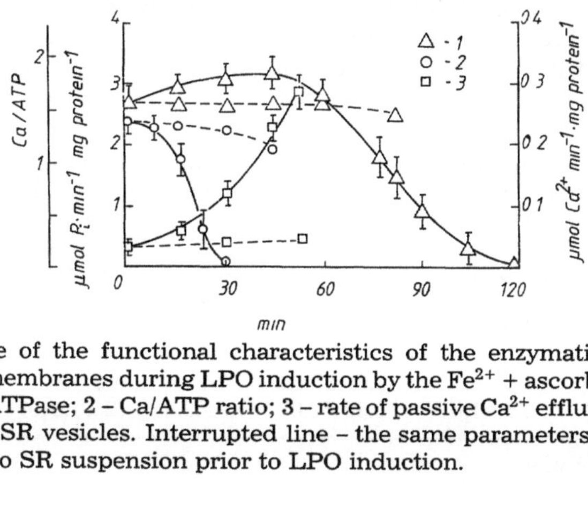

Fig. 3. Damage of the functional characteristics of the enzymatic Ca-transport system in SR membranes during LPO induction by the Fe^{2+} + ascorbate system. 1 – activity of Ca-ATPase; 2 – Ca/ATP ratio; 3 – rate of passive Ca^{2+} efflux from calcium oxalate-loaded SR vesicles. Interrupted line – the same parameters obtained after BHT addition to SR suspension prior to LPO induction.

strating the efficiency of Ca^{2+} pump operation is rapidly decreased. The catalytic activity of Ca-ATPase is far more stable. The main possible causes of Ca^{2+} transport system damage in SR induced by LPO are as follows: i) decrease of the Ca-ATPase activity and increase in the membrane permeability due to impaired complementarity of protein-lipid interactions and, ii) increase of passive Ca^{2+} permeability through the lipid bilayer. These causes of Ca^{2+} transport inhibition were subjected to further analysis.

In the next series of experiments we investigated the changes in passive permeability of SR membranes for Ca^{2+} ions. It appeared that the introduction of Ca^{2+}-loaded vesicles into the incubation medium causes Ca^{2+} efflux as recorded by a Ca^{2+}-selective electrode, the rate of this efflux being nearly directly proportional to the amount of LPO products accumulated by the membrane (fig. 3). We assumed that the increased permeability through the lipid bilayer is due to the formation of the so-called "peroxide clusters". This hypothesis was confirmed by spin probing studies (table 2), which demonstrated that LPO increases both the polarity and the rigidity of the SR lipid bilayer.

In experiments similar to those performed earlier by Lee et al. (10), we made an attempt to determine the number of lipid peroxide clusters in SR. The percentage of lipids involved in cluster formation at 37 °C after LPO amounts to 20 %. Our concept on peroxide cluster formation has been described in a recently published paper (11). In addition it is of interest to mention that according to Levitsky et al. (12) the peroxide-formed channels are Ca^{2+}-selective.

The predominant substrates of LPO are polyunsaturated phospholipids. This indicates that in SR membranes exposed to LPO the polyunsaturated fatty acids are accumulated in peroxide clusters, whereas the other regions of the membranes, e.g., lipid bilayer and microenvironment of Ca-ATPase, are almost devoid of them. Meanwhile numerous reports from other laboratories suggest that Ca-ATPase requires a fluid lipid matrix for its function. In other words, the deficiency of polyenoic lipids resulting from lipid redistribution induced by LPO should cause inhibition of the enzyme.

We may then expect that the addition of polyenoic lipids to a membrane suspension will induce reactivation of the enzyme. The next experimental data illustrate this phenomenon. Unsaturated lipids, e.g., egg lecithin, can

Table 2. Changes of hydrophobicity constant (h) and percentage of lipids in three regions of sarcoplasmic reticulum membrane under lipid peroxidation.

Conditions	nmole MDA*. $min^{-1} \cdot mg$ of $protein^{-1}$	h	Percentage of lipids		
			liquid in bilayer	ordered in bilayer	immobilized by protein
Control	1.6±0.2	0.65±0.03	65.0±5.4	2.0±0.1	36.0±3.0
LPO induction	16.4±1.8	0.39±0.02	49.0±3.8	25.0±1.4	22.0±1.9

* malonyldialdehyde

reactivate the enzyme in contrast to saturated ones, e.g., dipalmitoyl lecithin, that do not produce such an effect (not shown). Thus we may see that one of possible causes of Ca-ATPase inhibition is the deficiency of polyenoic lipids in the enzyme microenvironment; this inhibition is of a reversible type.

It should be emphasized that the reactivating influence of even the most unsaturated phospholipids is incomplete, since the activity of Ca-ATPase never reaches the original level. This indicates that there may be some other causes of the enzyme inhibition. For instance, LPO is known to give rise to formation of covalent intermolecular cross-links. The formation of these cross-links is mediated by the secondary products of LPO, i.e., by dialdehydes which interact with free amino groups of proteins and phospholipids. This is associated with an appearance of fluorescent pigments and occurs only after a certain lag period (fig. 2). It can easily be understood, therefore, that Ca-ATPase reactivation by unsaturated phospholipids is all the more complete, the less is the time elapsed from the onset of LPO induction to the moment of reactivation.

Hence LPO induces a loss of the Ca^{2+}-accumulating properties of SR as a result of the increased permeability of the membrane and inhibition of Ca-ATPase. The pathophysiological implications of LPO are obvious and consist in impairment of excitation-contraction coupling and, consequently, in impaired muscle contractility.

Sad as it may be, the accumulation of LPO products in muscle cells takes place in myocardial infarction, ischemia and in reoxygenation-induced lesions of the heart as well as in myopathies caused by alimentary vitamin E deficiency, aging, etc. The results of the present investigation demonstrate a high potency of free radical scavengers in preventing the accumulation of LPO products and in protecting the enzymic system of Ca^{2+} transport of SR vesicles against inhibition. We may thus conclude that the use of free radical scavengers as cardioprotectors opens new glamorous vistas for biochemists and cardiologists.

Conclusions

1. LPO is responsible for the damage of the Ca-transport system of heart SR under EPS.
2. Induction of LPO in SR membranes *"in vivo"* upon stress is associated with the same functional disturbances as take place during LPO induction *"in vitro"* in SR vesicles by the Fe^{2+} + ascorbate system.
3. The SR damage caused by LPO induction *"in vivo"* and *"in vitro"* can be prevented by the free radical scavenger, 4-methyl-2,6-di(tert-butyl)-phenol.
4. The damage of the Ca-transport system of SR during LPO is due to increased passive permeability of the membrane for Ca^{2+} caused by i) Ca^{2+} efflux from SR vesicles through the lipid bilayer mediated by "peroxide clusters" and, ii) impaired complementarity of lipid interactions with membrane-bound proteins.
5. Ca-ATPase is more resistant to LPO than the membrane permeability. The fall of the rate of ATP hydrolysis by the enzyme is caused by

simultaneous reversible (due to deficiency of polyenoic lipids in the enzyme microenvironment) and irreversible (due to formation of intermolecular cross-links) inhibition of Ca-ATPase.

References

1. Meerson, F. Z., M. V. Shimkovich, V. A. Khorunzhiy: Effect of emotional painful stress on cardiac muscle response to variation in calcium concentration. Bull. Exp. Biol. Med. **89,** 272–274 (1980).
2. Meerson, F. Z., V. V. Malyshev, V. E. Kagan, L. I. Treschuk, I. I. Rozhitskaya: Activation of lipid peroxidation and focal contracture injuries to the myocardium at emotional painful stress. Arch. Pathol. **42,** 9–12 (1980).
3. Desiderato, O., J. MacKinnon, H. Hisson: Development of gastric ulcers in rats following stress termination. J. Comp. Physiol. **87,** 208–214 (1974).
4. Martonosi, A., J. Donley, R. A. Halpin: Sarcoplasmic reticulum. III. The role of phospholipids in the adenosine triphosphatase activity and Ca^{++} transport. J. Biol. Chem. **243,** 61–70 (1968).
5. Gusev, N. B., V. B. Ritov: Study on membrane-myofibrills interaction with contractility model. Dokl. AN SSSR **208,** 1231–1234 (1973).
6. Danilov, V. S., M. V. Sitkovsky, V. E. Kagan, Yu. P. Kozlov: Study of lipid peroxidation in normal and pathological cases by polarographic method. Izv. AN SSSR, Ser. Biol. 574–579 (1972).
7. Bolland, J. L., H. P. Koch: The course of autoxidation reactions in polyisoprenes and allied compounds. Part IX. The primary thermal oxidation products of ethyl linoleate. J. Chem. Soc. **7,** 445–447 (1945).
8. Bidlack, W. R., A. L. Tappel: Fluorescence products of phospholipids during lipid peroxidation. Lipids **8,** 203–209 (1973).
9. Kohn, H. J., M. Liversedge: On a new aerobic metabolite whose production by brain is inhibited by apomorphine, emetine, ergotamine, epinephrine, and menadione. J. Pharm. Exp. Ther. **82,** 292–300 (1944).
10. Lee, A. G., N. J. M. Birdsall, J. C. Metcalf, P. A. Toon, J. B. Warren: Clusters in lipid bilayers and the interpretation of thermal effects in biological membranes. Biochemistry **13,** 3699–3705 (1974).
11. Meerson, F. Z., V. E. Kagan, Yu. P. Kozlov, L. M. Belkina, Yu. V. Arkhipenko: The role of lipid peroxidation in pathogenesis of ischemic damage and antioxidative protection of heart. Basic Res. Cardiol. **77,** No. 5 (1982).
12. Lebedev, A. V., D. O. Levitskij, V. A. Loginov: Oxygen as inducer of calcium translocation across lipid bilayer membranes. Dokl. AN SSSR **252,** 1494–1497 (1980).

Authors' address:

Dr. Yu. V. Arkhipenko, Institute of General Pathology and Pathological Physiology, U.S.S.R. Academy of Medical Sciences, Baltijskaya ul. 8, Moscow 125315, U.S.S.R.

Cardiac Adaptation to Hemodynamic Overload, Training and Stress
Dr. D. Steinkopff Verlag 265–266 (1983)

Changes of heart catecholamine levels, metabolism and adrenergic receptors in acutely and repeatedly stressed rats

R. Kvetňanský and T. Torda

Institute of Experimental Endocrinology, Centre of Physiological Sciences, Slovak Academy of Sciences, Bratislava (Czechoslovakia)

The activity of the adrenergic system in the myocardium was studied in rats exposed to stress immobilization (IMO) daily for 150 minutes.

Norepinephrine (NE) concentration in the myocardium was significantly decreased after the first IMO, and in the course of adaptation to repeated stress it kept gradually returning to values recorded in unstressed controls. Epinephrine (EPI) concentration in the heart displayed a manifold increase already after the first IMO and remained elevated also after repeated exposure to this stressor. The reduced NE level seen after the first IMO is conceivably caused by its release due to enhanced activation of noradrenalinergic neurons, which is a phenomenon common to all sympathetically innervated organs under stress. The unchanged NE concentration found in the myocardium of repeatedly IMO rats is presumably the result of increased synthesis of catecholamines (CA), as indicated also by the significantly increased activity of CA-synthesizing enzymes, tyrosine hydroxylase and dopamine-β-hydroxylase, determined in the myocardium of these animals. This unchanged NE concentration in repeatedly IMO rats may also be caused by its altered degradation. We determined the activity of CA-degrading enzymes, catechol-O-methyltransferase and monoamine oxidase, and found them to be decreased in the myocardium of repeatedly IMO rats, suggesting a possible involvement of degradation mechanisms in the increased NE levels.

The elevated EPI concentration in the myocardium of stressed rats appears to be the result of increased uptake from the circulation, as the plasma EPI level showed an up to 40-fold increase after the first IMO.

Thus the presented results show that the myocardium of repeatedly stressed rats has higher CA levels, compared to acutely stressed animals, and that is assumed to be due to their increased synthesis and decreased degradation. This phenomenon might represent one of the factors responsible for the development of hypertension found in some of the animals repeatedly immobilized.

On the one hand, then, we found higher CA levels in the myocardium, yet, on the other hand, repeatedly IMO rats which were pithed responded to EPI administration by a significantly diminished increase of blood pressure and heart rate. We therefore determined the number and affinity of beta and $alpha_1$ adrenergic receptors in the myocardium of IMO rats. In acutely IMO rats the receptors were found unchanged, whereas in repeatedly IMO rats the number of beta and $alpha_1$ receptors was decreased, yet their affinity remained unchanged.

On balance then, these results suggest that the adaptation of the adrenergic system in the myocardium to repeated stress occurs at the level of adrenergic receptors, whose desensitization might represent a defense mechanism protecting the organism from CA hyperproduction, and that particularly in repeatedly stressed

Abbreviations: MAO = monoamine oxidase, COMT = catechol-O-methyltransferase, PNMT = phenylethanolamine-N-methyltransferase animals. Thus hypertension induced by repeated stress might be the consequence of derangement of the mechanisms responsible for the desensitization of adrenergic receptors in sympathetically innervated organs.

Key words: rat, catecholamines, adrenergic receptors, myocardium, immobilization stress, hypertension, catecholamine-synthesizing and degrading enzymes, tyrosin, hydroxylase, dopamin-β-hydroxylase

Authors' address:

Dr. R. Kvetňanský, Institute of Experimental Endocrinology, Centre of Physiological Sciences, Slovak Academy of Sciences, Vlárska Str. 3, 833 06 Bratislava, Czechoslovakia

Cardiac Adaptation to Hemodynamic Overload, Training and Stress
Dr. D. Steinkopff Verlag 267–273 (1983)

Modulation of catecholamine synthesizing and degrading enzymes by swimming and emotional excitation in the rat

H. Rupp, A. R. Bukhari, and R. Jacob

Physiologisches Institut II der Universität Tübingen (FRG)

Summary

The activities of catecholamine enzymes have been determined in adrenal glands of Wistar rats following 2 and 6 weeks of intermittent swimming (max. 2 × 90 min daily in 35 °C warm water) and 6 weeks intermittent experimentally induced emotional excitation ("shock-induced aggression"). Following 2 weeks swimming, there was no significant change in activities of phenylethanolamine-N-methyltransferase (PNMT) and catechol-O-methyltransferase (COMT); monoamine oxidase (MAO) activity was significantly increased. In contrast, a swimming routine extending over 6 weeks resulted in significantly reduced activities of PNMT, COMT, and MAO. Intermittent emotional excitation of the same time-course extending over 6 weeks did not significantly affect the enzyme activities. Qualitatively similar changes were observed in the heart. It is concluded that the reduced activities of PNMT, COMT and MAO following 6 weeks swimming do not arise from stress elicited by the present swimming routine, but can be attributed to the effects of exercise, such as reduced sympathetic nerve activity.

In order to test the concept of altered enzyme levels, particularly of PNMT, as being diagnostic for changes in transmitter utilization, rats were treated with drugs known to interfere with normal catecholamine turnover. For this purpose, rats were chronically infused with isoproterenol and propranolol which are expected to induce a reflex increase in sympathetic activity. The expected effect on catecholamine enzymes would thus be opposite to that observed following swimming exercise. The rats were infused with isoproterenol (0.02 and 5 mg/kg daily) and propranolol (5 mg/kg daily) using osmotic minipumps. The lower dose of isoproterenol resulted in a significant increase of only PNMT activity in adrenal glands, whereas the higher dose of isoproterenol additionally increased significantly COMT and MAO activities. Propranolol induced a significant increase in COMT and PNMT activities in adrenal glands. In the heart, the activities of PNMT, COMT, and MAO were increased following isoproterenol and propranolol infusion. These results corroborate the above conclusions on 6 weeks' swimming-induced changes in catecholamine enzymes as arising predominantly from effects of exercise.

Key words: swimming, emotional excitation, stress, exercise, monoamine oxidase, catechol-O-methyltransferase, phenylethanolamine-N-methyltransferase, isoproterenol, propranolol

Introduction

In the framework of studies on reactions of the cardiovascular system to chronically altered functional demands (9), the role of the adrenergic system has been evaluated. In the present paper, activities of enzymes involved in catecholamine metabolism are described for functional states involving exercise and experimentally induced emotional excitation (also termed "shock-induced aggression" (8)). The catecholamine-synthesizing enzyme PNMT and the -degrading enzymes MAO and COMT can occur in different concentrations in a tissue. The tissue level of the enzymes provides a means of controlling long-term changes in adrenergic transmitter utilization. Chronically repeated sustained sympathetic nerve stimulation is known to result in increased levels of catecholamine synthesizing enzymes (22) for maintaining normal or increased adrenergic transmitter concentrations. In the present approach, the activities of PNMT, MAO, and COMT were determined in hearts and adrenals of Wistar rats following intermittent swimming and experimentally induced emotional excitation. In order to corroborate conclusions on transmitter turnover based on enzyme activities, the effect of interventions known to result in reflex increase of sympathetic nerve activity on PNMT, MAO, and COMT activities was investigated.

Methods

Animals and materials

15-week-old male Wistar (WU) rats were obtained from Ivanovas (Kissleg, FRG). Rats received a pellet diet (Ssniff, Soest, FRG) and tap water ad libitum. dl-propranolol hydrochloride was from EGA Chemie (Steinheim, FRG) and (±)-isoproterenol hydrochloride from Sigma (München, FRG), S-adenosyl-L-[methyl-^{14}C] methionine from CEA (Saclay, France) and tryptamine bisuccinate, [side chain-2-^{14}C]- from New England Nuclear (Boston, USA). All other chemicals were of analytical grade.

Experimental procedures

Protocols of intermittent swimming and emotional excitation extending over 6 weeks were as reported by Rupp et al. (20), with the exception that swimming was carried out with 30 rats/m^2 surface area. Chronic infusion of propranolol and isoproterenol in the conscious, unrestrained rat was carried out using ALZET model 2002 osmotic minipumps. The pumps released their content continuously at a rate of 0.46 ± 0.03 µl/h over 2 weeks. Minipumps were implanted containing propranolol (21) in a concentration corresponding to a daily release of 5 mg/kg. Isoproterenol concentrations were adjusted to result in a daily release of 5 mg/kg and 0.02 mg/kg. All solutions also contained 0.9 % NaCl and ascorbic acid (20 mg/l) as an antioxidant. The rats were killed by decapitation; rats subjected to swimming or the procedure resulting in emotional excitation were killed approximately 17–24 h after the last experimental procedure.

Assay of MAO, COMT, and PNMT

Left ventricles and adrenal glands were homogenized in 2 ml 0.9 % KCl, the homogenates were divided into two parts. The first part was diluted 1:10 (v/v) for determination of MAO activity, and protein determination according to Lowry et al. (15). The second part was centrifuged at 50,000 × g for 30 min at 1 °C. The supernatant was used for determination of COMT and PNMT activities. MAO was determined using tryptamine [^{14}C]bisuccinate, and COMT and PNMT were determined using S-adenosyl[methyl-^{14}C]methionine as described by Parvez and Parvez (19). The activities of MAO, COMT, and PNMT were expressed in cpm/mg protein. The extracted cpm was linearly proportional to the product formed.

Statistics

Results were expressed as means ± SE. The significance between two means was assessed with Student's t-test.

Body weight, left ventricular weight, and weight of adrenal glands

Compared to control rats, body weight was reduced by 14 % ($P < 0.001$) following 2 weeks of intermittent swimming, 19 % ($P < 0.001$) following 6 weeks of intermittent swimming and 17 % ($P < 0.001$) in rats subjected to a protocol resulting in intermittent emotional excitation (6 weeks). Left ventricular weight was not significantly affected by swimming, but was reduced by 8 % ($P < 0.01$) following the protocol resulting in emotional excitation. The weight of adrenal glands was not altered significantly by 2 weeks' swimming, but was increased by 22 % ($P < 0.01$) following 6 weeks' swimming. Intermittent emotional excitation (6 weeks) induced an 8 % increase ($P < 0.01$) in weight of adrenal glands. Chronic infusion of isoproterenol and propranolol only affected body weight in the case of infusion of 5 mg/kg isoproterenol: At sacrifice, body weight was increased by 10 % ($P < 0.05$). Left ventricular weight was also altered only by infusion of 5 mg/kg isoproterenol (+22 %, $P < 0.01$). Weight of adrenal glands was increased following propranolol infusion (5 mg/kg) by 36 % ($P < 0.01$). Infusion of isoproterenol had no significant influence.

Results

Enzyme activities of PNMT, COMT, and MAO were determined in adrenals of Wistar rats following a swimming routine extending over 2 and 6 weeks. Figure 1 shows activities of PNMT, MAO, and COMT related to control values of sedentary rats. Following 2 weeks' swimming, comprising 19 h total swimming time, MAO activity was significantly increased, not, however, COMT and PNMT activities. Within the next 4 weeks of swimming (2 × 90 min/day, 72 h total swimming time), a marked decrease in activities of the three enzymes was observed. It should be noted that activities of the adrenaline-synthesizing enzyme PNMT as well as of catecholamine-degrading enzymes COMT and MAO were reduced. In contrast, intermittent emotional excitation did not result in reduction of the three enzyme activities (not shown), although the time course was

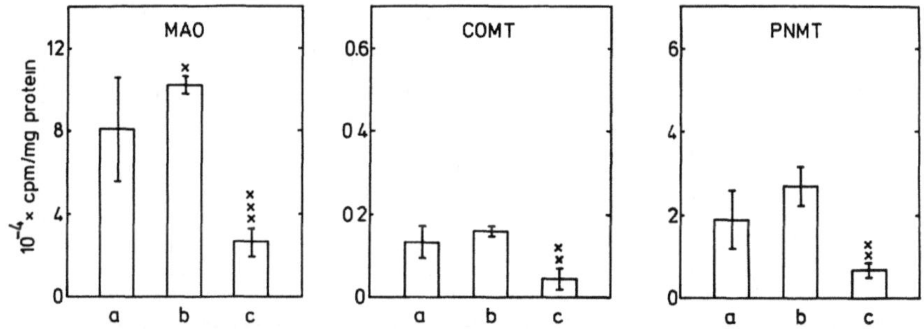

Fig. 1. Activities of MAO, COMT, and PNMT in adrenal glands of Wistar rats subjected to intermittent swimming (b) for 2 weeks ($n = 7$) and (c) 6 weeks ($n = 8$). x = $P < 0.05$, xx = $P < 0.01$, xxx = $P < 0.001$ compared to (a) the respective groups of age-matched control rats (same number of rats as in experimental groups).

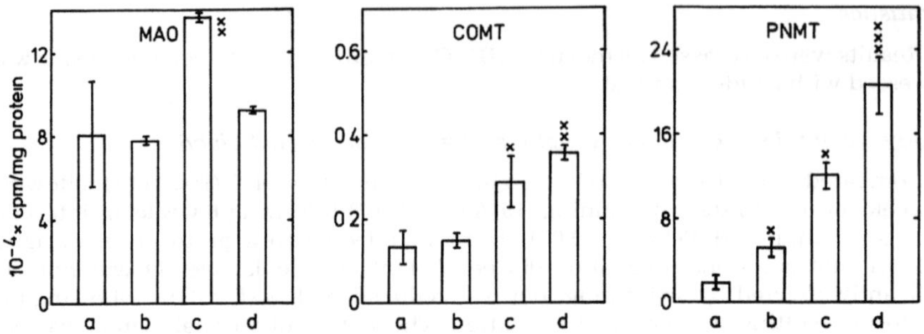

Fig. 2. Activities of MAO, COMT, and PNMT in adrenal glands of (a) Wistar control rats (n = 5) and Wistar rats following chronic infusion of isoproterenol corresponding to daily doses of (b) 0.02 mg/kg (n = 5), (c) 5 mg/kg (n = 5) and chronic infusion of propranolol (n = 5) corresponding to a daily dose of (d) 5 mg/kg. x = $P < 0.05$, xx = $P < 0.01$, xxx = $P < 0.001$.

identical. Qualitatively similar changes were observed in the heart (unpublished data).

In order to corroborate conclusions on transmitter turnover based on enzyme levels, Wistar rats were treated with propranolol (5 mg/kg daily) by continuous infusion over 2 weeks using osmotic minipumps. This treatment resulted in an increase in COMT and PNMT activities in adrenal glands as well as of MAO, COMT, and PNMT in the heart (fig. 2d and 3d). An increase in enzyme activities was also observed following chronic infusion of isoproterenol. The β-agonist was infused in 2 doses (daily 0.02 mg/kg and 5 mg/kg). In adrenal glands, the lower dose elicited a significant increase in PNMT activity (fig. 2b); the higher dose additionally induced increased activities of MAO and COMT (fig. 2c). In the heart, the activities of MAO, COMT, and PNMT were increased following infusion of 0.02 mg/kg (fig. 3b) and 5 mg/kg isoproterenol (fig. 3c).

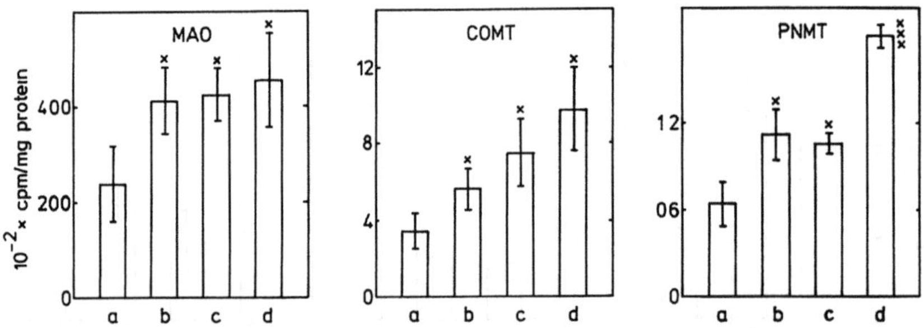

Fig. 3. Activities of MAO, COMT, and PNMT in left ventricles of (a) Wistar control rats and Wistar rats following chronic infusion of isoproterenol corresponding to daily doses of (b) 0.02 mg/kg, (c) 5 mg/kg and infusion of propranolol corresponding to a daily dose of (d) 5 mg/kg. Number of rats same as in figure 2. x = $P < 0.05$, xxx = $P < 0.001$.

Discussion

Chronically repeated, sustained sympathetic nerve stimulation results in increased synthesis of enzymes involved in catecholamine biosynthesis (22). For example, concentrations of tyrosine hydroxylase, dopamine β-hydroxylase, and PNMT were increased following forced immobilization (10–13). Also after psychosocial stimulation, tyrosine hydroxylase and PNMT activities were increased (1). These changes in enzyme activities can be considered as long-term adaptation to increased transmitter utilization. While concentrations of enzymes involved in biosynthesis are increased, degrading enzymes were found to be decreased. Examples of decreased enzyme levels are forced immobilization (12, 14) and exposure to strong environmental stimuli (16). The altered enzyme concentrations provide a mechanism for maintaining normal or increased adrenergic transmitter concentrations in functional states characterized by high transmitter turnover.

Although the present protocol induced the typical signs of aggressiveness and aggression (8), such as fighting, presenting flank and assuming the boxing position, and reduced the body weight, the activities of PNMT, COMT, and MAO were not significantly altered in adrenals. This indicates that the stressor was less severe than, for example, forced immobilization. In contrast, intermittent swimming over 5 weeks resulted in pronounced changes in the enzyme activities. When swimming was carried out under conditions which most probably avoided hypothermia and exhaustion (7), the activity of adrenal PNMT was decreased compared to sedentary control rats and was thus changed in a manner opposite to that generally assumed as resulting from severe stress. Furthermore, the activities of COMT and MAO were significantly reduced. These results suggest reduced transmitter turnover in adrenal glands. It can thus be concluded that the changes in catecholamine enzymes following 6 weeks of intermittent swimming arise from the effects of exercise, such as reduced sympathetic nerve activity.

The concept of enzyme levels as being diagnostic of transmitter utilization is supported by the effect of isoproterenol and propranolol on catecholamine enzymes: propranolol is expected to induce a reflex increase in sympathetic nerve activity as is the case with other drugs which interfere with post-ganglionic sympathetic transmission (2, 3). The expected effect would thus be opposite to that observed following 6 weeks intermittent swimming. As shown in figures 2 and 3, the activities of PNMT were indeed increased following chronic infusion of the β-adrenoreceptor blocking agent. In this respect, it is noteworthy that cardiac MAO, which is predominantly of extraneuronal origin, was increased, as was found also following bilateral adrenalectomy and which was attributed primarily to an increase in intraneuronal MAO (6). Similar results were obtained by chronically infusing isoproterenol, which probably results also in increased activity of the adrenergic system owing to its vasodilating action (4). Whether other mechanisms contribute to greatly increased enzyme activities after isoproterenol infusions requires further investigation, particularly in view of the finding that ganglionectomy did not prevent the effect of isoproterenol on MAO in salivary glands of the rat

(17). By extrapolating from the increased levels of MAO, COMT, and PNMT – attributable at least partially to chronically increased sympathetic nerve activity – to functional states characterized by the opposite change in enzyme levels, one has to assume reduced sympathetic nerve stimulation in rats following the above described swimming routine. Whether other factors, such as depletion of ACTH, contribute to the changes in catecholamine enzyme activities, particularly of PNMT (1, 5), remains to be clarified. In favour of the notion of reduced sympathetic nerve activity are the studies of Östman-Smith, who found reduced urinary excretion of catecholamines at rest and after swimming (18). In sum, there is good evidence that the changes in catecholamine enzymes following the swimming routine can be attributed to effects of exercise, such as reduced sympathetic nerve activity.

Acknowledgements

This study was supported by the Deutsche Forschungsgemeinschaft (Ja 172/13). The expert technical assistance of L. Schwarz is gratefully acknowledged.

References

1. Axelrod, J., R. A. Mueller, J. P. Henry, P. M. Stephens: Changes in enzymes involved in the biosynthesis and metabolism of noradrenaline and adrenaline after psychosocial stimulation. Nature **225,** 1059–1060 (1970).
2. Bhagat, B., W. J. Burke, J. W. Davis: Effect of reserpine on the activity of adrenal enzymes involved in the synthesis of adrenaline. Brit. J. Pharmacol. **43,** 819–827 (1971).
3. Bhagat, B. D.: Regulation of norepinephrine contents in cardiac sympathetic neuron during high impulse activity: alterations in monoamine oxidase activity. Recent Advan. in Studies on Cardiac Struct. Metabolism **3,** 343–356 (1973).
4. Bhagat, B. D., J. M. Sullivan, N. S. Dhalla: Alterations in norepinephrine pattern in the damaged myocardium in the rat. Recent Advan. in Studies on Cardiac Struct. Metabolism **6,** 159–165 (1975).
5. Ciaranello, R. D., G. F. Wooten, J. Axelrod: Regulation of rat adrenal dopamine β-hydroxylase. II. Receptor interaction in the regulation of enzyme synthesis and degradation. Brain Res. **113,** 349–362 (1976).
6. Clarke, D. E., S. S. Sampath: Neurogenic influences of bilateral adrenalectomy on monoamine oxidase. J. Pharm. Sci. **65,** 92–95 (1976).
7. Dawson, C. A., S. M. Horvath: Swimming in small laboratory animals. Medicine and Science in Sports **2,** 51–78 (1970).
8. Eichelman, B. S., Jr.: Effect of subcortical lesions on shock-induced aggression in the rat. J. Comp. Physiol. Psychol. **74,** 331–339 (1971).
9. Jacob, R., G. Kissling, G. Ebrecht, C. Holubarsch, I. Medugorac, H. Rupp: Adaptive and pathological alterations in experimental cardiac hypertrophy. In: Advances in Myocardiology, Vol. 4, Chazov, E., V. Saks, G. Rona (eds.), pp. 55–78. Plenum Medical Book Company (New York 1982).
10. Kvetňanský, R., V. K. Weise, I. J. Kopin: Elevation of adrenal tyrosine hydroxylase and phenylethanolamine-N-methyl transferase by repeated immobilization of rats. Endocrinology **87,** 744–749 (1970).
11. Kvetňanský, R., G. P. Gewirtz, V. K. Weise, I. J. Kopin: Enhanced synthesis of adrenal dopamine β-hydroxylase induced by repeated immobilization in rats. Mol. Pharmacol. **7,** 81–86 (1971).

12. Kvetňanský, R., T. Torda, E. Jahnová, N. Saleh: Activity of catecholamine degrading enzymes in rat adrenal medulla and cortex after acute and repeated stress. Endocr. Exp. **9,** 79–86 (1975).
13. Kvetňanský, R., I. Albrecht, T. Torda, N. Saleh, E. Jahnova, L. Mikulaj: Effect of stress on catecholamine synthesizing and degrading enzymes in control and spontaneously hypertensive rats. In: Catecholamines and Stress, Usdin, E., R. Kvetňanský, I. J. Kopin (eds.), 237–249. Pergamon Press (Oxford 1976).
14. Kvetňanský, R.: Recent progress in catecholamines under stress. In: Catecholamines and Stress: Recent Advances, Usdin, E., R. Kvetňanský, I. J. Kopin (eds.), 7–18. Elsevier North Holland, Inc. (Amsterdam 1980).
15. Lowry, O. H., N. J. Rosebrough, A. L. Farr, R. J. Randall: Protein measurement with the folin phenol reagent. J. Biol. Chem. **193,** 265–275 (1951).
16. Maura, G., A. Vaccari, A. Gemignani, F. Cugurra: Development of monoamine oxidase activity after chronic environmental stress in the rat. Environ. Physiol. Biochem. **4,** 64–79 (1974).
17. Mueller, R. A., J. de Champlain, J. Axelrod: Increased monoamine oxidase activity in isoproterenol-stimulated submaxillary glands. Biochem. Pharmacol. **17,** 2455–2461 (1968).
18. Östman-Smith, I.: Adaptive changes in the sympathetic nervous system and some effector organs of the rat following long term exercise or cold acclimation and the role of cardiac sympathetic nerves in the genesis of compensatory cardiac hypertrophy. Acta Physiol. Scand. Suppl. **477,** 1–118 (1979).
19. Parvez, H., S. Parvez: Microradioisotopic determination of enzymes COMT, PNMT and MAO in a single tissue homogenate. Clin. Chim. Acta **46,** 85–92 (1973).
20. Rupp, H., H.-R. Felbier, R. Jacob: Blood pressure and cardiac myosin heterogeneity in the rat as influenced by swimming and emotional excitation. This issue, p. 274–281.
21. Smits, J. F. M., H. van Essen, H. A. J. Struyker-Boudier: Cardiovascular effects of chronic infusion of propranolol in the conscious spontaneously hypertensive rat. J. Pharm. Pharmacol. **32,** 139–140 (1980).
22. Thoenen, H.: Trans-synaptic enzyme induction. Life Sci. **14,** 223–235 (1974).

Authors' address:

Physiologisches Institut II der Universität Tübingen, Gmelinstraße 5, 7400 Tübingen, FRG

Cardiac Adaptation to Hemodynamic Overload, Training and Stress
Dr. D. Steinkopff Verlag 274–281 (1983)

Blood pressure and cardiac myosin heterogeneity in the rat as influenced by swimming and emotional excitation

H. Rupp, H.-R. Felbier, and R. Jacob

Physiologisches Institut II der Universität Tübingen (FRG)

Summary

The influence of 6 weeks intermittent swimming or experimentally induced emotional excitation (also termed "shock-induced aggression") on blood pressure and cardiac myosin heterogeneity of male Wistar and spontaneously hypertensive (SH) rats was investigated. Swimming was carried out under conditions avoiding hypothermia and exhaustion. Emotional excitation was induced by subjecting rats in pairs to unpredictable electric stimulation. Daily swimming extending over 6 weeks resulted in significantly reduced systolic blood pressure in normotensive Wistar rats (70 ± 7 mm Hg vs. 83 ± 12 mm Hg of controls) and SHR (109 ± 5 mm Hg vs. 137 ± 16 mm Hg of controls). Experimentally induced emotional excitation of the same time course as swimming did not alter significantly blood pressure of Wistar rats and SHR. The reduction in blood pressure following swimming was accompanied by a shift of the left ventricular myosin isoenzyme population in favour of ventricular myosin (VM)–1 in Wistar rats (78.7 ± 3.9 % VM–1 vs. 59.4 ± 7.8 % VM–1 of controls) and SHR (60.9 ± 3.4 % VM–1 vs. 36.7 ± 5.2 % VM–1 of controls). Experimentally induced emotional excitation did not affect significantly the myosin isoenzyme population of Wistar rats, but led to a significant decrease in VM–1 in SHR (29.3 ± 4.8 % VM–1 vs. 36.9 ± 4.9 % VM–1 of controls). It is concluded that the changes following swimming cannot be attributed solely to stress, which may be elicited by the present swimming routine, but arise predominantly from the exercise component of swimming.

Key words: blood pressure, myosin isoenzymes, swimming, emotional excitation, stress, exercise

Introduction

Swimming of rats is generally used as a model of exercise. However, beside the exercise component of swimming, stress arising from failure of the escape reaction and from pronounced interactions of the rats in water has to be considered. Stress is probably unavoidable whenever a large number of rats are subjected to swimming in a limited area. The question therefore arose as to whether changes, particularly in blood pressure and cardiac myosin heterogeneity following swimming (14, 15), arise predominantly from the effect of exercise or from stressors inherent in the swimming procedure. For the present approach a procedure was, therefore, devised, which induced emotional excitation and led to aggressions [also termed "shock-induced aggression" (5)], without significant accompanying physical activity. This treatment was chosen, since it was accompanied by pronounced social interaction as encountered during the present swimming routine. If the effects on blood pressure and myosin heterogeneity were due to stress elicited by swimming, one would expect more marked alterations following experimentally induced emotional excitation of the same time course, since the severity of such elicited stress would appear to be greater compared to that arising from swimming. The influence of swimming and emotional excitation was studied in relation to blood pressure and cardiac myosin isoenzyme profile in normotensive and spontaneously hypertensive (SH) rats.

Methods

Animals and materials

15-week-old male Wistar (WU) rats and age-matched male SHR of the Aoki-Okamoto strain were obtained from Ivanovas (Kisslegg, FRG). Rats received a pellet diet (Ssniff, Soest, FRG) and tap water ad libitum. Reagents for polyacrylamide gel electrophoresis were from Serva (Heidelberg, FRG). All other chemicals were standard laboratory reagents of analytical grade whenever possible.

Experimental procedures

Swimming of rats was performed in a tub (95 × 60 cm) of approximately 40 cm water depth. Water temperature at the beginning of swimming was 35 ± 0.5 °C, it fell to 33 ± 0.5 °C after 90 min. Swimming was started with 10 min and was increased in daily 10 min steps. A swimming time exceeding 100 min was divided into a morning and afternoon routine of equal duration. Maximum swimming time was 2 × 90 min daily. On weekends swimming time was 90 min. Swimming was carried out with 32 rats. No attempts were made to interfere with the natural behaviour of rats in water. 2 rats died during the swimming routine. Aggressive behaviour was induced by subjecting rats in pairs to unpredictable electric stimulation. The design of the experimental chamber was similar to that described by Desiderato & Testa (3). It was modified to accommodate 8 pairs of rats. It consisted of a box with a 100 × 100 cm floor. In the centre of the box was a platform (50 × 50 cm) elevated 5cm from the floor. The chamber was surrounded by 80 cm high walls. The box was divided by 8 walls (80 cm high), which were fixed at the centre of the square, into 8 compartments of triangular shape. Both platform and floor were covered with metal grids which were connected to the negative outputs of 2 constant-current shock sources (Stimulator I, Sachs Hugstetten, FRG). To complete the circuit, a tail electrode, held against the base of the tail by a spring, was connected to the positive outputs of both shock sources. The tail electrodes were suspended from the top of the chamber to each triangular shaped compartment in a manner which allowed the rats to move freely. Floor and platform were charged independently. The stimulation pattern was for the floor: a pulse train of 20 sec duration consisting of 14 pulses of 2.5 mA intensity and 0.1 sec width delivered every 15 min. For the platform: 2 pulses of 0.5–1 mA intensity and 0.1 sec width with a 2 sec interval were delivered every 10 sec. A conflict due to the different stimulation pattern was unlikely to evolve in the present procedure, since 2 rats were in one compartment which resulted in aggressive behaviour and led to fighting. The complex stimulation pattern combined with the differently charged floor and platform grids resulted in unpredictable electric stimuli. All rats were killed approximately 17–24 h following the last experimental procedure.

Blood pressure recording

Rats were daily habituated to the procedure 1 week before the experiments started. Systolic blood pressure was measured using a plethysmographic method

(2), whereby the temperature of the tail was kept at 28 °C. The conscious rat was kept under a black cloth by hand and was restrained as little as possible. Effective cuff length was 21 mm; a pressure of approximately 15 mmHg was necessary for inflating total lumen of the cuff. Heart rate of rats during the measurements was increased typically by 5 % compared to values measured in the unhandled rat under normal cage activity. Blood pressure recording was carried out approximately 17–20 h following the last experimental procedure.

Pyrophosphate gel electrophoresis

Methods were as described by Rupp and Jacob (15).

Statistics

Results were expressed as mean ± SE. The significance between two groups of data was assessed with Student's t-test. Statistical significance was considered to be $P < 0.05$.

Changes in body weight and heart weight

Following 6 weeks intermittent swimming or experimentally induced emotional excitation, body weight of the experimental Wistar rats was reduced at sacrifice: swimming Wistar rats 268 ± 14 g vs. controls 351 ± 22 g ($P < 0.001$); stimulated Wistar rats 295 ± 12 g vs. controls 354 ± 23 g ($P < 0.001$); body weight of SHR at sacrifice was also reduced: swimming SHR 225 ± 10 g vs. controls 309 ± 15 g ($P < 0.001$); stimulated SHR 274 ± 16 g vs. controls 328 ± 12 g ($P < 0.001$). Swimming did not significantly affect ventricular weight. Emotional excitation reduced left ventricular weight of Wistar rats and SHR by 8 % ($P < 0.01$).

Results

Blood pressure

Blood pressure was measured on the tail of the conscious rat using a plethysmographic procedure. A swimming routine extending over 6 weeks resulted in reduction of blood pressure both in Wistar rats and SHR (fig. 1). In swimming SHR, reduced blood pressure did not reach levels typical for sedentary Wistar rats. Following 6 weeks of intermittent experimentally induced emotional excitation blood pressure was not significantly altered (fig. 1). In the present approach, no distinction was made between rats on the basis of dominant and subdominant behaviour.

Myosin heterogeneity

The representative stained pyrophosphate gels in figure 2 show myosins from left ventricles of normotensive Wistar rats and SHR. The quantitative changes in the myosin isoenzyme profile are shown in figure 3. The relative amount of VM–1 (given as a percentage) was determined from densitometric gel scans. The data correspond to average values of isoenzyme profiles of different rats which were analyzed separately. In 21-week-old sedentary Wistar rats, the VM–1 isoenzyme was predominant, whereas in the corresponding sedentary SHR the isoenzyme population was shifted towards VM–3. Swimming induced a shift towards VM–1, irrespective of the initial blood pressure and thus of initial pressure load of the heart. The isoenzyme VM–1 was the predominant isoenzyme both in

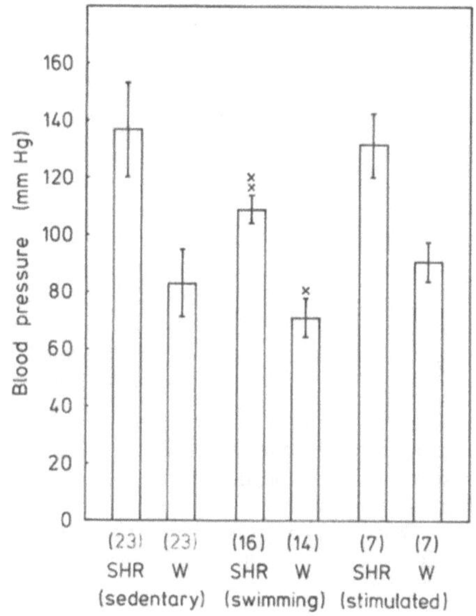

Fig. 1. Systolic blood pressure of Wistar rats and SHR subjected to intermittent swimming and emotional excitation. Number of rats is given in brackets. The blood pressure values of sedentary control rats were not significantly different for the 2 experimental groups and were combined. Statistical significance was, however, derived for the respective individual groups; x = $P < 0.005$, xx = $P < 0.001$ compared to the sedentary, age-matched control rats.

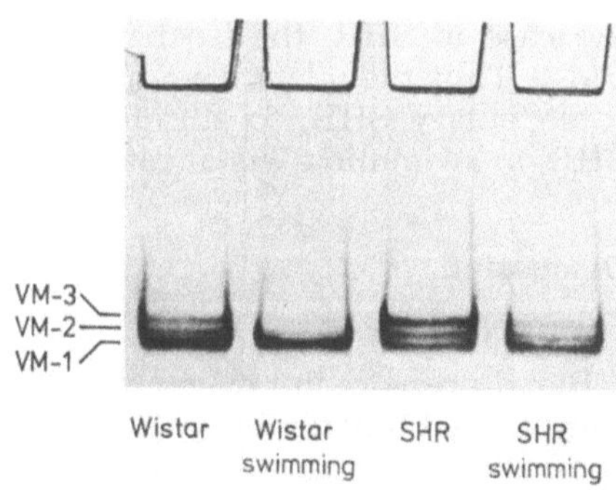

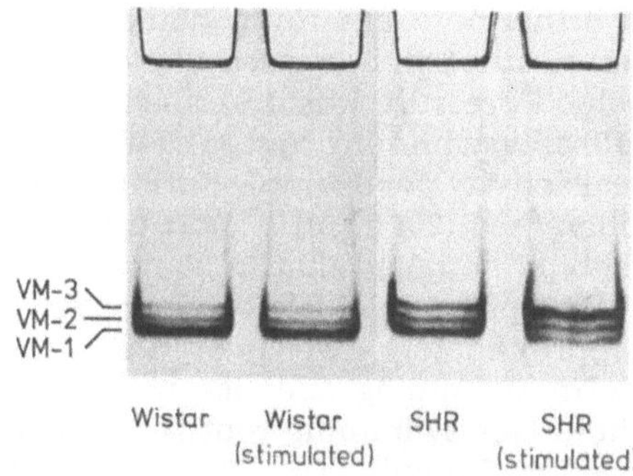

Fig. 2. Representative pyrophosphate gels of myosins isolated from individual rat left ventricles. VM-1, VM-2, VM-3 represent myosin isoenzymes differing in electrophoretic mobility based on the nomenclature proposed by Zak (21). A similar resolution was obtained for all cardiac myosins which were used for calculation of the proportion of VM-1 in figure 3.

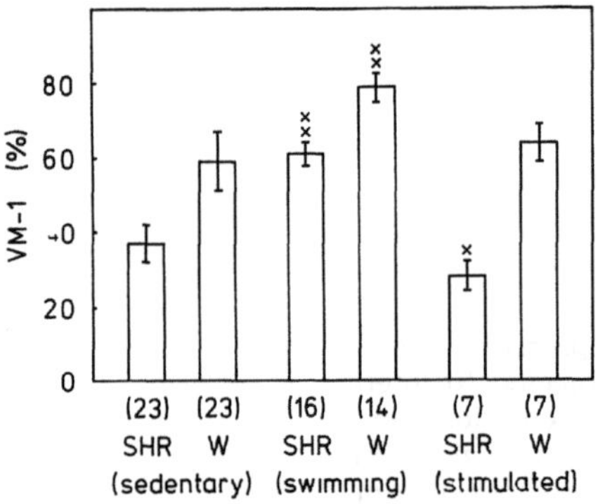

Fig. 3. Proportion of VM–1 given as a percentage for (n) rats. VM–1 did not differ significantly between control rats for the swimming and aggression groups, and the controls were combined. Densitometric gel scans were carried out two to three times on different positions for each sample. Typically, the variation was less than 1 %. Statistical significance was derived for the respective individual groups; x = $P < 0.01$, xx = $P < 0.001$ compared to the sedentary, age-matched control rats.

normotensive and SH swimming rats. SHR subjected to the swimming routine exhibited a myosin isoenzyme profile similar to that of sedentary Wistar rats. The myosin isoenzyme population of left ventricles of rats subjected to emotional excitation differed from sedentary controls only in the case of SHR: the isoenzyme population was changed in favour of VM–3. Thus the relative amount of VM–1 increased from stimulated SHR to sedentary SHR, to stimulated and sedentary Wistar and swimming SHR, to swimming Wistar rats.

Discussion

Blood pressure

Blood pressure in rats can be regarded as a sensitive marker of chronically altered functional states. Sustained increased blood pressure, on the one hand, was induced by different types of stressors in normotensive as well as hypertensive rats. A critical determinant of elevated blood pressure seems to be conflict evolving from operant conditioning (6–8, 11). Furthermore, environmental stimuli (17, 20) and psychosocial stimulation (1) resulted in increased blood pressure. On the other hand, reduction of blood pressure was described following different running procedures (4, 18) and swimming routines (15). When stress appeared with intense physical activity, for example during forced immobilization, blood pressure was increased (20) or on a short time scale reduced (10, 12). In this respect, it should be noted that in contrast to forced immobilization, which caused blood pressure of SHR to increase again to values of sedentary SHR after approximately 4 weeks of intermittent stress (12), SHR subjected to long-term swimming exercise maintain their reduced blood pressure. This holds for swimming routines extending over 6 weeks (present study) as well as 5 months (15). Thus, blood pressure reduction by swimming can hardly be attributed solely to stress elicited by swimming. This is corroborated by the unchanged blood pressure following experimentally induced emotional excitation. The lack of effect on blood pressure of the procedure resulting in emotional excitation is not unexpected, since firstly, it did not involve operant conditioning or strong physical stressors (as employed for example in ref. 9), secondly, it was not combined with marked physical activity.

Myosin heterogeneity

The marked influence of swimming on myosin isoenzymes was a contrast to the effect of aggressiveness. In the latter case, the isoenzyme profile was not altered in normotensive Wistar rats; and it was slightly shifted towards VM-3 in SHR. The changes seen following the swimming routine can thus hardly be ascribed merely to stress which may be elicited by swimming. In our opinion this conclusion is justified, since emotional excitation as induced by the present procedure represents such features also encountered during swimming as: emotional stress due to the failure of the escape reaction and strong psychosocial stimulation due to pronounced interaction of individual rats. Whereas fighting and dominant/subdominant behaviour evolved in the aggressive rats, signs of aggression were rarely observed in swimming rats as judged by tail bites. Stress elicited by the procedure leading to emotional excitation was thus most probably more severe compared to that arising from swimming.

As regards possible mechanisms responsible for the changes seen in the myosin isoenzyme population, the influence of thyroid hormones and of catecholamines should be considered. Although concentrations of circulating free thyroid hormones could be altered as a result of swimming, we tend not to consider them to be major contributing factors in the effects seen following swimming. This assumption is corroborated by an unaltered intrinsic rate of intact, isolated hearts from chronically swim-exercised rats (13). As regards altered catecholamine metabolism, there are indications that swimming reduces sympathetic nerve activity at rest as judged from bradycardia of swimming rats (16, 19). Repeated sustained sympathetic stimulation in the face of low sympathetic nerve activity at rest could thus be responsible for the redistribution of the myosin isoenzyme population towards VM-1 in swimming rats (15). In contrast, emotional excitation is expected to induce also increased sympathetic activity not, however, effects typical of lowered activity at rest, such as bradycardia. This point could be considered as a factor contributing to the further shift of the isoenzymes towards VM-3 in the case of the stimulated SHR which already exhibit hyperresponsiveness of the adrenergic system in the sedentary state. Whether or not other factors contribute to the changes observed in the isoenzyme population as a result of exercise and stressors leading to emotional excitation has yet to be established. In this respect it should be noted that normalized blood pressure in SHR does not necessarily result in normalized isoenzyme profile. Blood pressure reduction by the vasodilator hydralazine, for example, does not reverse the isoenzyme population in favour of VM-3, which is characteristic for pressure-loaded hearts. This is probably due to reflex increase in sympathetic nerve activity and withdrawal of parasympathetic tone following vasodilation, which would not occur in swimming rats. Findings on the differential effect of various antihypertensive agents with respect to blood pressure and cardiac myosin isoenzyme population will be reported elsewhere.

Acknowledgements

This study was supported by the Deutsche Forschungsgemeinschaft (Ja 172/13). The expert technical assistance of L. Schwarz is gratefully acknowledged.

References

1. Alexander, N.: Psychosocial hypertension in members of a Wistar rat colony (38063). Proc. Soc. Exper. Biol. & Med. **146,** 163–169 (1974).
2. Byrom, F. B., C. Wilson: A plethysmographic method for measuring systolic blood pressure in the intact rat. J. Physiol. (London) **93,** 301–304 (1938).
3. Desiderato, O., M. Testa: Shock-stress, gastric secretion and habituation in the chronic gastric fistula rat. Physiol. Behav. **16,** 67–73 (1976).
4. Edwards, M. T., J. N. Diana: Effect of exercise on pre- and post-capillary resistance in the spontaneously hypertensive rat. Amer. J. Physiol. **234,** H439–H446 (1978).
5. Eichelman, B.: Biogenic amines and their metabolism in the study of aggressive behaviour in rats. In: Frontiers in Catecholamine Research, Usdin, E., S. Snyder (eds.) 709–710 Pergamon Press (Oxford 1973).
6. Falk, J. L., M. Tang, S. Forman: Schedule-induced chronic hypertension. Psychosom. Med. **39,** 252–263 (1977).
7. Friedman, R., L. K. Dahl: The effect of chronic conflict on the blood pressure of rats with a genetic susceptibility to experimental hypertension. Psychosom. Med. **37,** 402–416 (1975).
8. Friedman, R., J. Iwai: Genetic predisposition and stress-induced hypertension. Science **193,** 161–162 (1976).
9. Hudak, W. J., J. P. Buckley: Production of hypertensive rats by experimental stress. J. Pharm. Sci. **50,** 263–264 (1961).
10. Kvetňanský, R., R. McCarty, N. B. Thoa, C. R. Lake, I. J. Kopin: Sympatho-adrenal responses of spontaneously hypertensive rats to immobilization stress. Amer. J. Physiol. **236,** H457–H462 (1979).
11. Lawler, J. E., G. F. Barker, J. W. Hubbard, R. G. Schaub: Pathophysiological changes associated with stress-induced hypertension in the borderline hypertensive rat. Clin. Sci. **59,** 307s–310s (1980).
12. Nagatsu, T., T. Kato, K. Fujita, H. Takahashi, T. Inoue, R. Teradaira, H. Beppu, K. Kawai, K. Maruta, S. Yagyu, T. Sato: Catecholamine synthesizing enzymes of spontaneously hypertensive rats under stress. In: Catecholamines and Stress: Recent advances, Usdin, E., R. Kvetňanský, I. J. Kopin (eds.) 339–348 Elsevier North Holland, Inc. (Amsterdam 1980).
13. Östman-Smith, I.: Adaptive changes in the sympathetic nervous system and some effector organs of the rat following long term exercise or cold acclimation and the role of cardiac sympathetic nerves in the genesis of compensatory cardiac hypertrophy. Acta Physiol. Scand. Suppl. **477,** 1–118 (1979).
14. Rupp, H.: The adaptive changes in the isoenzyme pattern of myosin from hypertrophied rat myocardium as a result of pressure overload and physical training. Basic Res. Cardiol. **76,** 79–88 (1981).
15. Rupp, H., R. Jacob: Response of blood pressure and cardiac myosin polymorphism to swimming training in the spontaneously hypertensive rat. Can. J. Physiol. Pharmacol. **60,** 1098–1103 (1982).

16. Schaible, T. F., J. Scheuer: Effects of physical training by running or swimming on ventricular performance of rat hearts. J. Appl. Physiol. **46,** 854–860 (1979).
17. Smookler, H. H., J. P. Buckley: Effect of drugs on animals exposed to chronic environmental stress. Fed. Proc. **29,** 1980–1984 (1970).
18. Suzuki, S., S. Oshima, M. Higuchi: Influence of physical exercise and nutrition on blood pressure of SHR. Jap. Heart J. **20,** Suppl. I, 365–367 (1979).
19. Tipton, C. M.: Training and bradycardia in rats. Amer J. Physiol. **209,** 1089–1094 (1965).
20. Yamori, Y., M. Matsumoto, H. Yamabe, K. Okamoto: Augmentation of spontaneous hypertension by chronic stress in rats. Jap. Circulation J. **33,** 399–409 (1969).
21. Zak, R.: Contractile function as a determinant of muscle growth. In: Cell and Muscle Motility, Vol. 1, Dowben, R. M., J. W. Shay (eds.) 1–33 Plenum Publishing Corporation (New York 1981).

Authors' address:

Physiologisches Institut II der Universität Tübingen, Gmelinstraße 5, 7400 Tübingen, FRG

Cardiac Adaptation to Hemodynamic Overload, Training and Stress
Dr. D. Steinkopff Verlag 282–287 (1983)

Calcium-antagonism: A new therapeutic access to hypertensive heart disease

W. Motz and B. E. Strauer

Medizinische Klinik I, Klinikum Großhadern, Ludwig-Maximilians-Universität München (FRG)

Summary

We studied in spontaneously hypertensive rats (SHR) whether a chronic antihypertensive treatment with the calcium antagonist nifedipine can prevent later deterioration in left ventricular (LV) function as frequently seen in sustained arterial hypertension. After treatment (60 weeks) with nifedipine (30 mg/kg body weight and day), LV pumping function was considerably augmented (cardiac index: + 25.7 %; LV ejection fraction: + 13 %) due to a marked systolic unloading of the left ventricle (systolic wall stress: −22.9 %) in comparison to untreated animals. Myocardial isometric function, which was assessed by the maximum actively developed LV systolic wall stress when totally occluding the proximal aorta, remained preserved in the nifedipine group whereas it decreased by 10.9 % in the untreated subjects. We conclude that in SHR later LV dysfunction can be prevented by an early onset of antihypertensive treatment with nifedipine.

Key words: nifedipine, left ventricular function, myocardial contractility, left ventricular afterload, left ventricular hypertrophy, left ventricular systolic wall stress, left ventricular systolic wall stress reserve

Introduction

Due to its distinct potency to relax arteriolar vascular smooth muscle, the calcium antagonist nifedipine is used successfully in the treatment of arterial hypertension (1, 2). In the course of long-standing arterial hypertension, impairment in cardiac function is frequently observed (3–5). Hence it was the goal of the study to investigate whether left ventricular (LV) function and myocardial contractility can be preserved by an early begin of an antihypertensive treatment with nifedipine.

Methods

Experiments were performed in spontaneously hypertensive rats (SHR, Okamoto-strain), after 20, 40 and 60 weeks of treatment with nifedipine. Therapy was started at the age of 4 to 5 weeks. Nifedipine (30 mg/kg body weight and day, Bayer AG, Wuppertal, Federal Republic of Germany) was mixed with standard rat food and given as a substitute for normal food.

Left ventricular hemodynamics

Central hemodynamics were measured under ether anesthesia. Cardiac output was determined by means of an electromagnetic flow probe around the ascending aorta, LV pressure by directly puncturing the left ventricle at the apex with a fluid-filled steel cannula connected to a Statham pressure transducer (P23DB). After having completed the hemodynamic recordings (Hellige recording system), the heart was arrested in diastole by means of adenosine solution (2). On the basis of a passive pressure-volume curve, each end-diastolic pressure was related to its corresponding end-diastolic volume. Using this pressure-volume relationship, LV ejection fraction was determined from end-diastolic volume and stroke volume. Systolic wall stress was calculated from the peak systolic LV pressure, and the diastolic LV dimensions using a spherical model according to LaPlace (2). Maximum attainable systolic wall stress was determined by totally occluding the ascending aorta with a silk thread.

Left ventricular hypertrophy

LV hypertrophy was determined by means of the LV muscle mass related to body weight (LV/BW).

Statistical evaluations

Statistical calculations were made by using Student's t-test for unpaired data. Differences at the 95 % level were considered significant. The p-values denote statistical significant difference from untreated SHR. All values in the table and figures are means ± standard deviations (SD) (6).

Results

The table lists LV peak systolic pressure (P_{LV}), LV peak systolic wall stress (T_{syst}), cardiac index (CI), LV ejection fraction (EF), heart rate (HR), LV filling pressure (P_{LVED}) and LV muscle mass related to body weight (LV/BW) after a 60-week-long treatment with nifedipine in comparison to untreated animals.

Figure 1 displays ejection fraction, figure 2 maximum developed systolic wall stress (T_{max}) when occluding totally the ascending aorta and figure 3 systolic wall stress reserve, i.e., the quotient of maximum systolic wall stress (T_{max}) and instantaneous systolic wall stress (T_{syst}).

Discussion

The results demonstrate that blood pressure control by nifedipine can prevent later cardiac dysfunction as observed in untreated animals.

The peripheral vasodilating properties of nifedipine (7) are reflected in its marked LV systolic unloading and antihypertensive efficiency as shown by the lower LV afterload expressed as wall stress in the nifedipine-group in comparison to the untreated animals.

An inverse relationship between wall stress, i.e., afterload and LV ejection fraction, was found in patients with essential hypertension as well as aortic stenosis and aortic incompetence (5, 8). With an increase in systolic wall stress, LV ejection fraction progressively decreased (5, 8, 9). Accordingly, the considerably enhanced pumping function (by 20–30 %) after

Table

		P_{LV}	T_{syst}	CI	EF	HR	P_{LVED}	LV/BW
		mm Hg	10^3 dyn/cm^2	ml/min kg	%	l/min	mm Hg	mg/g
SHR, untreated	$\bar{x}$	171	214	175	54	307	5.8	2.76
n = 10	SD ±	26.9	36.3	32.8	7.8	25	3.3	0.16
SHR, treated with	$\bar{x}$	116	165	220	61	325	5.0	2.37
nifedipine, 60 weeks. n = 7	SD ±	26.8	51.8	27.4	6.3	26	0.9	0.27
	p	< 0.001	< 0.05	< 0.01	< 0.05	n.s.	n.s.	< 0.01

The values are means ($\bar{x}$) ± standard deviation (SD). The p-values denote statistical significance from the untreated control group. Abbreviations used: P_{LV} = LV systolic pressure; T_{syst} = LV systolic wall stress; CI = cardiac index; EF = LV ejection fraction; HR = heart rate; P_{LVED} = LV end-diastolic pressure; LV/BW = LV muscle mass/body weight.

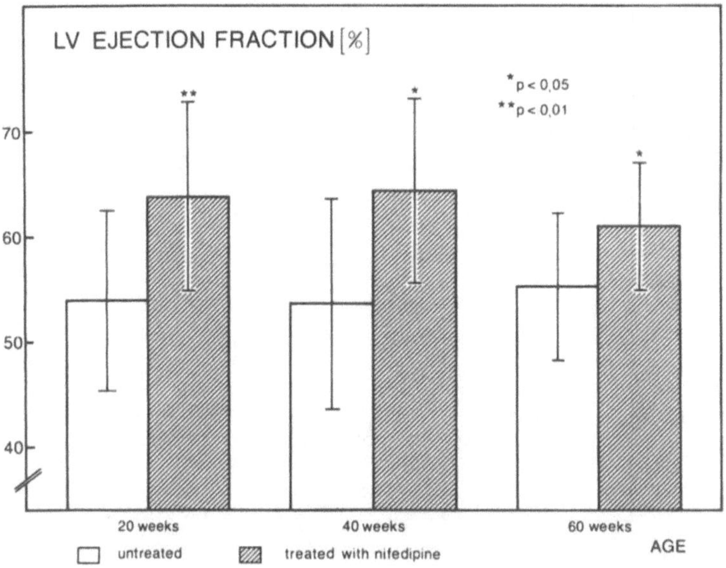

Fig. 1. LV ejection fraction of the group treated with nifedipine (hatched bars) and the untreated control group (open bars). Values are means ± standard deviations.

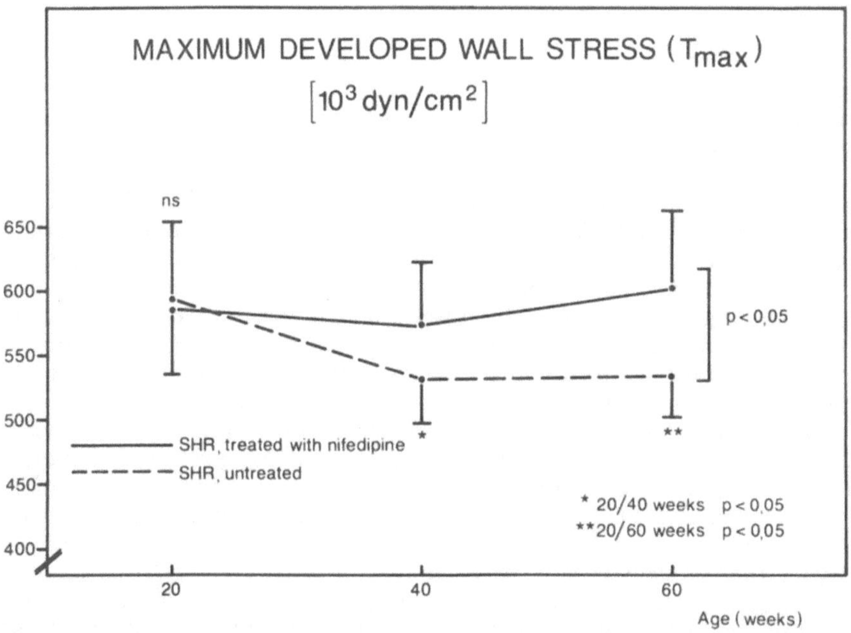

Fig. 2. Maximum developed systolic wall stress when occluding completely the proximal aortic arch (T_{max}). Values are means ± standard deviations.

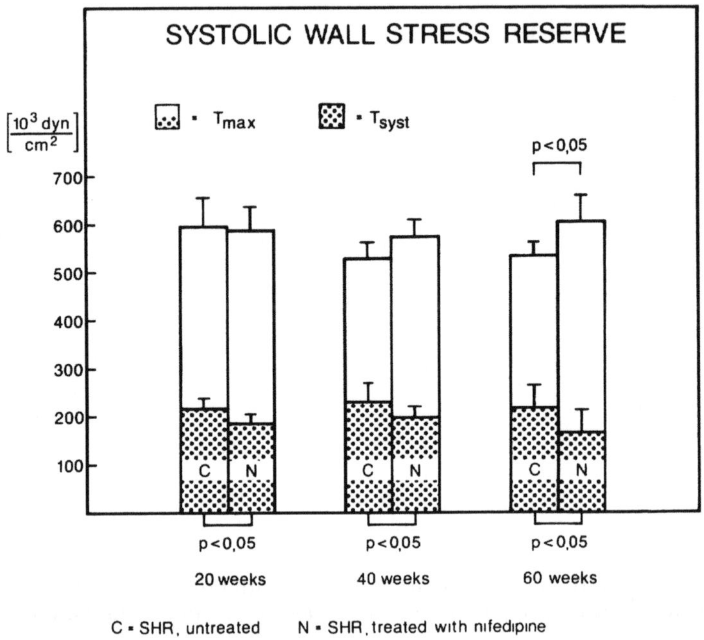

Fig. 3. Systolic wall stress reserve (T_{max}/T_{syst}). Notice that after 60 weeks of nifedipine treatment wall stress reserve is augmented duo to both an increased maximum developed wall stress (T_{max}) and a reduced instantaneous wall stress (T_{syst}). Values are means ± standard deviations.

nifedipine in this study (fig. 1) can be attributed to the easier systolic ventricular emptying due to the lower LV afterload.

Maximum developed systolic wall stress when occluding totally the aortic arch corresponds well to the maximum isometric tension development of the isolated LV papillary muscle, and can be used as a parameter of myocardial contractility (8, 9). Since maximum wall stress remained preserved in the treated animals (fig. 2), it can be concluded that a long-term blood pressure control by nifedipine can prevent later deterioration in myocardial contractility as seen in the untreated SHR. Furthermore, the higher myocardial contractility may also contribute to the augmented LV ejection fraction besides afterload reduction (fig. 1).

Instantaneous systolic wall stress is, on the one hand, a force opposing LV contraction and, on the other hand, a force being generated actively by the ventricular myocardium. Thus the quotient of maximum attainable systolic wall stress (T_{max}) and instantaneous wall stress (T_{syst}), i.e., systolic wall stress reserve (T_{max}/T_{syst}) can be regarded as a measure for the LV myocardial contractility reserve capacity (8). Due to both higher maximum wall stress and lower instantaneous wall stress, systolic wall stress reserve was increased in SHR treated with nifedipine (fig. 3). That indicates that in hypertensive heart disease the reserve capacity of myocardial contractility can be considerably improved by nifedipine.

The beneficial effects of nifedipine upon the myocardial function seem to be mainly the consequence of the long-term systolic relief of the left ventricle due to its extracardiac arteriolar vasodilating effects (7). A direct positive inotropic action by a calcium antagonist is unlikely due to its typical mechanism of action (7). However, specific nifedipine effects such as an improved LV relaxation (10), agumented LV compliance (11), or direct coronary artery dilating effects (12) may also contribute to the improved cardiac function. Moreover, one could argue that the lower extent of LV hypertrophy after nifedipine treatment itself might causatively contribute to the raised contractility reserve. However, previous studies (5, 8, 9) revealed that LV hypertrophy in SHR as such is not connected with a decrement in myocardial contractility.

Acknowledgement

The technical assistance of Monika Ploeger is gratefully acknowledged.

References

1. Guazzi, M. D., C. Fiorentini, M. T. Olivari, T. Bartorelli, G. Neechi, A. Polese: Short- and long-term efficiency of a calcium-antagonistic agent (nifedipine) combined with methyldopa in the treatment of severe hypertension. Circulation **61**, 913–919 (1980).
2. Motz W., M. Ploeger, G. Ringsgwandl, N. Goeldel, B. Garthoff, S. Kazda, B. E. Strauer: The influence of nifedipine on ventricular function and myocardial hypertrophy in spontaneously hypertensive rats. J. Cardiovasc. Pharmacol. **5**, 55–61 (1983).
3. Meerson, F. S.: Hyperfunktion, Hypertrophie und Insuffizienz des Herzens, VEB Volk und Gesundheit (Berlin 1969).
4. Alpert, N.: Cardiac hypertrophy Academic press (New York 1971).
5. Strauer, B. E.: Myocardial oxygen consumption in chronic heart disease. Role of wall stress, hypertrophy and coronary reserve. Amer. J. Cardiol. **44**, 730 (1979).
6. Sachs, L.: Angewandte Statistik. Springer (Berlin-Heidelberg-New York 1974).
7. Fleckenstein-Grün, A. Fleckenstein: Calcium-Antagonismus, ein Grundprinzip der Vasodilatation. In: Calcium-Antagonismus, edited by Fleckenstein, A., H., Roskamm, p. 191 Springer (Berlin-Heidelberg-New York 1980).
8. Strauer, B. E.: Hypertensive Heart Disease. Springer (Berlin-Heidelberg-New York 1980).
9. Bürger, S., B. E. Strauer: Left ventricular hypertrophy in chronic pressure load due to essential hypertension. I. Left ventricular function, left ventricular geometry and wall stress. In: The Heart in Hypertension, edited by B. E. Strauer, p. 13 Springer (Berlin-Heidelberg-New York 1981).
10. Ludbrook, P. A., A. J. Tiefenbrunn, B. E. Sobel: Influence of nifedipine on left ventricular systolic and diastolic function. Relationship to manifestions of ischemia and congestive heart failure. Amer. J. Med. **71**, 683 (1981).
11. Motz, W., B. E. Strauer: The influence of nifedipine on left ventricular compliance and myocardial stiffness. J. Amer. College Cardiol. (1983) in press.
12. Kaltenbach, M., W. Schulz, T. Kober: Effects of nifedipine after intravenous and intracoronary administration. Amer. J. Cardiol. **44**, 832 (1979).

Authors' address:

Dr. Wolfgang Motz, Medizinische Klinik I der Universität München, Klinikum Großhadern, Marchionistraße 15, D-8000 München 70, FRG

Cardiac Adaptation to Hemodynamic Overload, Training and Stress
Dr. D. Steinkopff Verlag 288–294 (1983)

Magnesium as the physiologic calcium antagonist: its vascular effects and therapeutic use

H. Nguyen Duong and K. Brecht †

Abteilung für Allgemeine Physiologie Universität Ulm (FRG)

Summary

Clinical studies have demonstrated that the unstable or primary angina attacks are caused by severe spastic occlusion of morphologically healthy or partially sclerotic segments of coronary vessels. The suggestion, expressed by some authors, that these spasms may be induced by hypomagnesemia is controversial. The present in-vitro experiments, carried out in isolated strips of coronary vessels (dogs and pigs) and other peripheral blood vessels (bovine facial arteries and veins) do not contradict the conclusion that the increase in basal tone observed after treatment of the vessel preparations with magnesium-free physiologic solutions may possibly represent one triggering factor for the induction of vasospasms, but they favour the concept that these spasms are primarily due to rhythmic contractions initiated by potential pacemaker cells occurring in the wall of the coronary vessels after degenerative processes. They show furthermore that an elevation of Mg_o (from 0.5 to 10 mmol/l) can reduce significantly the basal, physiologic tone as well as the tone resulting from an increased transmembrane Ca-ion movement taking place during membrane depolarization or after receptor stimulation. Since magnesium probably represents the most adequate blocker of calcium fluxes, there seems to be no argument against its prophylactic and therapeutic use.

Key words: vascular smooth muscle, magnesium ions, calcium antagonism, vascular pacemaker cells, coronary spasms

Introduction

Spasms of the coronary arteries are known to be responsible for the manifestation of stable and unstable angina pectoris, of acute myocardial infarction, and of sudden cardiac death. They are defined as a sudden increase in vascular tone associated with localized or multifocal vasoconstriction and may be superposed on a variable degree of sclerosis. Although several hypotheses have been advanced, nothing is actually known about the mechanisms underlying their etiology. The objective of this paper is to propose a possible chain of events leading to coronary spasms in human and to make clear that the preventive and therapeutic use of magnesium, as the physiologic Ca-antagonist, may be helpful for people with high risk of sudden cardiac death.

Materials and methods

Helical strips were prepared from approx. 70 blood vessel segments of different origin: swine coronary arteries; bovine facial arteries and veins (BFA, BFV); canine coronary arteries; human saphenous veins, obtained from patients undergoing surgical operations. The vessel strips were mounted vertically in a thermostat chamber and superfused continuously with physiologic salt solution (PSS) as described elsewhere (16). Some preparations were investigated in thermostatically controlled organ baths containing PSS. The vessel strips were prestretched by 1–10 mN, depending on their size. The mechanical reactions were followed isometrically or isotonically. The PSS employed contained (millimolar concentration): NaCl 136.9; KCl 2.7; $CaCl_2$ 1.4; $MgCl_2$ 0.5; $NaHCO_3$ 11.9; NaH_2PO_4 0.3; glucose 8. Isoosmotic conditions were observed throughout, when necessary by equimolar replacement of NaCl. The solutions were gassed with 95 % O_2 and 5 % CO_2 and maintained at 37 °C. An equilibration period of 1 h was allowed to elapse before starting the experiments.

Drugs used in this study included $BaCl_2$ and acetylcholine (E. Merck, Darmstadt).

Results

1 Spontaneous mechanical activity of bovine facial vessels

Spontaneous phasic activity in bovine facial veins (BFV) occurred with a cycle length of about 2 minutes (fig. 2 C). The vessels in these experiments had a diameter of about 8 millimetres. The rhythmic contractions developed immediately after the strips were mounted and became maximal 1 to 2 h after their onset. They disappeared transiently when the external Ca ion concentration was reduced from 1.4 to 1 mmol/l and completely in Ca-free PSS; the phasic contractions reappeared after reintroduction of 1.4 mmol/l Ca in the bath fluid, though with reduced amplitude and higher frequency (not shown in the figures).

Approximately 20–30 % of the isolated vessel preparations investigated in our laboratory exhibit this type of mechanical oscillations (which otherwise represents a disturbing phenomenon, when changes in mechanical tension under external stimuli are investigated).

The mechanical oscillations described above are occasionally superposed by additional rhythms of lower frequency (cycle length of 10 minutes) and higher amplitude (fig. 1 A, B).

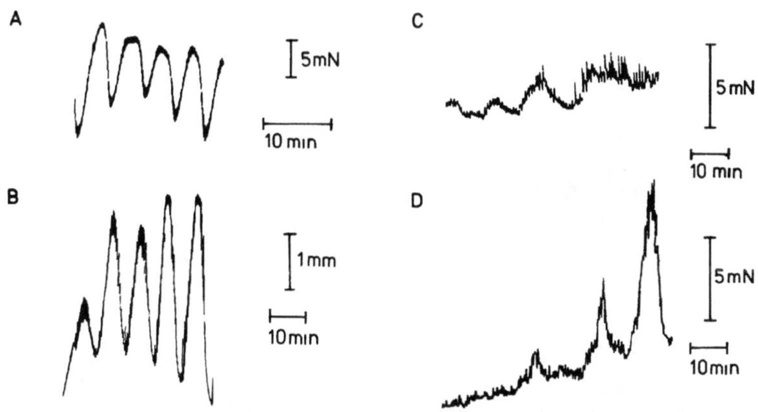

Fig. 1. Spontaneous mechanical activity of isolated peripheral vessel preparations: A and B: bovine facial veins; C and D: human saphenous veins.

2 Spontaneous mechanical activity of human vessels

Spontaneous rhythmic contractions were also observed in isolated, large-sized human saphenous veins (fig. 1 C, D). The mechanical oscillations, which developed 1–2 h after the preparations, have been mounted in the apparatus, were irregular at the beginning, became thereafter more regular and had a cycle length of 15 minutes. In one experiment the preparations, which were taken from the same saphenous vein of a patient at 3 different levels (knee, shank, and knuckle), showed that the rhythms occurred preferentially in the proximal segments (unpublished).

3 Dose-dependent relaxations of canine coronary arteries to increasing external magnesium ion (Mg_o) concentration

Increase in extracellular Mg from 0.5 to 6 mmol/l resulted in relaxation of the basal tension of canine coronary artery (fig. 2 A). This effect is not specific for coronary arteries, but is also observed with most vessel preparations, the EC_{50} values varying with the vascular strip investigated (17).

4 Effect of withdrawal of extracellular Mg in porcine coronary arteries

Exposure of the coronary strips to Mg_o-free PSS resulted in a sustained increase in basal tone (fig. 2 B). These effects were also observed with BFA and BFV.

5 Effect of increasing Mg_o concentration on phasic mechanical activity induced by treatment with 0.5 mmol/l Ba on BFV

Phasic contractions of BFV (diameter 8 mm) induced by addition of 0.5 mmol/l Ba were partly abolished by 5 mmol/l Mg_o and completely by 10 mmol/l Mg_o (fig. 2 D). The rhythms reappeared after gradual elevation of

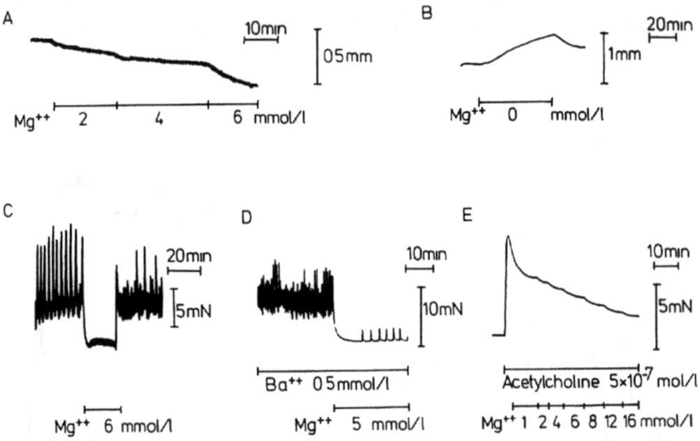

Fig. 2. A: Effects of magnesium on the basal tone of canine coronary artery; B: Effect of Mg-free solution on the basal tone of porcine coronary artery; C: Effect of 6 mmol/l Mg on spontaneous contractions of BFV; D: Effect of 5 mmol/l Mg on phasic contractions of BFV induced by 0.5 mmol/l barium ions; E: Effect of increasing Mg_o concentrations (1–16 mmol/l) on contractions of porcine coronary artery induced by 5.10^{-7} mmol/l acetylcholine.

Ca_o from 1.4 to 5 mmol/l, though with a changed frequency and amplitude (not shown in the figure).

6 Effect of increasing Mg_o on BFV precontracted by 5.10^{-7} mol/l Acetylcholine

Figure 2 E shows the dose-dependent relaxations in response to increasing Mg_o concentrations of porcine coronary arteries precontracted by 5.10^{-7} mol/l acetylcholine. The contractions were depressed by 80 % of their maximal values at a concentration of 16 mmol/l Mg_o. The EC_{50} values resulting from 8 experiments amounted to 3 mmol/l Mg_o.

Discussion

The etiology of the coronary spasms, which represent the most probable trigger mechanism in the variant form of angina pectoris (15), is not elucidated. It has been assumed, for instance, that altered sympathetic activity may directly trigger spasms in the coronary arteries. However, the observations by two groups of clinicians (2, 3) which were able to detect spasms in the coronary arteries of denervated, transplantated human hearts, seem to exclude this possibility. Obviously a different, more direct cause for the coronary spasms needs to be looked for, although it remains possible that a spasm, regardless how it may be triggered, could be exacerbated by the modulating activity of the autonomic nervous system (cf. fig. 3). Humoral factors have been taken into account, too (6, 14). Since high circulating thromboxane A_2 levels are found in patients with variant angina (14), this potent vasoconstrictor, which is released by platelets, is also a putative triggering factor. However, there is some evidence that this release represents only a secondary phenomenon produced by the injury of platelets (10). Nevertheless, this release could favour a vicious cycle leading to a potentiation of every preexisting contriction of the vessel wall (cf. fig. 3). On the other side, since epidemiologic and clinical studies have suggested that magnesium deficiency may also be implicated in the pathogenesis of sudden cardiac death in patients with coronary disease (1, 4, 11), it has been speculated that hypomagnesemia is the main and direct cause of the coronary spasms (20). This theory seems to be controversial, since recent clinical investigations indicate that in patients with coronary heart disease lowered serum magnesium concentrations are generally found only when left ventricular function is reduced. Thus they should be considered more a consequence than a cause of the disease. Furthermore, with respect to the whole coronary vascular tree, the contractions induced in isolated coronary vessels by withdrawal of the magnesium ions from the organ bath (fig. 2 B) are too unspecific an effect to account for the spasm observed during angiography, which are generally localized at a certain, clearly defined region.

The assumption that the human coronary spasms are primarily due to rhythmic contractions initiated by potential pacemaker cells occurring in the wall of the coronary vessels after degenerative processes seems to be more plausible. Spontaneous phasic contractile activity is usually seen in

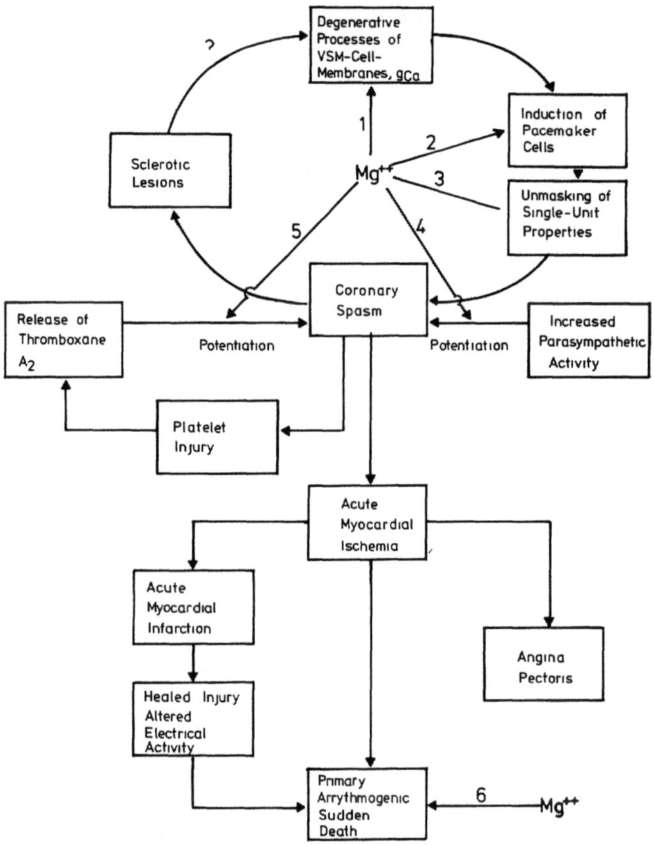

Fig. 3. Multiple influence of magnesium on the mechanism of induction of acute myocardial ischemia.

small arteries and in the portal mesenteric veins. In the literature there is general consensus that such oscillations of the mechanical activity do not occur in large resistance or capacitance vessels. Figures 1 A–D demonstrate the contrary to be true. Phasic activity has been reported in isolated coronary arteries of rabbits, cats, and rats (5), and in human coronary vessels (8, 9, 12, 19).

Which mechanisms are responsible for these phasic contractions? It is well known that they are initiated by bursts of spikes, having their origin in vascular pacemaker cells depolarizing and repolarizing rhythmically at a relatively slow rate. The frequency of this phasic activity is determined by the frequency of bursts; the amplitude depends partly on the degree of synchronization between the groups of cells, i.e., on the number of effective nexuses or gap-junctions between the cells. In vessels whose function does not consist in a peristaltic-like propulsion of the blood content, the regenerative production of action potentials is prevented by a potential-dependent increase in potassium conductance. In normally quiescent vascular cells, which have become leaky to Ca because of damage to the cell surface, K efflux is not sufficient for maintaining the resting membrane potential, which begins to oscillate reaching periodically the threshold value, thus inducing a burst of spikes. It is not surprising, therefore, that the treatment of the vessel preparations with tetraethylammonium or Ba ions, which are known to inhibit the outward K current, leads to the induction of rhythmic activity quite similar to the spontaneously occurring one. As shown in this report and in previous studies (17, 18), the magnesium ions are able, in virtue of their Ca antagonistic property, to inhibit the spontaneous mechanical activity as well as the induced one.

It is conceivable that the coronary spasms observed clinically are not caused solely by these vascular pacemaker-induced mechanical fluctuations, and that they may be further influenced by the autonomic nervous system. It was demonstrated 75 years ago by Langendorff that the large coronaries relax under the influence of catecholamines while contracting to acetylcholine (13). Since the activity of the parasympathetic part of the autonomic nervous system may increase during rest, sleep, or after a copious meal, the resulting contractions of the coronary arteries could possibly shift the phasic contractions described above to a higher level of tone. This mechanism may possibly be effective during the coronary spasm attacks at rest experienced by patients with variant agina (7). In figure 3 A a scheme summarizing the multiple effects of Mg on the sequence of events leading to acute myocardial ischemia induced by spasms is presented.

In summary, following conclusion can be drawn: It is undeniable that Mg is the "physiologic Ca antagonist". Since it is recognized now that coronary spasms play a role not only in variant angina but also in other, more common forms of ischemic heart disease, the spasmolytic effect of Mg could well be of benefit in the treatment or in the prevention of coronary heart diseases. The use of Mg should attract more attention in the clinical world.

References

1. Abraham, A. S., U. Eylath, M. Weinstein, E. Czaczkef: Serum magnesium levels in patients with acute myocardial infarction. New Engl. J. Med. **296,** 862 (1977).
2. Buda, A. J., R. E. Fowles, J. S. Schroeder: Coronary artery spasm in the denervated transplantated human heart. A clue to underlying mechanisms. Amer. J. Med. **70,** 1144–9 (1981).
3. Clark, D. A., R. A. Quint, R. L. Mitchell, W. W. Angell: Coronary artery spasm. Medical management, surgical denervation and autotransplantation. J. Thorac. cardiovasc. Surg. **73,** 332 (1977).
4. Dyckner, T.: Serum magnesium in acute myocardial infarction. Acta Med. Scand. **207,** 59 (1980).
5. d'Hemecourt, A., R. Detar: Possible physiological basis for locally-induced "spasm" of large coronary arteries. In: Maseri, A., G. H. Klassen, M. Lesch, eds.: Primary and secondary angina pectoris, Grune and Stratton Inc. (New York 1978).
6. Ellis, E. F., O. Oelz, R. L. Jackson: Coronary arterial smooth muscle contraction by a substance released from platelets: Evidence that it is thromboxane A_2. Science **193,** 1135–7 (1976).

7. Fleckenstein-Grün, G., A. Fleckenstein: Calcium-Antagonismus, ein Grundprinzip der Vasodilatation. In: Calcium-Antagonismus, A. Fleckenstein, H. Roskamm, eds, p. 196, Springer-Verlag (Berlin–Heidelberg–New York, 1980).
8. Ginsburg, R., M. R. Bristow, D. C. Harrison, E. B. Stinson: Studies with isolated human coronary arteries. Some general observations, potential mediators of spasm, role of calcium antagonists. Chest **78,** 180–6, Suppl. (1980).
9. Golenhofen, K.: Activation mechanisms in smooth muscle of human coronary arteries and their selective inhibition. Naunyn-Schmiedeberg's Arch. Pharmacol. **302,** R36, Suppl. (1978).
10. Hellstorm, H. R.: The injury-spasm (ischemia-induced hemostatic vasoconstrictive) and vascular autoregulatory hypothesis of ischemic disease. Resistance vessel-spasm hypothesis of ischemic disease. Amer. J. Cardiol. **49,** 802–10 (1982).
11. Johnson, C. J., D. R. Peterson, E. K. Smith: Myocardial tissue concentrations of magnesium and potassium in men dying suddenly from ischemic heart disease. Amer. J. Clin. Nutr. **32,** 967 (1979).
12. Kawasaki, K., K. Seki, S. Hosoda: Spontaneous rhythmic contractions in isolated human coronary arteries. Experientia **37,** 1291–2 (1981).
13. Langendorff, O.: Über die Innervation der Koronargefäße. Zentralbl. Physiol. **21,** 551–57 (1907).
14. Levy, R. L., L. Wiener, P. Walinsky: Thromboxane release during pacing-induced angina pectoris: possible vasoconstrictor influence on the coronary vasculature. Circulation **61,** 1165–71 (1980).
15. Maseri, A., R. Mimmo, S. Chierchia: Coronary artery spasm as a cause of acute myocardial ischemia in man. Chest **68,** 625 (1976).
16. Nguyen Duong Hoang, R. Rüdel, U. Voss: Effects of AR-L-115 on arterial and venous muscle tone in vitro. Arzneim.-Forsch./Drug Res. **31,** 197–9 (1980).
17. Nguyen Duong Hoang, K. Brecht: Experimentelle Studien über die Wirkung von Magnesium auf isolierte Blutgefäße und ihre therapeutischen Aspekte. Magnesium-Bulletin **2,** 33–41 (1980).
18. Nguyen Duong Hoang, K. Brecht: Über die Wirkung von Magnesium-Ionen auf isolierte Blutgefäße und ihre therapeutische Bedeutung bei Koronarspasmen. Med. Welt **32,** 964–6 (1981).
19. Ross, G., E. Stinson, J. Schroeder, R. Ginsburg: Spontaneous phasic activity of isolated human coronary arteries. Cardiovasc. Res. **14,** 613–8 (1980).
20. Turlapaty, P. D. M. V., B. M. Altura: Magnesium definiciency produces spasms of coronary arteries: relationship to etiology of sudden death ischemic heart disease. Science **208,** 198–200 (1980).

Authors' address:

Priv.-Doz. Dr. Nguyen Duong, Universität Ulm, Abteilung für Allgemeine Physiologie, Oberer Eselsberg, 7900 Ulm/Donau, FRG

Reactions at the tissue level

Cardiac Adaptation to Hemodynamic Overload, Training and Stress
Dr. D. Steinkopff Verlag 297–303 (1983)

Effects of hemodynamic load on myocardial fibre orientation

B. Korecky and K. Rakusan

Department of Physiology, Faculty of Medicine, University of Ottawa, Ottawa, Ontario (Canada)

Summary

We studied the relationship between long-term changes in haemodynamic loads and orientation of myocardial fibres in the free wall of the left ventricle (LV) of the rat. Pressure overload was induced by aortic banding in 3-week-old animals, which resulted in a twofold hypertrophy 5 months later. No significant difference in fibre orientation could be observed when compared to LV of control animals of the same or other strains of rats. Reduction of load leading to cardiac atrophy was induced by transplanting the heart into the abdominal cavity of an inbred recipient, producing an "in vivo" Langendorf preparation. Considerable restructuring of fibre orientation could be observed in the beating transplants. Initially the subepi- and subendocardial fibres changed their orientation from longitudinal to oblique and consequently the portion of circumferential fibres that are parallel to the equatorial plane increased. Later an increasing tortuosity of the long fibre axis could be observed. When the net loss of cardiac mass became more prominent (about 25 %), complete fibre disorientation was observed. We conclude that pressure overload does not induce demonstrable changes of fibre orientation in the LV. However, reduction of load with practical elimination of ejection leads to restructuring of fibre orientation and to their ultimate disarray.

Key words: heart, hypertrophy, atrophy, fibre orientation, overload, transplanted heart

Introduction

The left ventricular mammalian myocardium may be viewed as a series of interconnected shells, each composed of discrete fibres oriented in a single direction. When examined in series of histological sections, the orientation of fibres gradually shifts in a fan-like fashion between the outer and inner shells. When referenced to the equatorial plane, the spectrum of these angular changes was found to be specific for a given species and characteristic for a sampling site (Hort 1960, Streeter and Bassett 1966, Streeter and Hanna 1973). The predominant number of fibres is oriented circumferentially (midwall) while in the outside and inside layers the fibres become more obliquely oriented and may even become longitudinally oriented, i.e., perpendicular to the equatorial plane.

Supported by Ontario Heart Foundation and MRC of Canada

This rather specific array of long fibre axis throughout the wall may be either genetically predetermined or induced by the distribution of myocardial stresses during the life span. If the latter is correct, then unusual stresses imposed upon the heart should alter the orientation of fibres, since the power output of the three-dimensional cardiac muscle pump is ultimately related to the mechanics of individual muscle fibres, which develop force and shorten parallel to their long axis.

We therefore studied the relationship between unusual hemodynamic loads and the fibre orientation of the left ventricle in rat, first by inducing long-term pressure overload by gradually narrowing the aorta in growing animals and secondly by suddenly reducing the work load, by removing the heart from the body and transplanting it into the abdominal cavity of an inbred recipient.

Methods

Pressure overload

Aortic constriction was produced by banding the abdominal aorta of 21–25-day-old male Sprague Dawley rats with 000 surgical silk thread placed snuggly around the vessel with no visible narrowing while the sham-operated animals served as controls. The animals were kept for the subsequent 4–6 months on a standard diet while the arterial pressure in the upper torso was used as indicator of overload. For more details see Korecky et al. (1967).

Reduction of load

Rat hearts were transplanted into the abdominal cavity of recipients in adult male Lewis inbred rats (Microbiological Associates). The aorta and pulmonary artery of the transplants were attached end to side to the abdominal aorta and vena cava, respectively. Since the arterial blood of the recipient served to perfuse the beating transplanted heart this transplant may be considered as an in-vivo Langendorf preparation, i.e., an empty beating heart with preserved coronary flow. It ceases to grow and loses about 30 % of its initial mass in three weeks after surgery. For more details see Tolnai and Korecky (1981), Korecky and Rakusan (1982).

Collection of tissue samples

The rats were anesthetized with Nembutal (5 mg/100 g body weight), the abdominal cavity opened, 0.1 mg/100 g of heparin injected into the inferior vena cava followed by 0.1 ml/100 g of saturated KCl solution to produce diastolic ventricular arrest (Lin et al. 1977). The heart was removed, its aorta cannulated and the coronaries perfused with 5 ml saline followed by Bouin's fixative (~5 ml) and then immersed in this fixative overnight. The subsequent steps follow the principles outlined by Streeter (1979). The heart was trimmed, the longitudinal axis defined by passing i.v. needle through the mitral valve and out the apex, and oriented in a plexiglass box, which was filled with 15 % warm gelatine, and refrigerated overnight. The gelatine block was then removed, the i.v. needle extracted and the heart cut perpendicularly to the long axis at the point of greatest circumference, thus defining the equatorial plane against which fibre angles were measured. The transverse dimensions of the LV were then measured under dissecting microscope (10×). The heart was then cut longitudinally at the center of the left ventricular lumen at right angle to the equatorial plane and longitudinal dimensions of the LV measured. The two halves were then realligned and a third cut made approximately

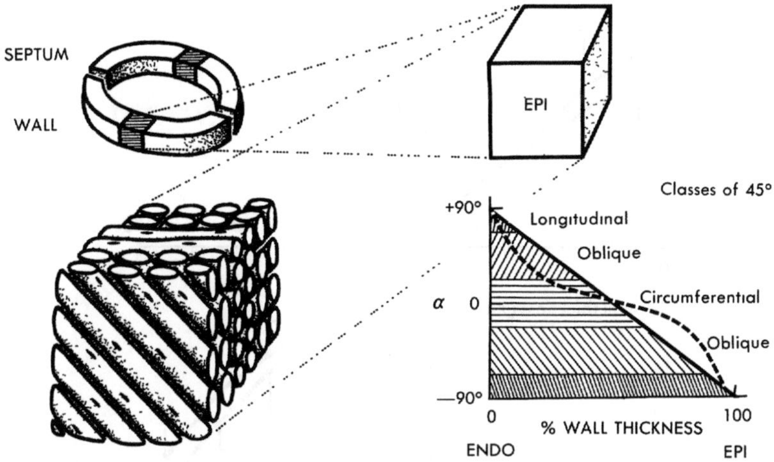

Fig. 1. Graphical description of the tissue sampling for serial sectioning in the free wall of the left ventricle. The helical angles α are plotted as a function of the wall thickness. The solid line indicates smooth gradual transition of fibre angles from endocardium to epicardium. Dashed line depicts a situation when majority of fibres are arranged circumferentially.

2 mm below and parallel to the equator. Sample blocks were taken from middle of the free LV wall (see fig. 1).

The samples were then processed by standard histological procedure, imbedded in parafin, mounted and cut so that the microtome passed at right angles to the equatorial plane throughout the wall. Sections 10 μm thick were retained at regular intervals, mounted on slides, stained and the angles of the fibres were measured relative to the reference plane using a light microscope with a viewing screen with 90× magnification (see fig. 1). Tortuosity of the rod-like fibres was estimated by dividing the length of their long axis by the distance between the ends of the respective fibres. Unless otherwise stated, data are expressed as mean ± SEM. Student's t-test is used to test the significance of differences between respective groups of data.

Results

Pressure overload

Control (sham-operated) rats and rats with aortic bands that showed significant elevation in arterial pressure were sacrificed on the average 4–6 months after surgery. Average body weights of eight controls were 576 ± 23 g while the experimental group (n = 7) weighed 547 ± 29 g. The average heart weights were 1140 ± 46 mg and 2060 ± 98 mg, respectively ($p < 0.01$). The distribution of fibre angles (α) throughout the wall is displayed as a function of percentage of LV wall thickness in figure 2. The transition of α in the controls (dashed line) from endocardium to epicardium is rather gradual. It starts from the longitudinal fibres of the subepicardial layer (−87°) and terminates as oblique fibres (+64°) in the endocardium. The distribution of α in the samples of LV free wall taken from hypertrophic

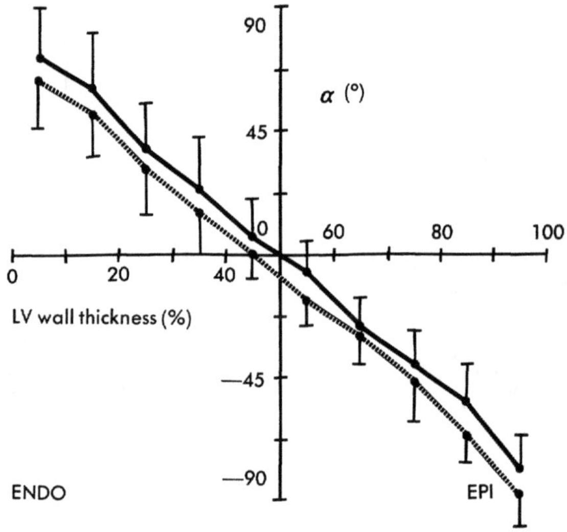

Fig. 2. Comparison of helix angle (shown as α) distribution through left ventricular (LV) free wall taken from transmural samples at the equator of the rat LV in diastole. The equatorial plane serves as a reference and was assigned the value of 0°. Percentage of wall thickness is measured from the average endocardial location to the epicardium of the sample. Mean value ± SD is shown for each decile of wall thickness. Dotted line: control hearts (n = 8), solid line: hypertrophic hearts (n = 7).

hearts shows a similar trend. There was no significant difference in any decile throughout the free wall of the LV between the two groups.

Reduction of load

The recipient rats with viable transplants in their abdomen were sacrificed between 14 and 45 days after surgery. The average weight of the heart was 890 ± 36 mg in the recipient hearts and 730 ± 46 mg in the transplanted hearts ($p < 0.01$). The distribution of α in the free wall of the LV is shown in figure 3. Dashed line represents mean values of the recipient hearts (n = 14), the dotted line represents mean values of transplants that showed atrophy less than 15 % as compared to their own recipients (n = 5). The solid line represents transplants with atrophies between 16 and 24 % (n = 6).

These data indicate a gradual diminishing of longitudinal and oblique fibres and increase in number of fibres, which lie close to parallel with the equatorial plane, i.e., circumferentially oriented fibres. In addition, the fibres in hearts showing greater atrophy exhibited increasing tortuosity of the long axis in contrast to straight line long axis of the fibres in the recipient hearts (1.35 as compared to 1.07). The degree of tortuosity increased as atrophy progressed and led ultimately to disarray of fibres, which could not be quantitated by the technique of serial sectioning.

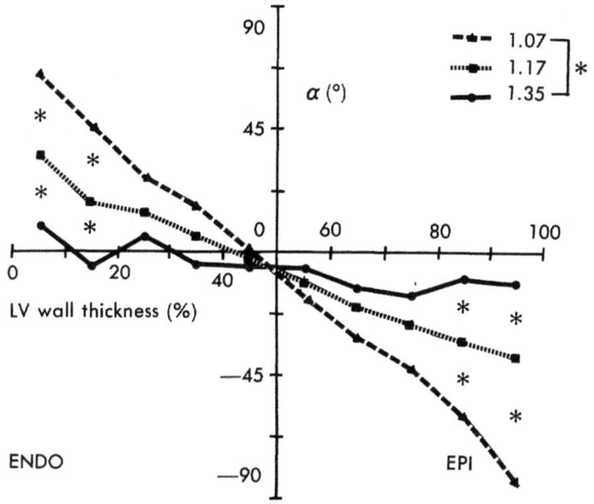

Fig. 3. Comparison of helix angle (shown as α) distribution through left ventricular (LV) free wall taken from transmural samples at the equator of the rat LV in diastole. The equatorial plane serves as a reference and was assigned the value of 0 °. Percentage of wall thickness is measured from the average endocardial location to the epicardium of the sample. Mean value is shown for each decile of wall thickness. Dashed line: recipients (N = 14), dotted line: transplants with up to 15 % atrophy (N = 5), solid line: transplants with atrophy between 16 and 24 % (N = 6) as compared to recipient hearts. Note the gradual disappearance of vertically arranged longitudinal fibres in the subepicardial and subendocardial regions. The numbers in upper right corner indicate average degree of tortuosity. Transplants with higher degrees of atrophy then above show fibre disorientation and cannot be evaluated by this technique. * indicates statistically significant difference, at $p < 0.05$.

Discussion

The data from hypertrophic hearts indicate that no changes in fibre orientation could be observed in the diastolic-like potassium arrested rat left ventricle. Since the pressure overload represents primarily an increased resistance to flow, the wall stress must have increased to develop greater transmural pressure. In our rats with pressure-hypertrophied hearts, the internal radii remained unchanged while the external radii and wall thickness were significantly increased. These results are in agreement with similar data reported by Lin et al. (1977) who also found that external dimensions increased, while luminal dimensions remained unchanged in pressure-hypertrophied ventricles of adult rats.

In hearts of hypertensive patients Jean et al. (1972) found an increased range of fiber angles as compared to normal cadaver hearts, however, this could have been at least partly caused by changes of eccentricity. Carew et al. (1973) could not find any changes in fibre angle distribution in exercise hypertrophy in dogs. However, the same authors (1979) reported a slight increase (7.3 %) in number of fibres oriented longitudinally in hypertrophic dog hearts after aortic stenosis. They speculated that this may have been an adaptation to increased meridional stress.

In general, it seems that no major changes in fibre orientation could be demonstrated as a consequence of increased afterload. This may be due to the fact that the fibres are optimally oriented in the ventricular wall under normal conditions (Manasek 1970). The produced force is thus translated into pressure due to optimal curvature of fibres which then shorten and eject adequate stroke volume. In case of overload they may essentially perform the same kind of work except they do more of it. Therefore there may be no need for individual fibres to rearrange their long axis with respect to the equatorial plane in pressure induced hypertrophy.

In case of unloading, the situation may be quite different. The transplant beats empty provided the aortic valve is competent and no coronary blood is drained into the left ventricle. In case of some drainage, several beats may be isovolumic and when the end-diastolic volume becomes sufficient, an ejection beat will follow. The fibres therefore contract isometrically either all the time or most of the time. This situation represents not only a decrease in load but also a considerable change in its character. Consequently, the long axis of the fibres might not have the best array for the altered loading conditions and they start to rearrange their positions within the wall.

Myocardial fiber disarray has been observed under several clinical situations (Wigle and Silver 1978) probably due to anatomically predisposed changes in wall stresses related to isometric contraction. This situation may have been caused either by cavity obliteration (Bulkley et al. 1977) or catenoid shape of the left ventricular septum (Hutchins and Bulkley 1978) or in cases of extreme outflow tract gradients when isometric contraction occurred at end systole even in absence of cavity obliteration (Wigle and Silver 1978). In all the above clinical situations, the preeminence of isometric contraction and disappearance of directional stresses may represent a possible loss of stimulus for orderly fiber arrangement. Since similar conditions exist in the heterotopically isotransplanted rat heart in our experiments, similar outcome, i.e., fiber disarray was observed.

Acknowledgement

The authors wish to thank Mrs. L. Jui for her technical assistance and Mrs. J. Parker-Parent for her secretarial help.

References

1. Bulkley, B. H., M. L. Weisfeldt, G. M. Hutchins: Isometric cardiac contraction. A Possible Cause of the Disorganized Myocardial Pattern of Idiopathic Hypertrophic Subaortic Stenosis. New Engl. J. Med. **295,** 135–139 (1977).
2. Carew, T. E., I. M. Birhett, M. G. Joseph, J. W. Cowell: Myocardial Fibre Angle Distribution in Chronic Exercise Hypertrophy and Chronic Cardiac Dilatation in the Dog. Fed. Proc. **32,** 433 (1973).
3. Carew, T. E., J. W. Covell. Fibre Orientation in Hypertrophied Canine Left Ventricle. Amer. J. Physiol. **236,** H487–493 (1979).
4. Hutchins, G. M., B. H. Bulkley: Catenoid Shape of the Interventricular Septum: Possible Cause of Idiopathic Hypertrophic Subaortic Stenosis. Circulation **58,** 392–397 (1978).
5. Hort, W.: Makroskopische und mikrometrische Untersuchungen am Myokard verschieden stark gefüllter linker Kammern. Virchows Arch. (Pathol. Anat.) **333,** 523–564 (1960).

6. Jean, C. F., D. D. Streeter, D. D. Reichenbach: Fibre Orientation in the Normal and Hypertensive Cadaver Left Ventricle. Circulation **45/46** (Suppl. II), II–44 (1972).
7. Korecky, B., K. Rakusan, O. Poupa: Experimental Cardiomegaly. Meth. Achiev. Exp. Pathol. **2,** 15–171 (1967).
8. Korecky, B., K. Rakusan: Physiological and Morphological Aspects of Cardiac Atrophy. In: Biology of Cardiac Hypertrophy and Failure, Raven Press, N. Alpert, ed. pp. 293–309 (1983).
9. Lin, H. L., V. Katele, A. F. Grimm: Functional Morphology of the Pressure - and the Volume - Hypertrophied Rat Heart. Circulat. Res. **41,** 830–835 (1977).
10. Manasek, F. J.: Histogenesis of the Embryonic Myocardium. Amer. J. Cardiol. **25,** 149–168 (1970).
11. Streeter, D. D., D. L. Bassett: An Engineering Analysis of Myocardial Fiber Orientation in Pigs Left Ventricle in Systole. Anat. Rec. **155,** 503–512 (1966).
12. Streeter, D. D., W. T. Hanna: Engineering Mechanics for Successive States in Canine Left Ventricular Myocardium. I. Cavity and Wall Geometry. Circulat. Res. **33,** 639–655 (1973).
13. Streeter, D. D.: Gross Morphology and Fiber Geometry of the Heart. In: Handbook of Physiology, Section 2, Vol. I, pp. 61–112, Editor R. M. Berne (1979).
14. Tolnai, S., B. Korecky: Lysosomal Hydrolases in Heterotopically Isotransplanted Heart Undergoing Atrophy. J. Molec. Cell. Cardiol. **12,** 869–890 (1980).
15. Wigle, E. D., M. D. Silver: Myocardial Fiber Disarray and Ventricular Septal Hypertrophy in Asymmetrical Hypertrophy of the Heart. Circulation **58,** 398–402 (1978).

Authors' address:

B. Korecky, M.D., Ph.D., Department of Physiology, Faculty of Health Sciences, University of Ottawa, 451 Smyth Road, Ottawa, Ontario K1H 8M5

Cardiac Adaptation to Hemodynamic Overload, Training and Stress
Dr. D. Steinkopff Verlag 304–313 (1983)

Biochemical characteristics and cellular mechanisms of fibrotic processes

J. Rauterberg, B. Voß, and G. Pott

Institut für Arterioskleroseforschung an der Universität Münster und Medizinische Klinik der Universität Münster (FRG)

Summary

Fibrosis can occur as systemic disease or restricted to single organs; it is characterized by pathologic new-formation of connective tissue. Most fibrotic processes are characterized not only by proliferation but also by changes in the composition of the extracellular matrix and by qualitative changes of single components. There is no general tendency concerning the properties of the newly formed tissue, but there are considerable organ-specific differences. One reason for this diversity may be the participation of different cell types. In addition to typical connective tissue cells (fibroblasts, smooth muscle cells, "myofibroblasts"), cell types may be involved which have been shown to take up synthesis of connective tissue components under cell culture conditions.

Activation of connective tissue producing cells, resulting in proliferation and enhanced biosynthetic activity, may occur as direct reaction to injury; but a more common mechanism involves the induction by mediators which are, in the course of inflammation, released by invading phagocytes, lymphocytes, or thrombocytes. Antifibrotic therapy may be directed either towards inhibition of collagen synthesis or towards intervention in processes leading to the activation of connective-tissue-producing cells.

Key words: fibrosis, connective tissue, collagen(s), proliferation, activation of connective tissue cells

Fibrosis as a general phenomenon can occur as systemic disease or rather restricted to single organs. In each organ, fibrosis has its own characteristics; but there are, on the other hand, common features of fibrotic processes, so that gaining more knowledge about fibrosis in one organ may provide better understanding of the mechanisms involved in the emergence and development of fibrosis in others.

Corresponding to its diversity, the definition of fibrosis cannot be very accurate. In all events the term fibrosis includes the new-formation of connective tissue. This may be

(1) proliferation of already existing connective tissue (as in scleroderma or in keloid formation)
(2) invasion of connective tissue into parenchymal tissues (as in liver fibrosis)

Table 1. Systemic and organ-specific fibrotic processes.

Systemic fibrotic processes		Examples:
Idiopathic fibrosis		Systemic fibrosis
Fibrosis due to metabolic diseases		α1-antitrypsin deficiency
Fibrosis due to immunpathologic processes		SLE
Fibrotic processes in organs		
Liver	Liver fibrosis	
Pancreas	Pancreas fibrosis	
Lung	Idiopathic lung fibrosis	
	Asbestosis and other reactive fibrotic processes	
Blood vessels	Atherosclerosis	
Heart	Heart fibrosis	
Muscle	Myositis ossificans	
Tendon	Dupuytren's disease	
Fibrotic neoplasias		

(3) a qualitative change in the kind of connective tissue (such as the replacement of cartilage in fibrotic joint diseases).

No fibrotic disease represents a pure form of one of these aspects. Table 1 summarizes some of the most important systemic and organ-specific fibrotic processes.

To understand the diversity of fibrosis, we have to consider the diversity of connective tissue itself: There is, on the one hand, the interstitial connective tissue as extends through all organs, providing and protecting their integrity and often contributing essentially to their architecture. There are, on the other hand, specialized connective tissues like tendon, bone, cartilage, skin, vessel wall, and others. But in spite of its diversity there may be a justification for speaking of connective tissue as a common term. Each of the tissues mentioned above possesses an extracellular matrix, which essentially is composed of the same components. (For review see 1.)

It has very recently become clear that we may speak of three families of connective tissue components; they may be called: the "interstitial family", the "basement membrane family", and the "cartilage family". The first certainly is the most prominent one, forming the interstitial and most of the specialized connective tissues. The chemically defined components of this family are:

(1) collagens type I and III (fibril-forming collagens)
(2) structural glycoproteins, e.g., fibronectin
(3) elastin
(4) proteoglycans.

Cartilage has developed its own system of collagens; besides the well-known type II collagen a number of further cartilage-specific collagenous proteins have recently been discovered (2–6). There seems also to exist a cartilage-specific glycoprotein, chondronectin, which has possibly similar functions to fibronectin (7).

Basement membranes are widespread throughout the organism: mostly they are tightly linked to certain cell types (endothelial cells, epithelial

Table 2. Post-translational steps in collagen biosynthesis.

Step	Enzyme involved	Biological significance	Disorder: Genetic	Disorder: Others
Removal of hydrophobic N-terminal "Pre"-peptide	ER-membrane bound protease	Transport through membrane of ER		
Hydroxylation of proline	Prolylhydroxylases	Stability of tripelhelix Tripelhelix formation at 37 °C		Scurvy
Hydroxylation of lysine	Lysylhydroxylase	Stability of crosslinks Essential for glycosylation	Ehlers-Danlos VI	
Glycosylation of hydroxylysine	Galactosyl-transferase Glucosyltransf.	Stability of crosslinks (?) Interaction with matrix components (?) Regulation of fibrilformation		Diabetes
Assembly; disulfide bonding Tripelhelix formation	– –	Essential for secretion Stops hydroxylation and glycosylation		
Cleavage of procollagen peptides	Procollagen-peptidases	Essential for fibre formation	Dermatosparais Ehlers-Danlos VII	
Aldehyde formation	Lysyloxidase	Essential for crosslink formation	Ehlers-Danlos V	Lathyrism
Crosslinking	–	Strength and stability of fibrils	Homocysteinuria Menke's Syndrome	(Ageing?)

cells) on the one hand and to interstitial connective tissue on the other. Collagen type IV represents the collagenous component of basement membranes; a structural glycoprotein (laminin) and a basement membrane-specific proteoglycan (a heparan sulfate) are further integral components of basement membranes (for reviews see 8, 9).

Within these "families", especially among the "interstitial" connective tissue components, widely varying morphologic and chemical characteristics can be recognized, corresponding to the variations in properties and functions of the tissue, as for instance in skin, bone, tendon, or cornea.

These differences are introduced and regulated by several mechanisms

(1) The components are synthesized in different quantitative ratios; for instance the percentage of type III collagen in the fibrillar collagen of a tissue varies between nearly zero in bone and tendon to ca. 40 % in vessel walls.

(2) Post-translational modifications represent an essential step in the biosynthesis of collagens, and tissue specific differences can be introduced at this level. A number of enzymes are involved in the intra- as well as in the extracellular steps of collagen processing, and differences in their activity may influence the properties of the final product, the extracellular collagen fibril.

Table 2 comprises the most important intra- and extracellular steps of collagen processing. Tissue-specific differences do for instance occur in the degree of hydroxylation of lysine, thus essentially determining the stability of intermolecular crosslinks in collagen fibrils. Other extracellular components influence the last steps of collagen processing. Especially fibril thickness seems to be regulated to a great extent by other extracellular components.

Due to the complexity of regulative processes in connective tissue formation, it is quite understandable that fibrotic processes are not only connected to enhanced production of connective tissue but that they also imply changes in the quantitative ratio and in the qualitative properties of single components. The ratio of type I and type III collagens in the normal and atherosclerotic vessel wall as well as in the normal and fibrotic liver may serve as an example.

In the vessel wall the ratio of type I to type III shows a typical age-related development. The type III portion in the aorta of adults is enhanced considerably as compared to the aortas of new born or very young individuals (10). In the fibrotic intima of the atherosclerotic aorta the reverse development occurs: there is a decrease in the portion of type III (11).

In the liver there is an opposite effect: fibrotic processes are connected with a relative increase of type III collagen (12). A similar tendency has been reported for skin collagen: the relatively low portion of type III collagen in normal skin (ca. 10 %) has been found enhanced in hypertrophic scars (13).

Another interesting feature of fibrotic changes in the artery and in the liver is the behaviour of basement membrane-related components, as for instance collagen type IV and laminin. Figure 1 shows immunfluor-

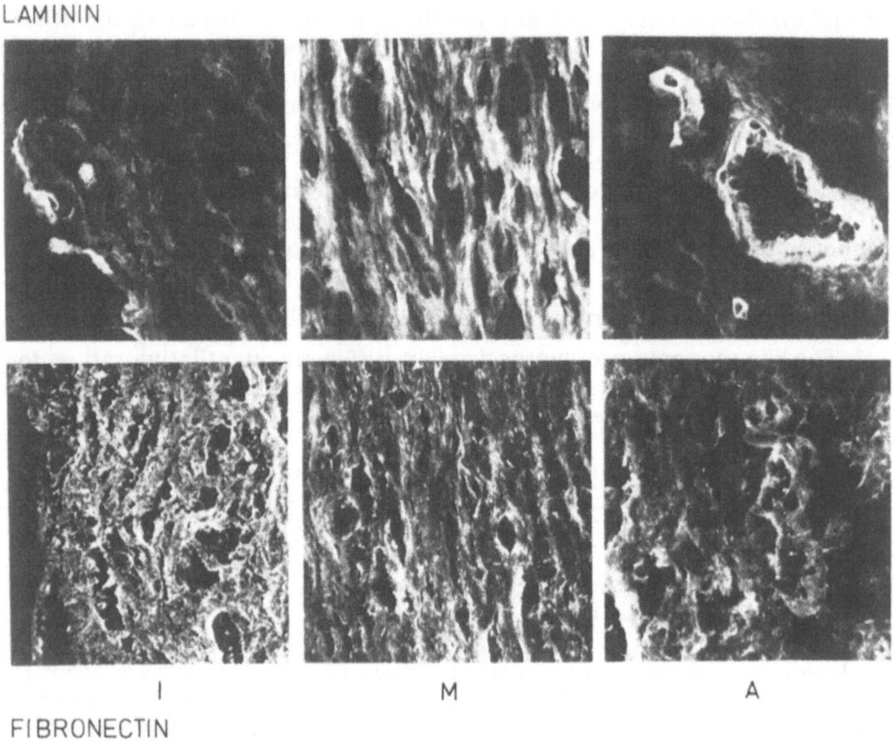

Fig. 1. Immunfluorescence microscopic detection of fibronectin and laminin in the three layers of an atherosclerotic human aorta.

escence detection of laminin (as a representative for basement membrane components) and of fibronectin (as a representative for the "interstitial family") in the three layers of an atherosclerotic human aorta. The intima – the main site of the fibrotic process – is rich in fibronectin, but very poor in laminin. On the other hand, in the normal aorta there is an especially high concentration of laminin and type IV collagen in the intima. In the parenchyma of the liver occurrence of basement membrane components is extremely low. The fibrotic liver, however, shows a remarkable increase in type IV collagen.

Both examples show that qualitative changes occur together with connective tissue proliferation, and that these changes are not uniform, but differ in dependence of the organ affected. There is no general tendency in the composition of the newly formed extracellular matrix, but there are typical organ-specific differences.

One possible reason for this diversity in the composition of fibrotic tissue could be that different cell types are responsible for the production of connective tissue components.

In recent years we have learned that, besides fibroblasts which have been recognized as the main producers of connective tissue components, a number of other cell types are able to produce extracellular matrix proteins. The upper part of table 3 lists those cell types, which are known to play an important role in connective tissue formation.

Smooth muscle cells and myofibroblasts produce a pattern of connective tissue components very similar to that of fibroblasts: Type I ist the main collagen component, together with varying amounts of type III collagen. Smooth muscle cells are responsible for the production of most of the extracellular matrix components in vessel walls, and they are known to occur in atherosclerotic lesions in a biosynthetically active form. Occurrence of myofibroblasts, which in their morphology resemble smooth muscle cells rather than fibroblasts, have been described mainly for pathologic conditions; apparently they play an important role in liver fibrosis (14) or in the formation of granuloma tissues (15).

In their normal functioning form, chondrocytes and endothelial cells reveal a complete different biosynthetic pattern. The main collagenous product of chondrocytes for instance is type II collagen together with other cartilage-specific collagens. Endothelial cells in culture produce relatively low amounts of collagens (mainly type IV, III and V) but large quantities of fibronectin. Both cell types, however, can change their biosynthesis of connective tissue proteins to a more fibroblast-like pattern. Especially chondrocytes are known to undergo a complete change under certain conditions, taking on a fibroblast-like appearance and producing mainly type I and type III collagens (16). This change, which is reversible in cell culture experiments, probably plays an important role in the development fo fibrotic joint diseases.

The cell types mentioned in the lower part of table 3 usually produce, if any, only small amounts of collagens or other connective tissue proteins, but they have been shown to acquire this ability under cell culture conditions (17, 18, 19, 20). It is not known so far whether the potentiality of these cells to take up connective tissue production plays a role in certain fibrotic processes.

There remains an essential question: Why do connective tissue cells change their behaviour, why do they proliferate more than usual and produce more or qualitatively different collagens? A number of authors

Table 3. Cell types which synthesize connective tissue components.

		Collagens	Other connective tissue proteins
"Professionals"	Fibroblasts	I, (III, V)	FN
	Myofibroblasts	I, III, V	FN
	Smooth muscle cells	I, III, V	FN
	Chondrocytes	II, (I, III)	Chondronectin
	Endothelial cells	III, IV, V, SC	FN
"Amateurs"*	Several epithelial cells	IV, I	FN
	Hepatocytes	I	FN
	Several neural cells	I	?
	Myocytes/myotubes	I, III, V	FN
	Macrophages	(I, III, V)	FN

* Synthesis of connective tissue components under cell culture conditions.

agree in the hypothesis that the onset of fibrosis is essentially a process of repair as reaction to an injury. A skin wound, for instance, causes an inflammative reaction followed by connective tissue activation, finally leading to scar formation.

R. Crystal (21) has emphasized the idea that in fibrosis it is not the reaction of connective-tissue-producing cells that is pathologic – they react in the normal way as they should do in the case of injury and inflammation. But there is a decisive quantitative difference in the degree of injury, which is not limited to a small area, but may involve the whole organ, e.g., alcoholic intoxication of the liver. The damage caused by this injury is too great for the repair process to lead to a normally functioning tissue. The persistent dysfunction of the organ may cause further cell necrosis and new inflammative reaction, thus leading to a self-perpetuation of the fibrotic process.

There are several mechanisms by which injury can result in connective tissue activation. Though in some cases connective-tissue-forming cells may be activated directly, e.g., by a toxic agent, the more common mechanism will be that inflammation-specific cells produce mediators, which activate connective tissue cells.

A number of different substances have been identified as mediators in connective tissue activation in a more or less specific way. Three main groups may be mentioned here:

(1) Chemotactic substances: they attract fibroblasts or other cells towards the area of inflammation.

(2) Growth factors: they induce proliferation of connective tissue synthesizing cells.

(3) Proteases: enhanced proteolytic activity is mostly found in inflammative processes and several invading phagocytes produce actively a number of extracellular proteases; they contribute to connective tissue activation in a complex manner that is often not fully understood.

Proliferation is probably the most important reaction in the course of connective tissue activation. It has even been doubted that fibroblasts can be activated to produce more collagen per cell (21). On the other hand, smooth muscle cells are known to change from a quiescent form to a biosynthetically active form (22, 23).

Figure 2a gives a general scheme of connective tissue activation following injury. Figure 2b and 2c present two important variants of this process. Activation in connection with hemostasis (fig. 2b) is an important part of the wound healing process, but may contribute essentially also to the appearance of fibrotic lesions in atherosclerosis (24). In figure 2c the role of immunologic processes in connective tissue activation is emphasized, which probably play a role in most fibrotic processes and contribute – via autoimmune reactions – essentially to the self-perpetuation of fibrotic diseases.

There are in principal two ways of intervening therapeutically in fibrotic processes. The first is the inhibition of collagen production. Several steps in the course of collagen biosynthesis can be inhibited: possibilities of special therapeutic interest are

(1) to inhibit proline hydroxylation by proline analogues, which are built into the polypeptide chains. The underhydroxylated chains cannot

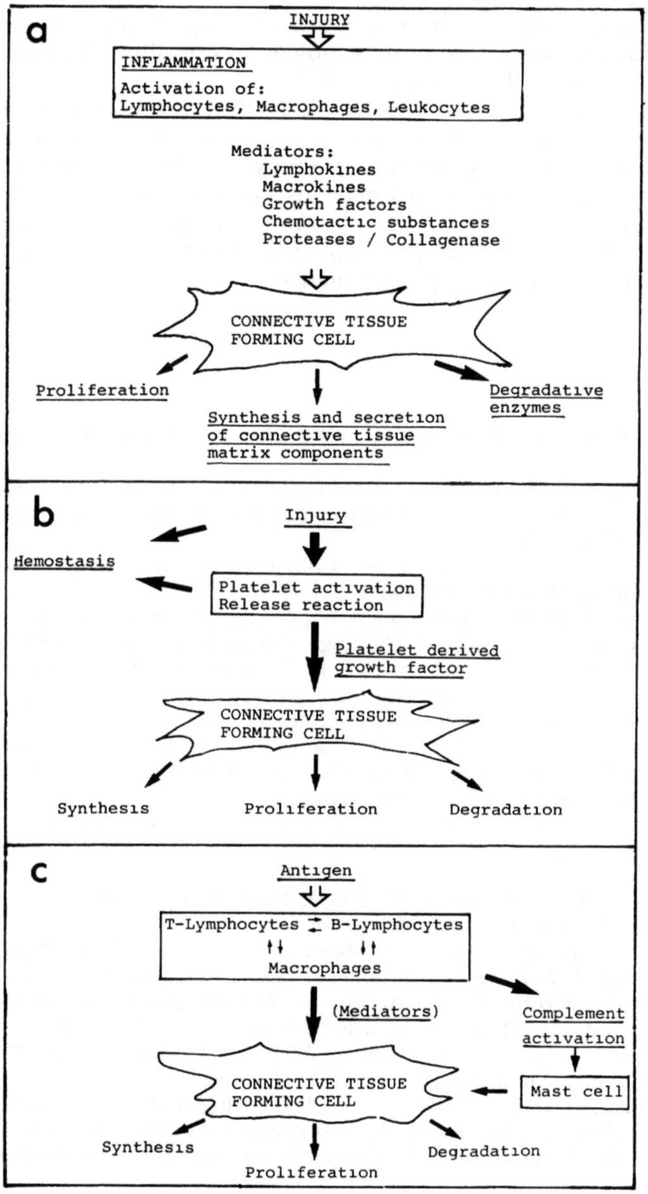

Fig. 2. Mechanisms of connective tissue activation. (a) General mechanism of connective tissue activation as response to injury. (b) Connective tissue activation in connection to hemostasis. (c) Connective tissue activation as response to immunologic processes.

form the triple helical collagen structure and are degraded within the cell,
(2) to inhibit secretion by tubulin-interfering agents like colchicin,
(3) to inhibit the formation of intermolecular crosslinks by agents like D-penicillamine or β-aminopropionitrile.

The second way is to inhibit the activation of connective tissue cells. Inhibition of the mediator-synthesizing activity of inflammatory cells may be more successful in antifibrotic therapy than the specific inhibition of collagen synthesis. The widespread use of cortison and related steroid hormones in antifibrotic therapy shows the importance of this way, and better knowledge of the single steps in connective tissue activation may lead to more specific therapeutic agents.

References

1. Hay, E. D. (editor): Cell Biology of Extracellular Matrix. Plenum Press (New York 1981).
2. Burgeson, R. E., D. W. Hollister: Collagen Heterogeneity in Human Cartilage: Identification of Several New Collagen Chains. Biochem. Biophys. Res. Com. **87,** 1124–1131 (1979).
3. Reese, Ch. A., R. Mayne: Minor Collagens of Chicken Hyaline Cartilage. Biochemistry **20,** 5443–5448 (1981).
4. von der Mark, K., M. van Menxel, H. Wiedemann: Isolation and Characterization of New Collagens from Chick Cartılage. Europ. J. Biochem. **124** (1), 5762 (1982).
5. Ricard-Blum, S., D. J. Hartmann, D. Herbage, C. Payen-Meyran, G. Ville: Biochemical Properties and Immunolocalization of Minor Collagens in Foetal Calf Cartilage. FEBS-Letters **146** (2), 343–345 (1982).
6. Burgeson, R. F., P. A. Hebda, N. P. Morris, D. W. Hollister: Human Cartilage Collagen. Comparison of Cartilage Collagens with Human Type IV Collagen. J. Biol. Chem. **257** (13), 7852–7856 (1982).
7. Hewitt, A. T., H. K. Kleinman, J. P. Pennypacker, G. R. Martin: Identification of an Adhesion Factor for Chondrocytes. Proc. Nat. Acad. Sci. US-Bio. Sci. **77,** 385 (1980).
8. Kuehn, K., H. H. Schoene, R. Timpl: New Trends in Basement Membrane Research. Raven Press (New York 1982).
9. Sage, H.: Collagens of Basement Membranes. J. Invest. Derm. **79,** 5159 (1982).
10. Rauterberg, J., S. Allam: Occurrence of Type I and Type III Collagen ın Normal and Atherosclerotic Human Aortas. In: Atherosclerosis IV. Schettler, G., Y. Goto, Y. Hata, G. Klose (ed.), p. 368, Springer-Verlag (Berlin 1977).
11. Rauterberg, J., S. Allam, U. Brehmer, W. Wirth, W. H. Hauss: Das Kollagen der Arterienwand. Therapiewoche **29,** 2717–2737 (1979).
12. Rauterberg, J., H.-E. Schlief, G. Pott: The Collagen of the Normal and Fibrotic Liver. In: Connective Tissue of the Normal and Fibrotic Human Liver. Gerlach, U., G. Pott, J. Rauterberg, B. Voß (ed.), pp. 36–37, Thieme Verlag (Stuttgart 1982).
13. Weber, L., W. N. Meigel, W. Spier: Collagen Polymorphism in Pathologic Human Scars. Arch. Dermatol. Res. **261,** 63–71 (1978).
14. Rudolph, R., W. J. McClure, M. Woodward: Contractile Fibroblasts in Chronic Alcoholic Cirrhosis. Gastroenterology **76,** 704 (1979).
15. Gabbiani, G., M. LeLous, A. J. Bailey, S. Bazin, A. Delaunnay: Collagen and Myofibroblasts of Granulation Tissue. A Chemical, Ultrastructural and Immunological Study. Virchows Arch. B Cell Path. **21,** 133 (1976).

16. v. d. Mark, K., V. Gauss, H. v. d. Mark, P. Müller: Relationship between Cell Shape and Type of Collagen Synthesis as Chondrocytes Lose their Cartilage Phenotype in Culture. Nature, Vol. **267**, 5611, 531–32 (1977).
17. Voß, B., J. Rauterberg, K. Ullrich, V. Gieselmann: Primary Cultures of Rat Hepatocytes Synthesize Fibronectin. Biochem. Biophys. Res. Comm. **90,** 1348–1354 (1979).
18. Hata, R. J., Y. Ninomiya, Y. Nagai, Y. Tsukuda: Biosynthesis of Interstitial Types of Collagen by Albumin-Producing Rat Liver Parenchymal Cell (Hepatocytes) Clones in Culture. Biochemistry **19,** 169–176 (1980).
19. Hatahara, T., J. M. Seyer: Procollagen production by Rat Hepatocytes in Primary Culture. Biochim. Biophys. Acta **716** (3), 431 (1982).
20. Laurent, M., P. Kern, Y. Courtois, F. Regnault: Synthesis of Types I, III and IV Collagen by Bovine Lens Epithelial Cells in Long-Term Culture. Exper. Cell Res. **134,** 23 (1981).
21. Crystal, R. G., S. J. Rennard, P. B. Bittermann: Conformity and Diversity of Fibrotic Processes. In: Connective Tissue of the Normal and Fibrotic Human Liver. Gerlach, U., G. Pott, J. Rauterberg, B. Voß (ed.), pp. 3–7, Thieme Verlag (Stuttgart 1982).
22. Haust, M. D., R. H. More: Significance of the Smooth Muscle. Cell in Atherogenesis. In: Evolution of the Atherosclerotic Plaque, R. Jones (ed.), The University of Chicago Press (1963).
23. Staubesand, J.: Ein neuer Aspekt zur Pathogenese der Mediadysplasie: Myozytentransformation, Matrix-Vesikel und extrazelluläre Lysosomen in der Wand fehlbelasteter Blutgefäße. Münch. Med. Wschr. **121,** 57–64 (1979).
24. Ross, R.: Atherosclerosis: A Problem of the Biology of Arterial Wall Cells and Their Interactions with Blood Components. Arteriosclerosis **1,** 293 (1981).

Authors' address:

Dr. Jürgen Rauterberg, Institut für Arterioskleroseforschung, Domagkstraße 3, 4400 Münster, FRG

Cardiac Adaptation to Hemodynamic Overload, Training and Stress
Dr. D. Steinkopff Verlag 314–329 (1983)

Cardiovascular aging

J. Lindner and P. Schmiegelow*)

Department of Pathology, University of Hamburg (FRG)

Summary

Cardiovascular aging processes are demonstrated by combined morphological and biochemical methods.

It is shown that investigations on aging have to regard the phases of development, growth, and maturation. The prenatal and postnatal differentiation and development of the muscle and connective tissue cells of the myocard are important for aging of the heart.

The demonstrated reactions on stimuli and injuries, the increased ^{3}H-thymidine-labeling index, the enhanced DNA-synthesis and turnover, the compensatory hypertrophy and polyploidization – until the numerical hyperplasia of the heart muscle cells are indicators for the capacity of the human heart in regeneration after injury or loss of heart muscle cells (in humans as well as in experimental animals, especially after infarction, hypoxia, and ischemia).

Aging of heart and arteries is the aging of the cardiovascular connective tissue components.

Besides alterations in cells and proteoglycans/GAG, resp., the very important age fibrosis is investigated on the cardiovascular tissues. The comparability of the age-dependent changes investigated in human organs with corresponding findings obtained on organs from other species (rats) is demonstrated, with special references to comparable age groups from the period of postnatal maturation and its cessation through the period of aging until the senile age.

Age-dependent proteoglycan-alterations are frequently caused by reductions of synthesis, degradation and turnover, by changes of the chemical compositions, and the molecular weights of proteoglycans, by alterations of the glycosaminoglycans (GAG)-distribution patterns, of the relative and absolute amount of the individual GAG and by alterations of the proteoglycan aggregate-sizes.

Then the appropriate results of the age-related alterations of synthesis, degradation, turnover, half-life, total content and type patterns of collagen in cardiovascular aging of humans and rats are demonstrated and discussed.

Failures of transcriptions and translations can increase with disturbed DNA repair mechanisms in connective tissue cells with aging. This is why the danger of faulty synthesis processes grows with aging, regarding especially the less precise proteoglycan/GAG-synthesis, the GAG patterns (the microheterogeneity of GAG), the increasing synthesis of non-collagen proteins with aging, the alterations of the collagen type patterns, the amyloid formation, etc. with cardiovascular aging. But the normal synthesis processes are difficult to distinguish from the synthesis processes due to pathological conditions or diseases!

The adaptation capacities of the cardiovascular organs, especially of the heart, become smaller with aging. The number of diseases increases and grafts more strongly on the heart as well as on arteries in cardiovascular aging.

*) This work was supported by the Deutsche Forschungsgemeinschaft, Bonn-Bad Godesberg.

The clinical term of "aging heart" is to be considered newly, using the new data of the connective tissue research in heart aging. An aging atrophy of the heart does not exist, but an aging insufficiency and more a polypathy of the heart in aging of humans and other species.

Older organs are more diseased than younger ones. This is especially true for the cardiovascular system. So these investigations on the cardiovascular aging have practical importance especially regarding the so-called polypathy, i.e., the increase in the number of diseases with aging.

Key words: cardiovascular aging, connective tissue aging, collagen content, collagen pattern, ^{3}H-thymidine-labeling index, proteoglycan, glycosaminoglycan

During life the first cardiovascular reaction in humans and animals to several unspecific stimuli (and injuries) can be an increase of the division and performance metabolism of cardiovascular connective tissue cells (6, 15, 24, 25, 36). This is investigated by morphological and biochemical methods (details see: 23–25, 29, 36–38).

The increased proliferation rates are determined by ^{3}H-thymidine-autoradiographs of human vascular smooth muscle cells and endothelia as well as by assays of the specific DNA-activity of cardiovascular tissues.

^{3}H-Thymidine Labeling Index (in %)

	1 day bef. birth	1.5 month	5.5 month
Hepatocytes	4.05	0.84	0.31
Kupffer + Sinusoid Cells	1.13	2.37	1.75
Portal Conn. Tissue Cells		2.45	2.00
Endothelia			
- Liver Central Veins		0.88	1.15
- Endocard		5.11	3.50
- Aorta		0.73	0.38
Smooth Muscle Cells			
- Aorta	11.00	8.10	5.05
- A.pulmonalis	13.11	9.02	7.11
- Small Intestine	12.74	10.00	8.04
- Colon	19.03	15.11	13.14
Joint Cartilage			
- Shoulder		0.58	0.10
- Knee		0.66	0.13
Epiphys. Cartilage			
- Shoulder		13.60	0.50
- Knee		15.17	0.58
Spinal Joint Cartilage		1.30	0.50
Nucleus pulposus		0.70	0.51
Anulus fibrosus		0.40	0.90
Rib Cartilage		0.53	0.20
- Perichondrium		0.46	0.33

Fig. 1. ^{3}H-thymidine-labeling index (in percent) of various cardiovascular and other connective tissue cells during development and maturation (further details, see text).

The ^{3}-H-thymidine-labeling indices of the several connective tissue cells decrease rapidly and significantly up to the end of the growth phase of rats and mice. These values are as low as the values (= ^{3}H-thymidine-labeling indices) of the most stabile parenchymal cells (hepatocytes etc.) (fig. 1). Contrary to that, the indices of the various endothelia and especially of the several smooth muscle cells are higher. There are differences, due to location and function; e.g. the ^{3}H-thymidine-labeling indices of aortic endothelia are 5 times lower than the values of endocardial endothelia of the heart after the end of maturation in adult rats and mice. The indices of gastro-intestinal smooth muscle cells are partly 2 times higher than those of the vascular ones during and after the end of maturation and growth (25, 36–38) (fig. 1).

So the most connective tissue cells, including aortic endothelia, react on several stimuli (irritations and injuries) "out of rest", but the smooth muscle cells react "out of run", because their growth fraction resp. proliferation pool is more extensive during life. Vascular smooth muscle cells

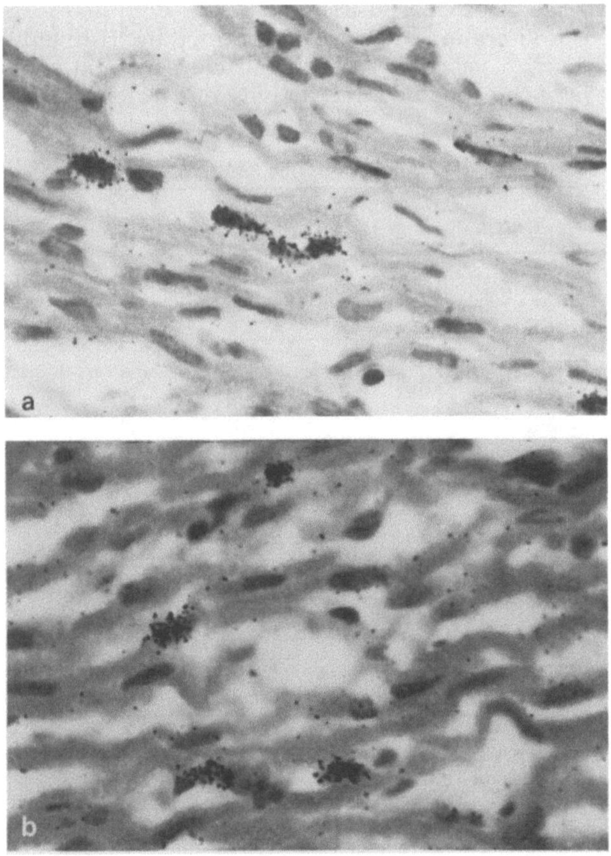

Fig. 2. a+b) Examples of ^{3}H-thymidine-autoradiographs of heart muscle cells and myocardial connective tissue cells during the first three postnatal weeks of rats.

and myocardial connective tissue cells can react very fast on stimuli and injuries during the whole life. These findings are important for disease, grafted on age-dependent changes (23–25).

Replications of heart-connective tissue cells, partly also of heart muscle cells, are found by ^{3}H-thymidine autoradiographs immediately after birth. The cell proliferation rates of smooth muscle cells and heart muscle cells are quantified autoradiographically (fig. 2).

The ^{3}H-thymidine-labeling index is used as a rough measure of the proliferation rates, for the DNA synthesis, and for the DNA turnover of muscle cells and of non-muscle cells (= connective tissue cells) of the heart and arteries.

The ^{3}H-thymidine indices and therewith the proliferation rates of muscle and non-muscle cells of the heart as well as of arterial smooth muscle cells can be influenced by several stimuli and injuries, especially by hypoxia (as a general unspecific pathogenetic factor) as well as by some drugs. This is demonstrated by examples. The mitogen Kallikrein elevates significantly the ^{3}H-thymidine-labeling indices of smooth muscle cells of arteries (and other organs) as well as of muscle and non-muscle cells of the heart by one single application (with dosis-dependent differences). This is shown in figure 3a, furthermore that the ^{3}H-thymidine-labeling indices of heart muscle cells of ventricles are higher than those of the atria. Both are significantly enhanced by Kallikrein (fig. 3a). This is also true for Kallikrein influences on the specific DNA-activity as well as on the DNA-content (= the sum of increase and decrease (= turnover) of cells) (36, 37).

The DNA-content of rat-heart (compared with kidney) is significantly increased by various Kallikrein-dosages, compared with controls, in 21-day-old rat embryos (= one day before birth) (fig. 3b).

The extent and the normalization of the increased labeling indices depend on kind and duration of the injury (hypoxia included) as well as on its localization in the heart (as well as in arteries).

The compensatory hypertrophy, the increased DNA synthesis – till the numerical hyperplasia of heart muscle cells, are indicators for their regeneration-possibilities in young, adult, and old animals.

The number of connective tissue cells increases 5 times during physiological heart growth and up to 10 times in markedly hypertrophied hearts. During normal heart growth in the first postnatal weeks and in cardiac hypertrophy, a numerical hyperplasia of myocytes and of myocardial connective tissue cells takes place (1, 11, 22, 23, 34).

The more increased DNA-synthesis of the connective tissue cells seems to be of functional importance for the muscle cells of the heart. There are morphological (structural) and functional (biochemical) relationships and interactions between muscle and non-muscle cells of the heart, which are to be investigated in future. Mitotic divisions of both cell types of rat myocardium are demonstrated in the prenatal and the early postnatal phase of development (till the 7th or the 14th postnatal day).

Mitotic processes of heart muscle cells are not accompanied by total dedifferentiation: the myofibrils and myofilaments are demonstrable in the myocytes during mitosis. The architecture of the myocytes of different animals is formed during the first few postnatal weeks. So no differences exist between this postnatal development and the adult phase of life. Most differentiation processes are completely

^{3}H-THYMIDINE LABELING INDEX (%)
Newborn Rat

	Expos. Time	NaCl	5 KU	25 KU
SMALL	2 weeks	8.28	13.96	11.26
INTESTINE	3 "	12.74	18.48	ø
S M C	4 "	14.37	21.63	ø
COLON	2 weeks	15.03	ø	18.16
S M C	4 "	21.88	ø	26.17
A. PULMON. S M C	2 weeks	3.93	ø	5.13
HEART MUSCLE C.				
ATRIUM	2 weeks	4.90	ø	6.97
VENTRICLE	2 "	7.65	ø	9.16

S M C = Smooth Muscle Cells

EINFLUSS VON KALLIKREIN BEI UNTERSCHIEDLICHER DOSIERUNG AUF DEN DNA-GEHALT VON NIERE UND HERZ BEI 21 TAGE ALTEN EMBRYONEN (RATTE)
INFLUENCE OF KALLIKREIN IN DIFFERENT DOSES ON THE DNA-CONTENT OF KIDNEY AND HEART ON 21 DAYS OLD EMBRYOS (RAT)

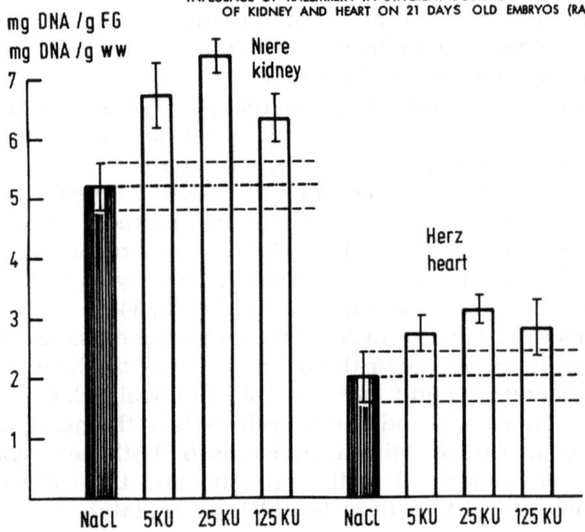

Fig. 3. a) ^{3}H-thymidine-labeling indices (in percent) of smooth muscle and heart muscle cells of newborn rats with significant increase by two doses of the mitogen Kallikrein (single application), compared with controls; b) increase of the DNA content of the heart (compared with kidney) by three Kallikrein doses (single applications) (further details, see fig. 3 and text).

finished after the first 3 to 4 postnatal weeks of development (regarding myofibrils, mitochondria, sarcoplasmic reticulum, glycogen, morphology of nuclei, etc.). There are some differences, especially between both the ventricles.

The volume densities of the heart muscle cells, of the non-muscle cells (= connective tissue cells), of the intercellular space, and finally of the capillary lumen and endothelia show some differences between both heart ventricles, vary during life, but are mostly the same in high age as at birth (11, 12, 15, 26, 28, 33, 34). Aging processes are more pronounced in the left than in the right heart.

The volume densities of the endothelial cells decrease in the right and remain constant in the left ventricle during life. The numerical density of the connective tissue cells is more than 2 times higher in the left than in the right ventricle, increasing about 20 % in the right and decreasing about 30 % in the left ventricle till the end of the growth phase (to the 6th month of rat life). This numerical density remains constant until high age. The same seems to be true in case of endothelial cells: At birth, their numerical density in the right ventricle is about 40 % of the value in the left ventricle, increasing till the 6th month, but remains constant till the high age.

During life, there is a particularly marked increase in the percentage of the intercellular space and in the non-muscle cell volume: in the right ventricle increasing from 25 to 51 % (duplication) at the end of 27th month of rats and in the left ventricle in that time from 35 to 58 % (less than in the right ventricle). The composition of the volume of heart muscle cells shows characteristic alterations during life, regarding the volume density of sarcoplasm, of myofibrils, of mitochondria, of the mitochondrial-myofibrillar ratio, etc., with differences between both ventricles (review: 11).

There are metabolic and structural relationships between heart muscle cells and non-heart muscle cells. This is demonstrated by morphological and biochemical investigations.

Age-related alterations of connective tissue cells and their products are decisive for aging of the cardiovascular system (3–5, 7–14, 16–19, 21–23, 30–32, 35, 43).

Age-dependent alterations of the content, performance, function, and efficiency of cardiovascular connective tissue cells are investigated during life, including the last prenatal as well as the first and following postnatal phases of development and maturation, the period of adult life *and* the senile age (20, 22, 23, 25, 29, 36–38). Therefore we compared the results of aging-investigations on arteries and hearts of humans and rats, with special reference to comparable age groups of these life periods.

The DNA-content of human and rat aorta and heart declines strongest during the first postnatal growth, less during the following maturation period. This depends mainly on the growth of cell cytoplasma and of intercellular substances, especially in humans. The DNA-content of the aorta of humans is nearly 4 times lower than that of rats at the end of the growth phase in comparable age groups as well as in the further life periods until high age. After the end of the growth period, the DNA-content of human and rat aorta and heart remains generally constant until advanced age. So we found a decrease of the DNA-content of the ventricles and atria of human left and right heart until the end of the growth phase, constant values until 60 years, after which a slight increase was observed in senium (especially through polyploidization (fig. not in press). There are also hearts without hypertrophy. The polyploidization of nuclei seems to be age-related, because it is observed in other aging mesenchymal and parenchymal cells, too. But polyploidization starts earlier in the heart than in other organs (1, 3, 5, 22, 23, 25, 26, 31, 33, 34, 41).

The absolute cell number of the heart can be estimated by means of assays of the pure myocardial weight, of the myocardial DNA amount, of the ploidy-grade of the nuclei, and of the ratio of the heart muscle cells to the myocardial connective tissue cells (1, 15, 34).

The constancy of the cell number is to be regarded as one of the signs for the end of maturation on the basis of the growth equilibrium achieved at cell level. The constancy of the DNA-content (or the cell number) is identical with achieving an overall constancy in the ^{3}H-thymidine-labeling indices. Heart, arteries, and other smooth muscular organs can be included in the group of the so-called stabile tissues and organs (22–25, 36–38).

Summarizing the results, it is shown that the DNA-content exhibits a statistically significant decrease to the level of about (or less than) 50 % of the initial values (of newborns) for aorta and heart as well as for the most human organs at the end of the maturation and growth phase. Significant age differences cannot be determined after this point under physiological conditions. This is also true for rats (7, 22, 23, 25). These results are particularly important because the DNA-content is the best parameter for investigations of cell performances, function, and metabolic rates during life, especially in connective tissue aging of the cardiovascular (and other) organs (7, 16, 23, 25, 31).

The specific DNA-activity of the aorta and the heart of mice and rats is higher than that of stabile mesenchymal (e.g., cartilage) and parenchymal organs (e.g., liver). But the specific DNA-activity of the cardiovascular organs decreases significantly 1. during postnatal maturation, 2. from the end of the growth phase until the 18th month and 3. from this age to senium (23, 25). This is an indication for the turnover-decrease of vascular smooth muscle and of myocardial cells during and after maturation, especially in senium (fig. 4).

The contents of uronic acids and hexosamines (the main components of connective tissue ground substance) are reduced in relation to the DNA-content in the cardiovascular connective tissue from the 3rd to the 18th month of a rat's life as well as in the comparable human age groups, more in aging (24, 25) (fig. 4).

The activities of glycosaminoglycan (GAG) synthesizing and degrading enzymes decrease during maturation and aging of aorta and heart in humans and rats (7, 13, 16, 23, 25). The same is true for the ^{35}S-sulfate-

Rat	Uronic Acid/DNA			Hexosamine/DNA			^{3}H-Thymidine/DNA		
Months	3	6	18	3	6	18	3	6	18
Aorta	0.56	0.51	0.48	0.50	0.51	0.44	6.35	3.89	2.71
Skin	0.29	0.23	0.17	0.48	0.53	0.31	7.74	7.98	2.79
Liver	0.11	0.04	0.10	0.16	0.13	0.22	0.43	0.27	0.18

underlined values : $p < 0.01$, 3 → 18 months

Fig. 4. Significant decline of the specific DNA-activity as well as of the uronic acid/DNA- and the hexosamine/DNA-ratio of the aorta (compared with skin and liver) between the 3rd and 18th month, of rat life (further details, see text).

incorporation, the indicator method for assays of the GAG synthesis. The specific activity of sulfated GAG of aorta and heart of humans and rats declines in maturation and aging, too. So the results of both methods are similar. The specific activity of sulfated GAG depends on the amount of GAG, synthesized per time unit, the transport velocity, the pool size of specific labeled precursors and the tissue concentration of the analyzed proteoglycans (7). The decline of this typical connective tissue performance is found in relation to the DNA-content as well as to the dry weight during life, especially in aging (7, 16, 22–25, 29) (fig. 5a). The same is true for the activities of enzymes of collagen synthesis and degradation. This is important for reactions of vascular (arterial) smooth muscle cells on applicated stimuli or injuries during life (14, 22, 23, 25).

There is a strong exponential decline in the ^{35}S-sulfate-incorporation with age (related to wet and dry weight), a weaker DNA-decrease and thus a decrease in the typical arterial performance related to the DNA-content or to the content of the smooth muscle cells responsible.

These relationships are similar, though not identical, to other connective tissues of rats (fig. 5a). Cartilage shows the same exponential decline in the ^{35}S-sulfate incorporation rate related to wet and dry weight. This decrease can be divided into 3 phases: very steep during postnatal development and maturation, far less steep during aging – as in other mesenchymal and so-called parenchymal organs. The specific performance of ^{35}S-sulfate incorporation increases at high age in cartilage, in contrast to aorta, skin, heart, etc. (fig. 5a).

This is also true for GAG synthesizing enzymes, in part for further anabolic and catabolic enzymes of cartilage, too. The heart shows constancy of the ^{35}S-sulfate incorporation rates related to the DNA-content, similar like the skin. The stability of this performance related to cell content means: fibroblasts of the skin have the same performance (measured quantitively) at high age as in youth (fig. 5a) (5, 22, 24, 31). These results are also found for collagen synthesis and for oxygen consumption – related to the cell content. The same comes true for the heart – in contrast to the lung (with this course until the 28th month of life) (fig. 5a).

The ^{35}S-sulfate incorporation-rates decline exponentially in intima and media (and both together) as the specific activity of sulfated GAG from birth to high age in human aorta (fig. not in press). Arteries react with this specific performance on stimuli (or injuries) at higher age, too, but significantly less from the younger to the older age-groups (also in atheroma as in unchanged parts of the same aorta, in intima and media, compared with each other) (fig. 5b). This special arterial function is highest in fresh edema lesions and significantly increased in comparison to unchanged parts of the same human aorta in all age-groups, more in the intima than in the media (in-vitro incubation and incorporation with the most suitable precursor for investigations of the synthesis of sulfated GAG = ^{35}S-sulfate). The significant differences are indicated in figure 5b. The values are always higher in the intima than in the media of unchanged parts as well as of edema and fibrous plaques and of atheroma of the same human aorta. There is a significant decrease in both layers in scarring of these edema plaques and a further significant decrease in the resulting atheroma, compared with edema plaques and with the unchanged parts of the same aorta (fig. 5b). The findings demonstrated are responsible for the fact that the hexosamine content is higher than the uronic acid content in early atherosclerotic edema lesions in all age-groups, decreasing during life (fig. 6a) (24).

There are differences between the hexosamine and the uronic acid contents. Hexosamine-assays measure the acid *and* neutral glycoproteins, in the serum and in fresh edema (again with highest level in the youngest age-group). The age-dependent increase of the uronic acid and of the hydroxyproline contents in unchanged

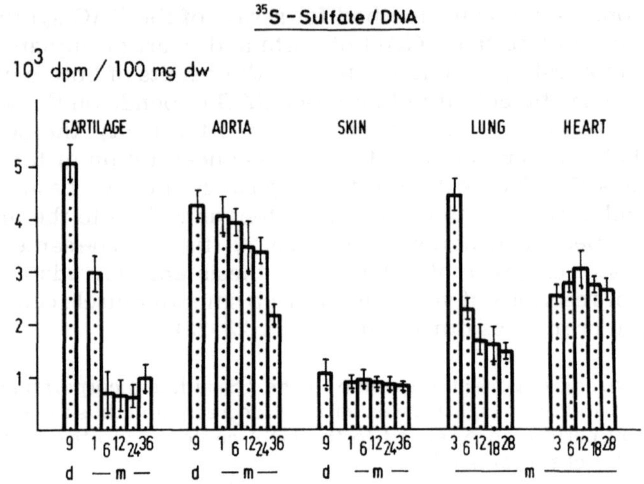

a)

S^{35}- SULFATE - INCORPORATION (cpm/mg dw) in vitro
in DEVELOPMENT and SCARRING of ATHEROSCLEROSIS

AORTA	AGE (in years)	MORPHOL. unchanged	EDEMA PLAQUES	FIBROUS PLAQUES	ATHEROMA
INTIMA	4o - 6o	51o2	7998	388o	2776
	61 - 8o	3441	5339	2449	1993
	81 - 9o	3oo1	ø	2333	1776
MEDIA	4o - 6o	2493	3447	2779	1882
	61 - 8o	1993	37o2	1424	899
	81 - 9o	1567	ø	2oo2	11o1

b) Significant values : ●●) = p < o.o1 ; ●) = p < o.o5

Fig. 5. a) Examples for the ^{35}S-sulfate incorporation rates in relation to the DNA-content: cardiovascular system (heart and aorta) compared with other mesenchymal and parenchymal organs of rats (from the 9th day (d) till the 28th or 36th month (m), resp.); b) Age-dependent differences in the results of this indicator assay for the synthesis of sulfated GAG in intima and media of several atherosclerotic plaques, compared with unchanged parts of the same human aorta (further details, see text).

Increase of Hexosamine Content and Decrease of Hydroxyproline Content in Developing Atherosclerosis (Early Lesions = E.L.)

Age (in years)	Hexosamine (mg/g dw)		Uronic Acids (mg/g dw)		Hydroxyproline (mg/g dw)	
	Norm.	E.L.	Norm.	E.L.	Norm.	E.L.
- 3o	13.8	15.1	4.5	5.3	4.2	3.9
4o - 6o	9.8	11.2	5.4	6.4	6.o	4.9
61 - 7o	7.8	1o.8	6.8	8.2	9.9	6.4
71 - 8o	7.o	7.4	7.o	5.1	12.7	8.2

a)

HEART-AGING : Water Content in %

	HEART	Lung	Xiphoid Cartilage	Aorta
R A T				
3 Months	77.46	79.51	52.46	68.34
6 "	77.79	79.86	46.83	72.21
12 "	77.41	77.85	57.90	67.30
22 "	76.09	78.90	48.37	64.20
31 "	76.73	78.42	∅	59.83
HUMAN				
- 5 Years	82.24	80.26	∅	78.90
11-15 "	79.40	77.98	69.07	71.99
30-39 "	80.30	82.23	62.79	77.08
50-64 "	76.02	80.26	57.27	73.27
75-79 "	77.89	80.28	63.13	73.56

b)

Fig. 6. a) Aging alterations of hexosamine, uronic acids, and hydroxyproline contents in unchanged human aorta, compared with so-called early lesions (E.L.) of atherosclerosis (see: fig. 5b and 6b); b) Percentual water content of the human and rat cardiovascular system (heart and aorta), compared with lung and cartilage during life (till high age: see text).

parts and in the early lesions in these age-classifications is demonstrated (fig. 6a). Early atherosclerotic lesions show a slight increase of uronic acids (only), but a significant decrease of the collagen content, due to the collagen-breakdown (fig. 6a) (23–25).

The changes of the GAG-patterns (= of the GAG-heterogeneity) – characteristic for the heart as well as for the different connective tissues – should be considered in heart aging, too – besides hybridizations, changes of sulfatation rates, of linkage regions, of chain lengths, molecular weights, of GAG-composition, -distribution, -pattern, -types, of aggregate sizes of proteoglycans, etc. (7). But all these age-dependent alterations of proteoglycans, GAG, resp., (and of collagen) do not influence the water content in rat and human heart with aging: comparing the water content of human and rat hearts, we found similarly the same water content in human as in rat heart, and no significant differences with aging for each species (fig. 6b). The constancy of water content exists until the 31st month for rat hearts, compared with the water content of the human heart until the 79th year of life, also with nearly constant values during this life period (without significantly differences between the compared age-groups of rats and humans). The same is true for the lung, consisting mainly of connective tissue, like the heart. Aorta and xiphoid cartilage, compared with the heart, show on the contrary percentual water contents in the rat which are partly significant lower than the values of the comparable age-groups of men. There is no evidence for a so-called "Altersaustrocknung" of the heart (nor of the compared mesenchymal and parenchymal organs) (fig. 6b), (8, 20, 22, 23, 25, 38).

In the human heart we found an initial decline of hexosamines and uronic acids in both atria, followed by a gradual rise during aging, especially of the uronic acid contents also in the left, but not in the right human ventricle in aging. Furthermore we found, as some other authors, a decline of the hexosamine and hexuronic-acid contents as well as of the hexosamine/hydroxyproline- and of the hexuronic acid/hydroxyproline ratios in heart aging of rats as well as in aging of human and rat aorta (fig. not in press). Similar results are reported by other groups in myocardial and arterial aging of human and other mammalians (10, 12, 15, 16, 22, 23, 25, 29–31, 35, 43).

Synthesis and degradation of collagen decrease, the content of soluble collagen fractions declines, the insoluble collagen fraction increases relatively and finally absolutely with cardiovascular aging. The collagen turnover decreases, the half-life increases in aging of heart and aorta. These results are summarized in a table (not in press), including age-related alterations of collagen types (= of the collagen heterogeneity) in the cardiovascular as well as in other connective tissues, which are discussed in detail by Rauterberg.

The collagen synthesis is reduced with cardiovascular aging (demonstrable by assays of protocollagen-prolylhydroxylase (PPH), of labeled hydroxyproline, of the specific activity of hydroxyproline, etc.). Measurement of the incorporations of radioactive proline into protein-bound hydroxyproline, although it is not entirely specific to collagen, is a widely used method for studying the synthesis rate of collagen (5, 9, 10, 14, 19, 22–25).

The high PPH-activity in young rats is due to the growth process (fig. 7a). The 1st and 2nd significant decreases after the end of maturation and during the further cardiovascular aging are similar to most organs investigated (as in aging rat aorta, combined with enhanced aorta and body weights: fig. 7a).

The collagen pool of organs increases with aging. So the specific activity of hydroxyproline (after a single injection of labeled proline) decreases with age from the 4-months-old to the 24-months-old (and older) rats, more so than does the incorporation of proline related to weight (23).

PPH - ACTIVITY OF RAT AORTA

age	body weight (g)	aorta (g)	PPH (dpm x 10^{-3}/ mg N)	
5 weeks	93.18 ± 7.44	0.111 ± 0.021	25.0 ± 6.2	
				> $p < 0.01$
4 months	378.30 ± 17.76	0.254 ± 0.025	9.8 ± 1.3	
				> $p < 0.01$
25 months	450.83 ± 51.05	0.315 ± 0.063	4.5 ± 0.7	

a)

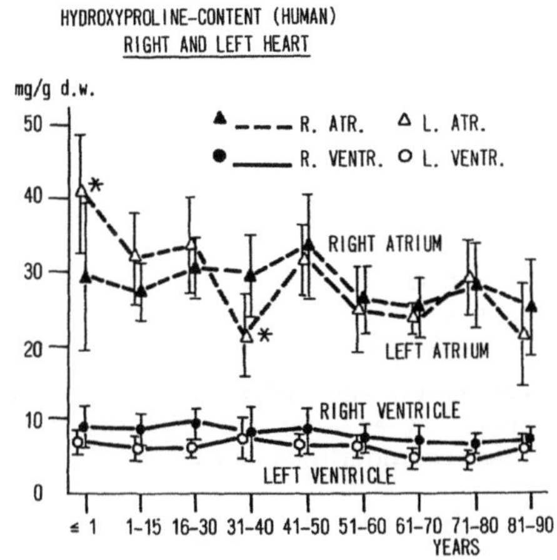

b)

Fig. 7. a) PPH-activity of rat aorta at various ages as well as body and aorta weights of rats (details see text); b) collagen (hydroxyproline) content of the right and left atria and ventricles of human hearts (* = statistically significant differences; d.w. = dry weight).

Metabolic activity (collagen turnover) is observed to be higher in younger than in older rats. Heart and arteries show higher values than the skin. Organs with a high collagen content have a low collagen turnover and vice versa: organs with a low collagen content have a higher collagen turnover (e.g. heart or liver: see fig. 8) (22–25, 29).

Age fibrosis can be found in the rat heart (both sexes), but no age fibrosis occurs in the two atria or in the two ventricles of human (male or female) heart (fig. 7b). The collagen (= hydroxyproline) values in the atria are about 3 times higher than in the ventricles of the human heart during life (fig. 7b).

So we find that the structurally and functionally noteworthy age fibrosis differs from organ to organ and within a single organ from species to species. Different results about the cardiovascular aging fibrosis are mainly due to the species investigated and to localizations as well as to the methods used (fig. 8) (17, 21–23, 29, 30, 35, 43).

The increase of collagen contents, the co-called aging fibrosis, can be due to an increased synthesis of collagen but also due to a decreased collagen breakdown or a decrease of the normally high collagen turnover in the heart. This is shown by appropriate methods mentioned above. Collagen precursors have a rapid turnover rate, but partly are degraded intracellulary before being processed extracellulary

Fig. 8. Aging: hydroxyproline content (mg/g d.w.) rat.

	3 months		12		36	31 m.
	male	female	male	female	male	female
Heart	5.25 t 0.33	5.64 t 0.67	4.76 t 0.54	5.51 t 0.45	6.72 t 1.21	7.85 t 0.76
Aorta	45.38 t 5.61	49.03 t 4.30	53.29 t 2.72	50.11 t 2.94	53.48 t 5.27	42.36 t 2.57
Liver	1.33 t 0.27	1.33 t 0.15	1.53 t 0.12	1.55 t 0.27	2.19 t 0.39	1.71 t 0.10
Kidney	4.42 t 0.49	5.01 t 0.58	7.58 t 0.60	7.54 t 0.74	12.81 t 0.83	12.74 t 0.99
Lung	17.13 t 2.34	18.90 t 2.51	21.36 t 2.43	19.69 t 1.54	27.98 t 3.44	26.93 t 2.70
Skin	92.88 t 9.40	82.37 t 4.53	114.99 t 3.51	103.13 t 3.49	112.73 t 8.92	105.64 t 6.76

Fig. 8. Hydroxyproline content in aging of the rat cardiovascular system: heart and aorta (compared with liver, kidney, lung, and skin), regarding the so-called aging-fibrosis (significant values are underlined: see text).

into the fibrous forms. Type III collagen precursors appeared to have a slower turnover rate than those of type I collagen (if the mature forms, too, is still unclear).

The absolute and the proportional increase of the collagen type I and the decrease of the collagen type III in maturation and aging of the cardiovascular system is discussed. The basement collagen types IV and V partly are responsible for the pericellular environment. These collagen types may participate in the cytoskeletal structure and function between cells and the intercellular matrix in the cardiovascular system. The connective tissue components of heart, arteries, and other organs play a significant role in development and aging, regarding their structural, biochemical, metabolic as well as biomechanical relationships. Ground substance and fibres are responsible for the cellular environment as well as for the tissue integrity in the cardiovascular development and aging.

The progressive stabilization of collagen during aging is a generalized phenomenon and is partly responsible for the decreased myocardial function in higher age: So the structural and chemical composition and properties of the connective tissue components are responsible for the aging of heart.

The question of overlapping of coronary sclerosis and scarring of myocard, on the one hand, and aging fibrosis, on the other hand, is still open, in rat strains like in humans (2, 8–12, 15–17, 21–27, 30–33, 42, 43). An aging atrophy of the heart does not exist, but an aging insufficiency and more a polypathy of the heart in aging of humans and other species (26, 27).

The fundamental mechanisms of differentiation, growth, and maturation of heart muscle cells but also of connective tissue cells of the several parts of the heart are to be clarified together and not separately: The connective tissue aging of the heart is the aging of the heart!

The knowledge about the morphological and biochemical alterations during development and aging as physiological processes, compared with pathological ones, is the prerequisite for measurements of aging processes and of age-dependent diseases, enhanced in aging, as well as their influences on each other.

The clarification of the pathogenesis of hypertrophy, of cardiovascular diseases, etc., is impossible without exact data about the physiological alterations of the several structural components of the heart during prenatal and postnatal development, maturation, and aging.

Cardiac muscle cells are formed by undifferentiated mesenchymal cells during differentiation, growth and maturation. Similarly the same processes seem to take place in the pathogenesis of hyperplasia, hypertrophy, and other heart diseases. So we investigate, like other groups, if the human heart is able to regenerate heart muscle cells by undifferentiated mesenchymal cells, beside heart muscle cell replication after loss (for example, by infarction, etc.).

The heart valves can show more age-related alterations than the myocardium: increase of the collagen content = fibrosis, combined with hyalinosis and elastosis, with reduction of the proteoglycan-content (as in any fibrosis); reduction of fibroblasts with polyploidization of the nuclei; thickenings of the valves with despositions of lipids and calcium. These alterations can start in early adult life, progress with aging and are strongest in high senium (2, 3, 5, 15, 26–28, 33).

They are summarized and overlapped partly also by the so-called atherosclerosis of mitral and aortic valves (42). The aging fibrosis is particularly marked at the insertion sites of the tricuspid and mitral valves. These age-related changes of heart valves are demonstrated in humans, but in some rat strains, too (2, 3, 8, 12, 15, 22, 26–28, 42).

Aging alterations of valves are similar to vascular intima aging, due to a similar structure and composition.

Regarding age-related alterations of the cardiovascular connective tissue, amyloid deposits are to be discussed, too. The amyloid formation includes proteoglycan synthesis processes by local connective tissue cells. The proteoglycan/GAG-content of amyloid is responsible for the so-called "metachromasia" of amyloid. Findings about the incidence of amyloid in cardiovascular aging are controversial. Some authors describe a relatively low frequency of amyloid in aging of human hearts being an unspecific finding for heart aging (frequency of 0.3–7 %) (2, 6, 12, 18), while other authors reported a frequency of amyloid in heart aging of 2.5–90 % (4, 8, 15, 26, 27, 32, 33, 39, 40). These differences depend mainly on the staining methods used for amyloid as well as on the number of cases investigated. At the time the meaning prevails that the incidence of amyloid in the heart is not typical for aging, but due to various other reasons. Furthermore the different findings can be caused by differences of the localization of amyloid deposits. Most authors investigated mainly the heart ventricles. Beneke et al. (1970) tested these differences of the localization carefully and did not find amyloid in the right ventricle; in the left ventricle they found amyloid in 9 %, a much more frequent occurrence in the atria: 45 % in the left one, and 18 % in the right atrium, resp., 91 % in the left auricle, and 36 % in the right one.

The accumulation of lipofuscin in cardiocytes during aging is described and discussed before: not typical for aging, but enhanced in higher age (residual bodies representing undigested residues from autophagic processes of mitochondria and other cell-membranes by lysosomal activities) (2, 3, 7, 15, 22, 23, 26, 33, 41).

References

1. Adler, C. P.: DNS-Gehalt und Zellzahl in alten Menschenherzen. Verh. dtsch. Ges. Path. **59,** 328 (1975).
2. Baskin, S. I., P. B. Goldberg, Z. V. Kendrick, J. Roberts, R. J. Montali, J. D. Strandberg: Age-related histopathologies of the Fischer 344 rat. Fed. Proc. **37,** 88 (1978).
3. Beneke, G., W. Schmitt: Altersveränderungen am Klappenapparat des menschlichen Herzens. Verh. dtsch. Ges. Path. **51,** 209 (1967).
4. Beneke, G., A. D. Rakow, L. Rakow, W. Schmitt: Nachweis von Fibrin und Amyloid mit morphologischen Methoden in Gewebeschnitten. Beitr. Path. **141,** 404 (1970).
5. Beneke, G.: Altersabhängige Veränderungen des Kollagens und der Bindegewebszellen. Altern und Entwicklung. Bd. 2. Schriftenreihe der Mainzer Akademie. Schattauer (Stuttgart–New York 1971).
6. Berg, E.: Über kardiales Amyloid. Z. Alternsforsch. **21,** 27 (1968).
7. Buddecke, E.: Pathobiochemie. 1. Aufl., de Gruyter (Berlin–New York 1978).
8. Bürger, M.: Altern und Krankheit als Problem der Biomorphose. 4. Aufl., Thieme (Leipzig 1965).
9. Chvapil, M., K. Rakusan, M. Wachtlova, O. Poupa: Collagen in the heart of wild and domesticated animals. Gerontologia **12,** 14 (1969).
10. Clausen, B.: Influence of age on connective tissue. Hexosamine and hydroxyproline in human aorta, myocardium and skin. Lab. Invest. **11,** 229 (1962).
11. David, H., A. Bózner, R. Meyer, G. Wassilew: Pre- und postnatal development and ageing of the heart. Ultrastructural results and quantitative data. Exp. Pathology, Suppl. **7** (1981).
12. Fairweather, F. A.: Cardiovascular disease in rats. In: Pathology of Laboratory Rats and Mice (E. Cotchin and J. C. Roe, eds.), pp. 397–421. Blackwell (London 1967).
13. Gerlach, U.: Über die Alternsabhängigkeit der Aktivität sulfataktivierender Enzyme im Herzen. Klin. Wschr. **41,** 873 (1963).
14. Grasedyck, K., J. Lindner: Aortic protocollagen proline hydroxylase (PPH). In: W. Manning, D. Haust (eds.): Atherosclerosis, pp. 758–761. Plenum Publ. (New York 1977).
15. Harris, R.: Cardiac changes with age. In: The Physiology and Pathology of Human Aging (R. Goldman and M. Rochstein, eds.), pp. 109–122. Academic Press (New York 1975).
16. Hauss, W. H., G. Junge-Hülsing, U. Gerlach: Die unspezifische Mesenchymreaktion. Thieme (Stuttgart 1968).
17. Jansen, H. H.: Über den Bindegewebsgehalt des Herzmuskels. Verh. dtsch. Ges. Path. **46,** 262 (1962).
18. Jones, R. S., D. B. Frazier: Primary cardiovascular amyloidosis: its clinical manifestations, pathology and histogenesis. Arch. Path. **50,** 366 (1950).
19. Kao, K. Y. T., D. M. Hilker, T. H. McGavack: Connective tissue. V. Comparison of synthesis and turnover of collagen and elastin in tissues of rat of several ages. Proc. Soc. exper. Biol. (N.Y.) **106,** 335 (1961).
20. Kewitsch, F., B. Schütte, R. Eurich, J. Lindner: Beitrag zur Frage des Wassergehaltes (mit Untersuchung von Frisch- und Trockengewicht) mesenchymaler und parenchymatöser Organe von Mensch und Ratte im Lebensablauf. akt. gerontol. **8,** 303 (1978).
21. Knieriem, H. J.: Über den Bindegewebsgehalt des Herzmuskels des Menschen. Arch. Kreisl.-Forsch. **44,** 231 (1964).
22. Lindner, J.: Altern des Bindegewebes. In: G. Holle (ed.) Handbuch der Allgemeinen Pathologie, Bd. IV/4, p. 245. Springer (Berlin–Heidelberg–New York 1972).
23. Lindner, J.: Zur Alterung der Organe. Verh. dtsch. Ges. Path. **59,** 181 (1975).

24. Lindner, J.: Morphologische und histobiochemische Befunde am Bindegewebe bei arteriosklerotischen Frühveränderungen. Z. ges. Inn. Med. **33,** 582 (1978).
25. Lindner, J.: Zur Entwicklung und Alterung von Binde- und Stützgeweben. Verh. Anat. Ges. **75,** 61 (1981).
26. Linzbach, A. J.: Das Altern des menschlichen Herzens. In: G. Holle: Handbuch der Allgemeinen Pathologie, Bd. IV/4, p. 150. Springer (Berlin–Heidelberg–New York 1972).
27. Linzbach, A. J.: Altern und Krankheit. Ableitung einer neuen Alternstheorie auf der Grundlage der Polypathie. Verh. dtsch. Ges. Path. **59,** 242 (1975).
28. McMillan, J. B., M. Lev: The aging heart. II. The valves. J. Gerontol. **19,** 1 (1964).
29. Mangold, I., B. Uhlenhop, B. Mester, J. Lindner: Untersuchungen zur Entwicklung verschiedener Bindegewebssysteme. akt. gerontol. **9,** 369 (1979).
30. Oken, D., R. J. Boucek: Quantitation of collagen in human myocardium. Circulat. Res. **5,** 357 (1957).
31. Platt, D.: Biologie des Alterns. Quelle & Meyer (Heidelberg 1976).
32. Pomerance, A.: The pathology of senile cardiac amyloidosis. J. Path. Bact. **91,** 357 (1966).
33. Pomerance, A.: Cardiac pathology in aged. Geriatrics **23,** 101 (1968).
34. Sandritter, W., C. P. Adler: Numerical hyperplasia in human heart hypertrophy. Experienta (Basel) **27,** 1435 (1971).
35. Schaub, M. C.: The aging of collagen in the heart muscle. Gerontologia **10,** 38 (1964/65).
36. Schröder, S., P. R. Bock, H. W. Schürmann, J. Setiawati, B. Zerbst, J. Lindner: ^{3}H-Thymidin-autoradiographische Untersuchungen zur Proliferation verschiedener Populationen glatter Muskelzellen prä- und postnatal (und ihrer möglichen Beeinflussung). Arzneim.-Forsch. (Drug Res.) **31,** 37 (1981).
37. Schütte, B., J. Eggert, J. Lindner: The effect of Kallikrein on the DNA-content and synthesis of embryonic and postembryonic development. In: G. L. Haberland et al.: Kininogenases. Kallikrein **3,** p. 148. Schattauer (Stuttgart–New York 1975).
38. Schütte, B., K. Ziebell, B. Zerbst, P. R. Bock, S. Bittmann, I. Mangold, J. Lindner: Untersuchungen von Gewichten und Wassergehalt sowie von DNA-Synthese und -Gehalt bindegewebiger und parenchymatöser Organe der Ratte prä- und postnatal. akt. gerontol. **9,** 527, 573; **10,** 37 (1979/80).
39. Schwartz, P., J. Kurucz: Amyloid deposits in the hearts of aged persons. J. Amer. Ger. Soc. **13,** 718 (1965).
40. Schwartz, P.: Amyloidosis, cause and manifestation of senile deterioration. Thomas (Springfield, Ill. 1970).
41. Strehler, B. L.: Time, Cells and Aging. Academic Press (New York–London 1962).
42. Walton, K. W., N. Williamson, A. G. Johnson: The pathogenesis of atherosclerosis of the mitral and aortic valves. J. Path. **101,** 205 (1970).
43. Wegelius, O., J. V. Knorring: The hydroxyproline and hexosamine content in human myocardium at different ages. Acta med. Scand. **175,** 233 (1964).

Authors' address:

Prof. Dr. med. Dr. med. vet. h. c. J. Lindner, Universität Hamburg, Universitäts-Krankenhaus Eppendorf, Pathologisches Institut, Martinistraße 52, D-2000 Hamburg 20, FRG

Cardiac Adaptation to Hemodynamic Overload, Training and Stress
Dr. D. Steinkopff Verlag 330–340 (1983)

Connective tissue alterations in coronary arteries of spontaneously hypertensive rats (SHR); electron microscopic and morphometrical investigation

H. Ziegler, H. Schmiebusch, M. Heisterkamp, and J. Staubesand

Anatomisches Institut, Universität Freiburg (FRG)

Summary

The coronary and testicular arteries of spontaneously hypertensive and Wistar rats of various ages (4–6 weeks, 4–6 months and more than 12 months) were subjected to morphological and morphometrical examination. Electron microscopy revealed marked changes in all layers of the investigated vessels as a result of hypertension and aging. The most pronounced alterations were observed in the tunica media, however. In both groups of animals, the intercellular space increases with aging, whereas the media myocytes, the nuclear component of the muscle cells, and the metabolic space decrease. These changes are more pronounced in the spontaneously hypertensive than in the Wistar rats. The alterations are generally more pronounced in the coronary than in the testicular arteries.

Key words: hypertension, coronary arteries, testicular arteries, 'k'-myocytes, 'm'-myocytes, electron microscopic, morphological and morphometric investigation

Introduction

Different injurious agents – such as haemodynamic and metabolic unphysiological stress (amongst others: hypertension, hypotension and diabetes mellitus) – can act as 'risk factors for the vessel wall'. Our own investigations have allowed us to recognise a 'risk factor of the first order' for the production of sclerotic change in a vessel: namely, arterial hypertension.

SHR have been used by our research team for a long series of experiments in which various types of 'metabolic and haemodynamic unphysiological stress' have been included (Okamoto and Aoki, 1963; Staubesand, 1976a, 1977, 1978, 1979a, 1979b, 1980, 1981).

The object of these studies is the morphological description of processes in the diseased vessel wall with the help of the electron microscope, and their morphometric quantification. We have been particularly concerned with the following questions:

1. How does a muscular artery react to hypertension, particularly with regard to the intima and media?
2. Do arteries of the muscular type show a relatively uniform reaction to systemic hypertension, or do different body regions with their vessels show specific reactions? To answer this question, we have used the coronary and testicular arteries as models.

Materials and methods

28 male rats were used for the combined morphological and morphometric investigation: 14 controls (Wistar) and 14 SHR. The animals were chosen so as to include three age groups, conforming to the hypertensive stages of SHR described by Ichijima (1969): first 4–6 weeks, second 4–6 months and third more than 12 months.

The transverse sections were investigated by an overall magnification of 33,300× (see table 1).

The morphological results in additional are based on the changes of vessels of 3 SH-rats in the age of 9, 10 and 15 months. In comparison to the vessels under blood pressure, these testicular arteries had – because of a ligation – 'null-function' (Staubesand, 1976b; Schmiebusch, 1979).

The photographs were examined with a MOP Digiplan desk computer which measures structural outlines electromagnetically. A number of measurements were made, the results were calculated with the Univac Computer belonging to the University of Freiburg, and significant differences obtained with an 'F'-test (Heis-

Table 1. Vascular changes of coronary and testicular arteries due to haemodynamic unphysiological stress materials (symbols see table 2).

age in months	Wistar RR	n	SHR RR	n	
1 – 2	~130	AT : 48 AC : 49	~160	AT : 39 AC : 40	> Σn = 176
4 – 6	~130	AT : 24 AC : 36	~180	AT : 23 AC : 32	> Σn = 115
> 12	~130	AT : 16 AC : 41	~190	AT : 15 AC : 29	> Σn = 101
		Σn = 214		Σn = 178	Σn = 392

n = sum of cross – sections

Table 2. Key to the symbols used.

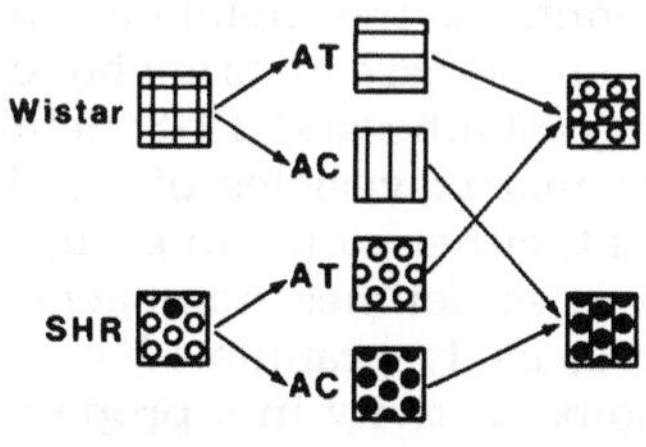

A.T. Testicular Artery
A.C. Coronary Artery

Signs in ✱✱✱ - high significant
✱✱ - significant
✱ - little significant

column – diagrams with:

1 dash	(\ )	Animals, aged	1 – 2 months
2 "	(\\ )		4 – 6 "
3 "	(\\\ )		> 12 "

terkamp, 1979). The results will be presented as column diagrams. For the marking of the columns, we have used several symbols, please compare table 2 with the key to the symbols.

Results

I Morphology

The following observations were made in the region of the endothelium: We have the impression that an increase in the number of micropinocytotic vesicles is to be seen. Both the rough and smooth endoplasmic reticulum are dilated. We have been able to recognise Weibel-Pallade bodies. Their quantity is discussed below.

We specially noted – particularly in the coronary vessels of SHR – smooth muscle cells lying between the endothelial layer and the internal elastic lamina. Heteromorphic 'detritus' (appearing as 'ghost bodies', lamellated corpuscles, granular vesicles or lysosomes) found in the vicinity indicates that the myointimal cells have a marked tendency towards degeneration and cell death. The internal elastic lamina (particularly in the Wistar rats) occasionally appears as a translucent band, although in the majority of haemodynamically stressed arteries it is electron dense and possesses an irregular border (Staubesand, 1979a). In the coronary arteries it is frequently seen to consist of several fragmented layers. 'Osmiophilic single-cell necroses' appear particularly in the coronary arteries of SHR, and are relatively frequent within the endothelial layer itself.

Changes in the vessel wall due to haemodynamic unphysiological stress are particularly to be seen in the media (Backwinkel et al., 1970; Massmann and Weidenbach, 1972; Backwinkel et al., 1973; Joris and Majno, 1974).

The smooth muscle cells in this layer show a reaction-pattern to hypertension that is in general uniform, but in which some specificity for region and age can also be detected. The most important of the non-specific changes in reactivity and structural alteration of the vessel wall is the transformation of the differentiated contractile smooth muscle cell, the 'k'-cell, into a metabolically modified variant, the 'm'-cell. Whereas the 'k'-cells have the ability to contract, the metabolic function of the 'm'-cell preponderates, and shows an increase in its anabolic and catabolic activity at the cost of its contractility (Staubesand, 1978; Schmiebusch et al., 1980).

The intercellular space: matrix vesicles of varying shapes, sizes and electron density are present; either alone, in groups or in larger foci. The content of these vesicles is sometimes homogeneous, but may also be heteromorphic, finely or coarsely granulated or multivesicular. It was possible to confirm lysosomal activity in a proportion of the vesicles by demonstrating the presence of acid phosphatase (Riede and Staubesand, 1977; Staubesand, 1978).

Collagen and elastic fibres can usually be found near the collections of 'detritus', the elements of which are extensively altered in shape and size. In the collagen fibrils we were able to recognise both intrafibrillar and interfibrillar dysplasia (Staubesand and Fischer, 1979, 1980), which is another way of saying that fibrils irregular in calibre or in arrangement could be seen.

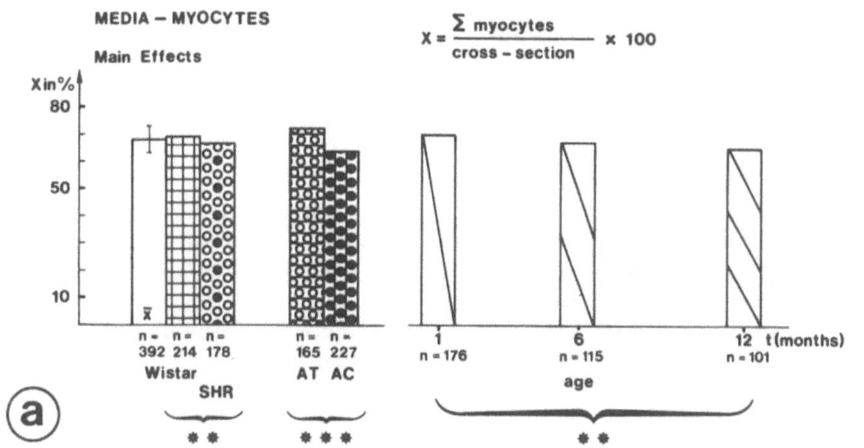

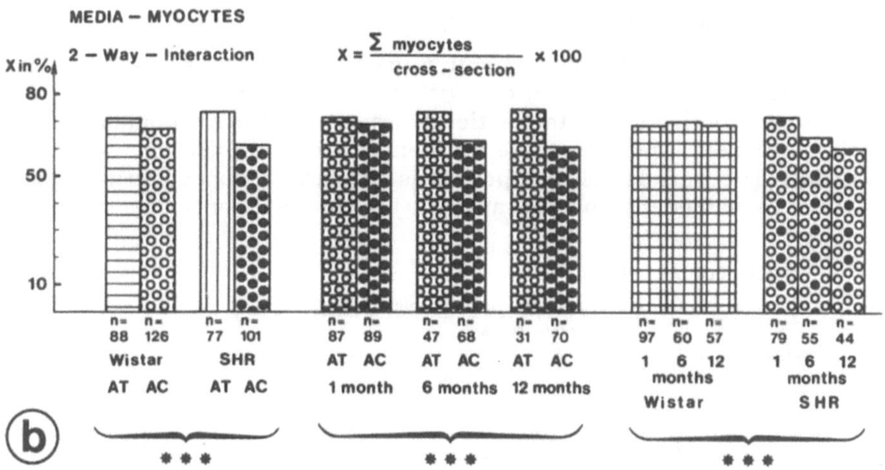

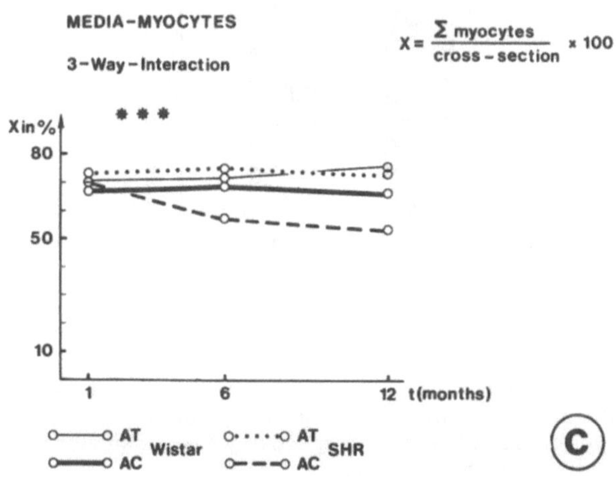

Fig. 1. The portion of the myocytes to the cross-section in %: a) the individual influence of the three parameters hypertension, kind of vessel and age; b) the influence of respectively two parameters combined; c) the influence of all three parameters combined.

Near the degenerating muscle cells and the internal elastic lamina, foci of strongly osmiophilic structures which can be identified as concretions of calcium salts are to be seen among the detritus (Kim, 1976; Kim et al., 1976).

II Morphometry

The morphometric work compares quantitatively the coronary and testicular arteries of normotensive Wistar animals with those of SH-rats, subjected to haemodynamic unphysiological stress. It allows conclusions to be drawn about the typical changes that occur with age (Ziegler, 1980) and under the influence of hypertension, and confirms the dependence of these changes on the vascular region concerned. Owing to important differences in their nature, the changes in the coronary vessel have been compared and contrasted with those in the testicular arteries.

Smooth muscle cells and intercellular space of the media – components per sections (fig. 1a, 2a)

Calculations involving the smooth muscle cells of the media show that the SHR in comparison with the Wistar vessels – and similarly the coronary in comparison with the testicular arteries possess a smaller muscle cell component, and that these differences are significant or highly significant. The muscle cell component is similarly reduced during aging. This is explained by the alteration in the intercellular space, since the

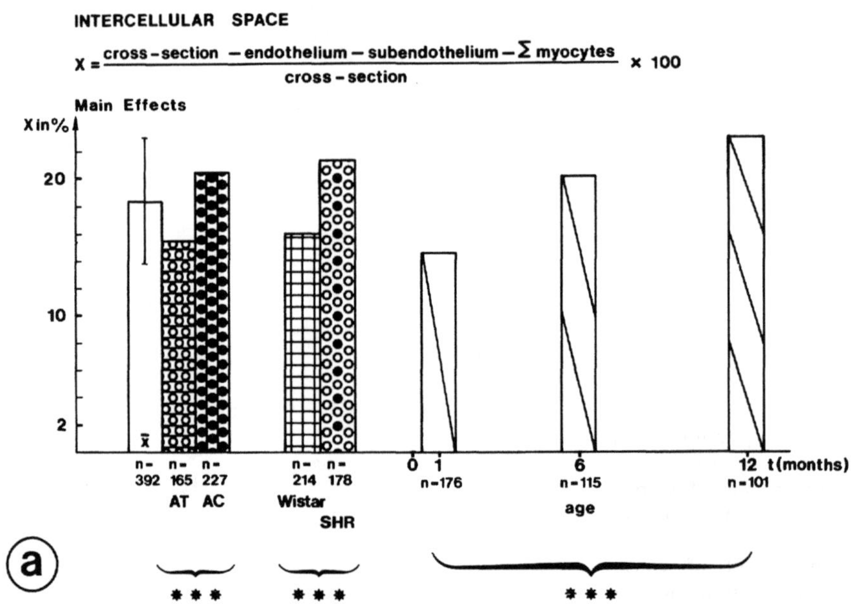

Fig. 2. The portion of the calculated intercellular space to the cross-section in %: a) the individual influence of the three parameters hypertension, kind of vessel, and age; b) the influence of respectively two parameters combined; c) the influence of all three parameters combined.

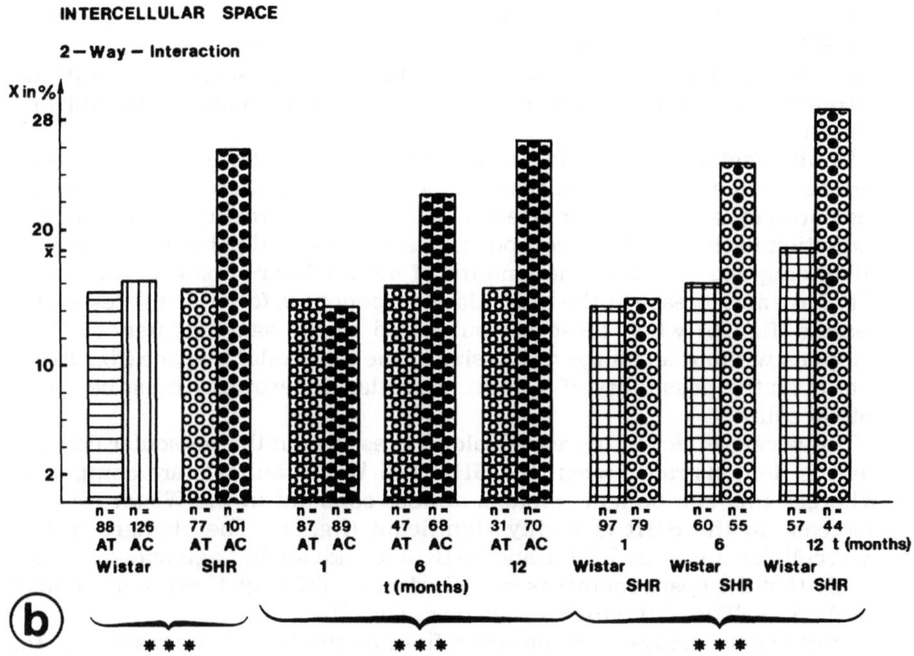
INTERCELLULAR SPACE
2 – Way – Interaction
X in%
28
20
x̄
10
2
n= 88 AT
n= 126 AC
Wistar
n= 77 AT
n= 101 AC
SHR
n= 87 AT
n= 89 AC
1
n= 47 AT
n= 68 AC
6
n= 31 AT
n= 70 AC
12
t (months)
n= 97
n= 79
1
Wistar
SHR
n= 60
n= 55
6
Wistar
SHR
n= 57
n= 44
12
Wistar
SHR
t (months)
b
***
***
***

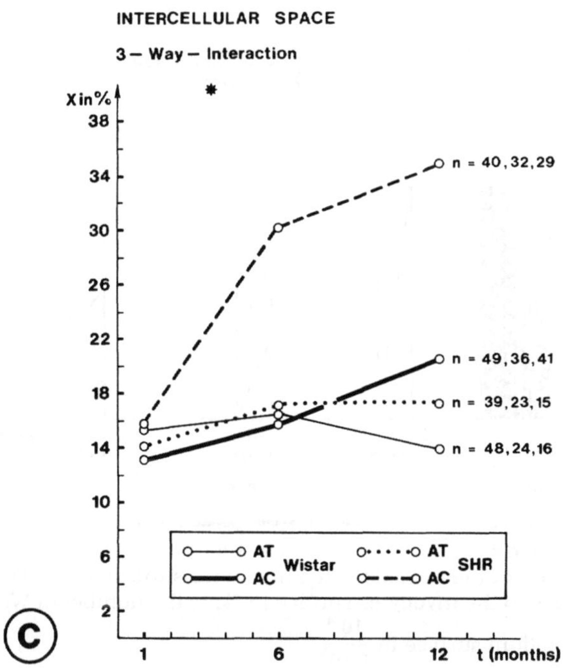
INTERCELLULAR SPACE
3 – Way – Interaction
*
X in%
38
34
30
26
22
18
14
10
6
2
n = 40,32,29
n = 49,36,41
n = 39,23,15
n = 48,24,16
AT
AC
Wistar
AT
AC
SHR
1
6
12
t (months)
c

reduction in the muscular component in all the coronary arteries and in all the SHR vessels – and also with aging – are principally brought about by the highly significant increase of the intercellular space, above all in the coronary arteries under the influence of hypertension and advancing age (fig. 2a).

Double factor analysis (fig. 1b, 2b) also reveal exactly parallel changes – indead, with a significant difference between the pattern of behaviour of the coronary and testicular arteries. Whereas the coronary vessels show a reduction in the muscular component as a result of high blood pressure or advancing age – so that the amount of intercellular substance increases (fig. 2b) – an increase of the muscular component is found in the testicular vessels (fig. 1b) when these are subjected to the same influences. This happens without a change in the size of the intercellular space (fig. 2b) so that even the possibility of a slight muscular hypertrophy must be taken into account.

The severe effect of increased blood pressure on the muscular component is demonstrated when the SHR and Wistar animals are compared. Whereas this component remains almost constant in the Wistar rats, its decrease in the SHR is highly significant (fig. 1b). The changes in the intercellular space in Wistar and SHR with advancing age show conclusively that the space increases in both strains, although this is particularly marked in SHR of the middle age class (fig. 2b).

Triple factor analysis enables even finer distinctions to be made (fig. 1c, 2c).

The muscular component of the media increases in the testicular arteries of the Wistar rats, owing to a decrease in the intercellular space. In

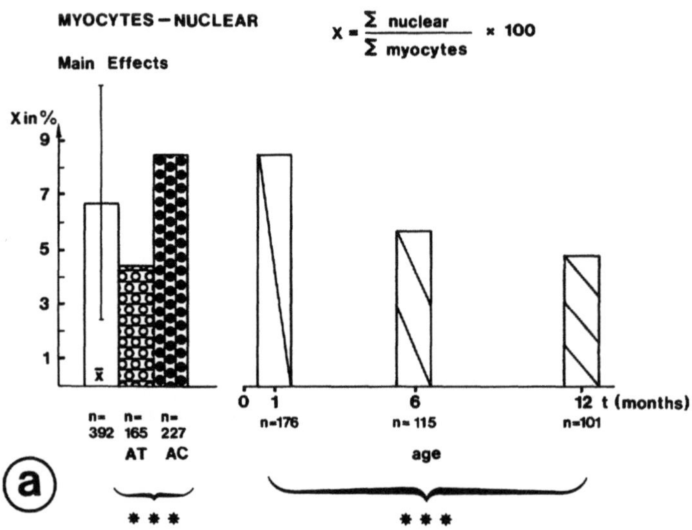

Fig. 3. a) The portion of the nucleus to the myocytes-surface in %; b) the portion of the metabolic space to the myocytes-surface in %; c) the number of Weibel-Pallade bodies per endothelium-surface in $\frac{10^{-4}}{mm^2}$.

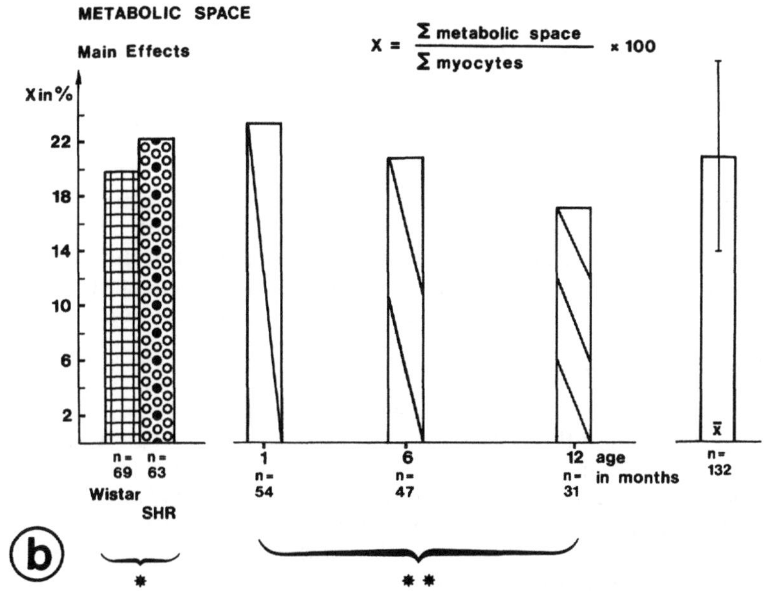

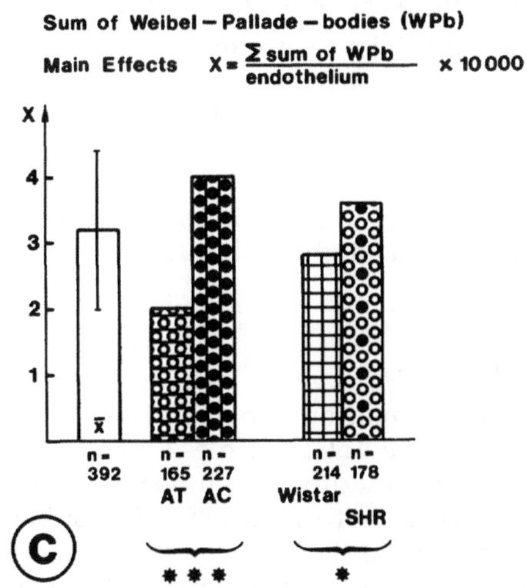

contrast, the muscular component in the coronary arteries of the same animals is reduced, in the latter case because of an increasing intercellular space.

In the SHR, the influence of high blood pressure produces almost no alterations in the muscular component of the testicular artery, although the intercellular space is here slightly increased. On the other hand, the reduction of the muscular component of the coronary vessels considerably accelerates, since in this case the size of the intercellular space is very markedly increased.

The coronary vessels are therefore extremely sensitive to raised blood pressure, as can be seen from the observed increase in the intercellular space.

Nuclear component of the muscle cells in the media (fig. 3a)

The separation of coronary and testicular vessels shows that the muscle cells of the coronary artery possess about twice as large a nuclear component as the others; and this allows one to infer considerably raised cellular activity. It is less surprising that the nuclear component of the muscle cells decreases with advancing age, since one might have expected aging to be accompanied by an increasing reduction in cellular function.

Component of the 'metabolic space' (fig. 3b)

This was investigated only in the testicular artery. Here, a highly significant reduction with increasing age in the 'metabolic space' indicates a reduced cell function, similar to the reduction of the nuclear component of the muscle cell with age. Only a slightly significant elevation of the size of the 'metabolic space' was observed in the SHR as compared with that seen in the Wistar rats. This correlates well with the increase of the intercellular space under the influence of high blood pressure.

Number of Weibel-Pallade bodies in the endothelium (fig. 3c)

The number of Weibel-Pallade bodies in the endothelium of all the vessels was counted. This led to the interesting and up to now unexplained finding that the count of these bodies in the coronary arteries is twice that found in the testicular vessels, a difference which is highly significant.

It has also been found that the count in the SHR vessels is higher than in the Wistar. This difference is slightly significant.

Discussion and conclusions

The morphological investigation shows in the endothelium an increase in the number of micropinocytotic vesicles and a dilatation of the smooth and rough endoplasmic reticulum. The internal elastic lamina is altered, and heteromorphic detritus is to be seen in the subendothelium. In the media it imports that the contractile smooth muscle cells are transformed into a metabolic modified variant. The explored lysosomal activity correlates with an increased number of matrix vesicles and a lot of altered collagen and elastic fibres (Schmiebusch, 1979).

The morphometric investigation shows that the action of high blood pressure on the wall of a blood vessel is expressed predominantly as an increase in the size of the intercellular space (Ziegler, 1980), especially seen at the coronary arteries of SHR. The theory that this damage is a sign of premature aging (Staubesand, 1977, 1979b) must be called into question, since a normal vessel like the testicular artery of normotensive Wistar rats can show a reduction in the size of the intercellular space with increasing age.

In addition, the great difference between the reaction of the testicular and coronary arteries to hypertension and aging leads one to suppose a response dependent on the location of the vessel, or on a testicular artery protecting mechanism. The increase in the size of the intercellular space per section in reaction to hypertension is again reflected in the enlarger metabolic space and in a nucleus/cytoplasm ratio that has been altered in favour of the nucleus. Additional differences between walls of vessels, which also depend on their location, are the raised Weibel-Pallade body count and the enlarger muscle cell nuclei in the coronary vessels.

References

Backwinkel, K. P., G. Schmitt, H. Themann, W. H. Hauss: Elektronenmikroskopische Untersuchungen über Frühveränderungen der Koronararterien bei experimenteller Hypertonie. Beitr. path. Anat. **141,** 374–391 (1970).

Backwinkel, K. P., H. Themann, G. Schmitt, W. H. Hauss: Elektronenmikroskopische Untersuchungen über das Verhalten glatter Muskelzellen in der Arterienwand unter verschiedenen experimentellen Bedingungen. Virchows Arch. path. Anat. **357,** 171–184 (1973).

Heisterkamp, M.: Statistische Methoden und Auswertungen mit SPSS 6. RZF-Bericht Nr. 2, Freiburg 11/1979.

Ichijima, K.: Morphological studies on the peripheral small arteries of spontaneously hypertensive rats. Jap. Circulat. J. **33,** 785–833 (1969).

Joris, I., G. Majno: Cellular breakdown within the arterial wall. An ultrastructural study of the coronary artery in young and aging rats. Virchows Arch. Abt. A. **364,** 111–127 (1974).

Kim, K. M.: Calcification of matrix vesicles in human aortic valve and aortic media. Fed. Proc. **35,** 156–162 (1976).

Kim, K. M., J. M. Valigorsky, W. J. Mergner, R. T. Jones, R. F. Pendergrass, B. F. Trump: Aging changes in the human aortic valve in relation to dystrophic calcification. Hum. Path. **7,** 47–60 (1976).

Massmann, J., H. Weidenbach: Die Reaktionen der glatten Mediamuskelzellen bei experimentellen Arterienveränderungen. Gefäßwand und Blutplasma **4,** 105–106 (1972).

Okamoto, K., K. Aoki: Development of a strain of spontaneously hypertensive rats. Jap. Circulat. J. **27,** 282–293 (1963).

Riede, U. N., J. Staubesand: A Unifying Concept for the Role of Matrix Vesicles and Lysosomes in the Formal Pathogenesis of Diseases of Connective Tissue and Blood Vessels. Beitr. path. Anat. **160,** 3–37 (1977).

Riede, U. N., J. Staubesand: Morphometrische Untersuchungen der Physio- und Pathosklerose. 1. Gem. Jahrestagung der Angiolog. Gesellschaften der BRD, Schweiz und Österreichs, Wien 9/1977, Verlag Gerhard Witzstrock (Baden-Baden–Köln–New York 1979).

Schmiebusch, H.: Zur Ultrastruktur der Arterienwand beim genetischen Hochdruck der Ratte. Inaug.-Diss. (Freiburg 1979).

Schmiebusch, H., J. Staubesand, F. Steel: Ultrastructural and Morphometric Investigations into the Arterial Wall of the Genetically Hypertensive Rat. Artery **8,** 294–304 (1980).

Staubesand, J.: Nachweis intra- und extrazellulärer Lysosomen in der hämodynamisch fehlbelasteten Arterienwand der Ratte. Verh. dtsch. Ges. Path. **60,** 148–155 (1976a).

Staubesand, J.: Beobachtungen an stillgelegten Arterien. Verh. anat. Ges. (Jena) 70. Vers. 715–721 (1976b).

Staubesand, J.: Lysosomen und lysosomale Enzyme in der Wand fehlbelasteter Arterien der Ratte. Res. exp. Med. **170**, 271 (1977).
Staubesand, J.: Matrix Vesikel und Mediadysplasie: Ein neues Konzept zur formalen Pathogenese der Varikose. Phlebol. u. Proktol. **7**, 109–140 (1978).
Staubesand, J.: Spezifische Ausprägungen, Fensterungen und Umbauvorgänge der Membrana elastica interna; experimentelle elektronenmikroskopische Untersuchungen an Arterien muskulären Typs. Verh. Anat. Ges. **73**, 767–770 (1979a).
Staubesand, J.: Ein neuer Aspekt zur Pathogenese der Mediadysplasie – Myozytentransformation, Matrix Vesikel und extrazelluläre Lysosomen in der Wand fehlbelasteter Blutgefäße. Münch. med. Wschr. **121**, Nr. 2 (1979b).
Staubesand, J.: Matrix Vesikel, extrazelluläre Lysosomen und Bindegewebsdysplasie bei Wundheilung und Narbenbildung. In: Wundheilung; Hgg. P. Eckert und R. Häring, Bibliomed 1981.
Staubesand, J.: Hämodynamische Fehlbelastung – Risikofaktor für die Gefäßwand. In: Ergebnisse der Angiologie, Bd. 20, Hgg. N. Klüken, I. Brändle, R. Stemmer. Schattauer (Stuttgart–New York 1980).
Staubesand, J., N. Fischer: Collagen dysplasia and the matrix vesicles. Researches with the electron microscope into the problem of the so-called "Weakness of the vessel wall". Path. Res. Pract. **165**, 374–391 (1979).
Staubesand, J., N. Fischer: The ultrastructural characteristics of abnormal collagen fibrils in various organs. Connective Tissue Res. **7**, 213–217 (1980).
Ziegler, R.: Vergleichend ultrastrukturell-morphometrische Analyse der juvenilen und adulten Hodenarterie der Ratte. Inaug.-Diss. Freiburg 1980.

Authors' adress:

Dr. Heidrun Schmiebusch, Anatomisches Institut der Universität Freiburg, 7800 Freiburg, FRG

Cardiac Adaptation to Hemodynamic Overload, Training and Stress
Dr. D. Steinkopff Verlag 341–348 (1983)

Myocardial mass and collagen content in Crotalaria spectabilis-induced pulmonary hypertension of young and adult rats*)

I. Medugorac and R. Jacob

Physiologisches Institut II der Universität Tübingen (FRG)

Summary

Right ventricular hypertrophy was produced in 5-week-old male Wistar rats by ingestion of Crotalaria spectabilis seeds (1 g seeds/kg food for ca. 4 weeks). The observed right ventricular hypertrophy was associated with a slight but significant decrease in collagen content per gram of hypertrophied right ventricular tissue. The changes in right ventricular weight and collagen concentration were more marked in young than in adult Crotalaria-fed rats.

In the course of 6–7 weeks following the removal of Crotalaria seeds from the diet of young rats, the absolute right ventricular weight did not begin to decrease, whereas the ventricular collagen concentration increased rapidly.

Key words: Crotalaria spectabilis intoxication, pulmonary hypertension, cardiac hypertrophy, collagen concentration

Introduction

The seeds and vegetation of the Crotalaria spectabilis plant contain monocrotaline, a toxic pyrrolizidine alkaloid (1). Ingestion of the seeds damages the liver of domestic animals (2, 3, 4). In addition, drinking a bush tea which contains a species of Crotalaria causes veno-occlusive disease of the liver in man (5). In various species, oral ingestion of Crotalaria seeds (6, 7) as well as intravenous (8) or intraperitoneal (9, 10) injection of monocrotaline pyrrole induces a change in pulmonary vasculature which is associated with increased pulmonary vascular resistance. The resulting hypertension enhances the work load of the right ventricle and leads to subsequent right ventricular hypertrophy. The interest of previous investigators (6–8, 10–12) has been focused on pathological changes in the pulmonary vasculature of Crotalaria-treated rats. Functional, morphological and biochemical alterations in the hypertrophied right ventricle of Crotalaria-fed animals have received scant attention.

Substantial (2–3-fold) enlargement of the right ventricle after Crotalaria ingestion is accompanied by a variety of marked alterations in functional, morphological and biochemical characteristics of right ventricular myocardium. As shown by earlier investigations of our group (13–16),

*) Supported by the Deutsche Forschungsgemeinschaft.

cardiac hypertrophy is frequently accompanied by changes in myocardial connective tissue which, in turn, may affect myocardial distensibility and, in some cases, even the supply of substrates to the myocardial cell. Systematic investigation of myocardial connective tissue alterations in Crotalaria-induced hypertrophy has not been reported to date.

The aim of the present study was to examine collagen content, represented by hydroxyproline concentration, in right and left ventricles of rats which were fed a diet containing Crotalaria spectabilis seeds. Furthermore, we were interested in knowing whether the effect of monocrotaline in inducing pulmonary hypertension, subsequent right ventricular hypertrophy and accompanying alterations in myocardial collagen content depends on the age of the experimental animals. Thus ventricular hypertrophy and cardiac collagen were examined in a group of young, postnatally developing rats and a group of adult rats maintained on a diet containing Crotalaria spectabilis seeds. The findings were compared with those obtained from control rats of the same age. In addition, we examined changes in collagen concentration and ventricular mass of young Crotalaria-fed rats 7 weeks after removing Crotalaria spectabilis seeds from the diet.

Materials and methods

44 ca. 5-week-old Wistar rats with an initial body weight of 80–100 g were divided into 12 control and 32 experimental animals. Both groups received a diet of water and cubes made with powdered rat food ("Sonderdiäten" from Altromin, D-4937 Lage, Germany) ad libitum. The pellets fed to the experimental animals (later referred to as "Crotalaria-fed rats") were made of powdered rat food and ground Crotalaria spectabilis seeds (kindly provided by the United States Department of Agriculture, USA) in a concentration of 1 g seeds/kg food. The first death of a Crotalaria-fed rat occurred on the 14th day. Another 14 Crotalaria-fed animals expired within the following 15 days.

The 17 surviving Crotalaria-fed rats were divided into two groups. A group of 6 animals was allowed to recover from Crotalaria intoxication by removing Crotalaria seeds from the diet (group 3). The remaining 11 animals (group 1) were sacrificed and used for investigation.

Group I animals

During the 4th week after the start of Crotalaria ingestion, 11 experimental and 12 control animals were sacrificed by intraperitoneal injection of urethane (2.5 g/kg body weight). The myocardium was carefully trimmed free of large vessels, auricles, fat and visible connective tissue. The free wall of the right ventricle was removed; weights of the right ventricular free wall, and the left ventricle with intraventricular septum were determined separately. Liver, kidney, and lungs were examined macroscopically for pathological changes.

Group II animals

18 ca. 3-month-old Wistar rats weighing 270–300 g were divided into 9 control and 9 experimental animals. The animals were fed as described above for the first group of animals. The experimental and control animals were sacrificed and examined as above (for the first group) during the 6th week after the start of Crotalaria feeding.

Group III animals

When the experimental rats of the first group were examined in the 4th week of Crotalaria feeding, 6 unexamined rats were set aside and allowed to recover by switching to standard rat food without Crotalaria spectabilis seeds. Within 14 days, 2 rats of this third experimental group had died of the aftermath of Crotalaria intoxication. Six weeks after the onset of recovery, the remaining experimental rats of this group were examined as above (for the first group). 9 animals of the same age served as controls.

Examination of collagen content

Collagen content was examined in both right and left ventricles of all experimental and control animals by analyzing hydroxyproline concentration (μg/mg dry tissue) with the procedure regulary employed in our laboratory (13).

Results

Pathological findings

The general condition of the Crotalaria-fed animals was poor, and their body weight reduced compared to age-matched controls. 15 of a total of 32 young Crotalaria-fed rats died of Crotalaria ingestion within 30 days. Not a single one of the 3-month-old Crotalaria-fed rats died within a period of 5–6 weeks. Liver damage accompanied by edema, ascites and pleural effusion; pulmonary infarction and atelectasis; and cyanosis was observed most frequently in the Crotalaria-fed rats of group I.

Weights

Group I: Crotalaria seed ingestion stimulated considerable absolute and relative increase in right ventricular weight: 105 % compared to right ventricular weight of controls. The mean weight ratio of the right ventricle, compared to the left ventricle plus intraventricular septum increased by 173 % in Crotalaria-fed rats. Body weight of the Crotalaria-fed young rats advanced at a slower rate than in the control animals; at the time of investigation (4th week after the onset of Crotalaria ingestion) the experimental animals therefore weighed only 70 % as much as the controls (table 1). Thus right ventricular hypertrophy would appear greater when expressed as a percentage of body weight.

Group II: In the adult Crotalaria-fed rats, the effect of Crotalaria ingestion was distinctly less rapid than in the young experimental rats. In contrast to the considerable enhancement of right ventricular weight of developing rats (group I), the increase (12 %) in right ventricular weight of adult Crotalaria-fed rats, as well as the increase relative to left ventricular (28 %) or body weight (21 %), was very slight compared to age-matched controls (table 1).

Group III: Six weeks after removing Crotalaria seeds from the diet, the difference in body weight between "recovered rats" and controls of the same age was markedly reduced in comparison to Crotalaria-fed and age-matched control rats in the first group (−13 % and −31 %, respectively). Though the absolute weight of both the right and left ventricles had increased during recovery, the rate of increase in the right ventricle was slower, and in the left ventricle greater, than in the control rats.

Table 1. Body and ventricular weights of young (I) and adult (II) *Crotalaria*-fed rats, and age-matched control rats. A group of 5-week-old (I) and a group of 3-month-old (II) Wistar rats received a diet with 0.1 % *Crotalaria spectabilis* seeds. Following 4 (I) and 6 (II) weeks of *Crotalaria* feeding, the body weights of the *Crotalaria*-fed rats and control rats were determined. Thereafter the rats were sacrificed and ventricular weights were determined.

	Weight of						RV/LV ratio (m/mg)		RV/Body wt. ratio (m/mg)	
	Body (g)		RV (mg)		LV (mg)					
	I	II	I	II	I	II	I	II	I	II
Crotalaria-fed rats	153 ±20 (12)	337 ±36 (9)	316 ±35 (12)	237 ±24 (9)	446 ±46 (12)	707 ±74 (9)	0.71 (12)	0.34 (9)	2.07 (12)	0.70 (9)
Control rats (age-matched)	223 ±19 (12)	364 ±31 (9)	154 ±13 (12)	211 ±19 (9)	584 ±52 (12)	805 ±77 (9)	0.26 (12)	0.26 (9)	0.69 (12)	0.58 (9)
Changes (%)	–31 p < 0.01	–7.4	+105 p < 0.001	+12	–24 p < 0.01	–12	+173	–28	+200	+21

RV = right ventricle; LV = left ventricle + septum. The data are expressed as means ± S.E.

Hydroxyproline analysis

Group I: The hydroxyproline content in μg/mg dried myocardial tissue was decreased slightly but significantly ($p < 0.001$) in the right ventricle of young Crotalaria-fed rats (3.61 ± 0.35 μg/mg) compared to the control value (4.19 ± 0.36 μg/mg) (fig. 1).

Group II: In the adult Crotalaria-fed animals, the concentration of right ventricular hydroxyproline was also decreased (4.31 ± 0.45 μg/mg) compared to control rats of the same age (4.62 ± 0.47 μg/mg) (fig. 1). However, the decrease was smaller in the adult than in the young rats (group I) and was not significant.

Group III: In contrast, the collagen concentration in right ventricular tissue increased remarkably (74 %) in those rats allowed to recover from Crotalaria intoxication (8.40 ± 0.91 μg/mg), in comparison to age-matched controls (4.62 ± 0.47 μg/mg) (fig. 1).

The collagen content per mg tissue in the contralateral nonstressed left ventricle of the young Crotalaria-fed rats (group I) was slightly increased after 4 weeks of Crotalaria intoxication (3.47 ± 0.34 vs. 3.10 ± 0.33 in controls) as well as after recovery (group III: 4.15 ± 0.42 vs. 3.38 ± 0.22 μg/mg in controls). In the adult Crotalaria-fed rats (group II) the left ventricular collagen content was unchanged (3.42 ± 0.33 μg/mg) compared to control animals of the same age (3.38 ± 0.22) (fig. 1).

Discussion

The data presented in this study are consistent with the findings of previous investigators (2–12) who have reported pulmonary hypertension

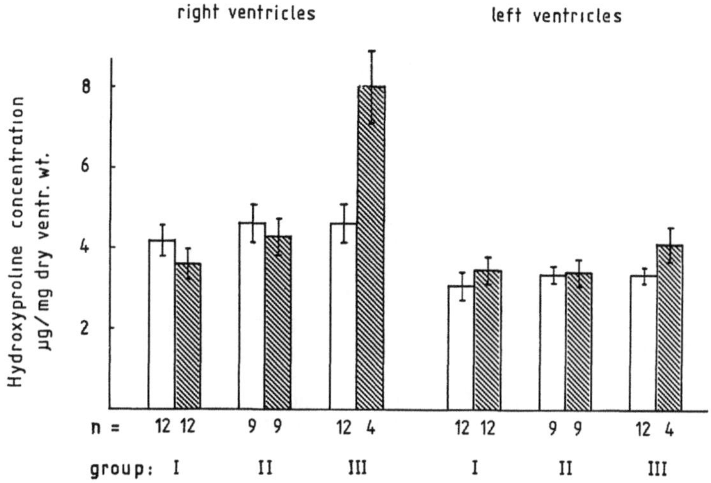

Fig. 1. Hydroxyproline content (µg/mg dry wt.) in the right and left ventricle of young *Crotalaria*-fed rats (group I), adult *Crotalaria*-fed rats (group II) and young *Crotalaria*-fed rats following 4 weeks of *Crotalaria* feeding and subsequent 6-week "recovery"; compared with age-matched control animals. Control values are represented by open bars, values of *Crotalaria*-fed rats by hatched bars. Data are expressed as means ± S.E. n = number of experimental animals.

and sequel right ventricular enlargement in the rat subsequent to ingestion of Crotalaria spectabilis.

Obviously, monocrotaline intoxication was more marked in young, ca. 5-week-old rats (80–100 g body weight at the beginning of experiments) than in mature, ca. 3-month-old rats (270–300 g body weight at the beginning of experiments). Furthermore, the difference in both body weight and ventricular weight of experimental and control animals was more marked in young rats than in rats which were mature at the start of Crotalaria feeding (table 1). Therefore, previously reported discrepancies between pathological changes in the rat following intoxication with monocrotaline (6, 8, 11, 12, 14, 17, 19) can probably be attributed to differences in the age of experimental animals. Indeed, investigators have often employed rats of diverse age as indicated by such body weights as 40 to 100 g (6, 17, 18) or 100 to 200 g (11, 19) or 200 to 300 g (8, 12).

It is interesting to note that absolute right ventricular weight did not begin to decrease in the course of 6–7 weeks of recovery, i.e., following the removal of Crotalaria seeds from the diet of young rats. In contrast, absolute right ventricular weight increased further, but not as quickly as in the respective control rats. At the same time, body weight of such "recovered rats" increased more rapidly than in the control animals. The degree of right ventricular hypertrophy would thus be reduced when ventricular weight is related to body weight. Nevertheless, comparison with the respective control values revealed that the ratios of right ventricular to left ventricular weight, as well as to body weight, remained significantly elevated 6 weeks after the onset of "recovery" (table 2). A more

Table 2. Body and ventricular weights of young *Crotalaria*-fed rats after "recovery" and control rats (group III). 5-week-old Wistar rats received a diet of powdered rat food and ground *Crotalaria spectabilis* seeds in a concentration of 1 g seeds/kg food for 4 weeks. Subsequently, the rats were allowed to recover by switching to rat food without *Crotalaria* seeds for six weeks. Thereafter the rats were used in the investigation. Data are expressed as means ± S.E. See also legend of table 1.

		Weight of			RV/LV ratio	RV/Body wt. ratio
	n	Body (g)	RV (mg)	LV (mg)	(mg/mg)	(mg/g)
Young Crotalaria "recovery" rats	4	318 ± 34	 ± 36	762 ± 81	1.11	0.46
Control rats	12	364 ± 32	211 ± 20	805 ± 75	0.58	0.26
Changes (%)		–13 N.S.	+67 $p < 0.01$	–5 N.S.	+91	+77

precise description of the recovery process would have required knowledge of the amount of, and any changes in pulmonary pressure.

The hydroxyproline content in μg/mg dried right ventricular tissue was decreased in young and adult Crotalaria-fed rats in comparison to control values (fig. 1). However, the difference in the adult rats was lower than in the young rats. In contrast, the hydroxyproline concentration in the right ventricle increased remarkably (74 %) in the rats recovering from Crotalaria feeding.

According to a previous report (14), the hydroxyproline concentration of hypertrophied left ventricular tissue is elevated during chronic pressure overload induced by experimental renal hypertension, as well as spontaneous hypertension. One reason for the alterations in collagen concentration in ventricular tissue in various models of hypertrophy has been discussed in detail in earlier publications (13, 14).

We cannot exclude that the pulmonary hypertension induced by Crotalaria feeding in young animals leads not only to muscle cell hypertrophy but also to myocardial cell hyperplasia. Indeed, the capacity for myocardial cell division at this age of the animals is retained to some extent. This would permit rapid increase in muscle cell mass. Hence, the cardiac hypertrophy induced by congenital anatomical defects of the heart of young animals may generally differ from myocardial hypertrophy which develops in the mature organism.

Furthermore, a direct effect of Crotalaria intoxication on connective tissue proliferation cannot be excluded on the basis of the present findings. During the initial period of hypertrophy the intoxication could cause a relative reduction in collagen protein synthesis, in the late stage a vigorously stimulated synthesis of collagen proteins.

In any case, the present results demonstrate that the age of experimental animals is one of the factors determining the relative rapidity of the increase in ventricular weight, as well as the change in connective tissue content induced by enhanced pulmonary hypertension following Crotalaria ingestion.

Cuttiletta et al. (21) observed that elevated collagen content in the hypertrophied left ventricle following constriction of the ascending aorta in rats does not return to normal following the relief of hemodynamic overloading. Collagen content per g tissue tends to be higher in the debanded animals than in those with persistent bands, because total ventricular mass decreases more rapidly than the collagen content during the regression of hypertrophy.

However, our findings on right ventricular hypertrophy of the recovered rats revealed that the collagen concentration, in μg/mg dry weight, increased markedly, although total ventricular mass continued to increase – though less than during Crotalaria ingestion. Proliferation of right ventricular connective tissue appears to be an essentially irreversible alteration; retrogression is substantially slower than that of cardiac muscle cells.

Finally, it is interesting to note that overloading of the right ventricle in young Crotalaria-fed rats was associated with slight inverse changes in ventricular weight and collagen content in the contralateral, nonstressed left ventricle. As a rule, overloading stresses on either the right or left ventricle are associated with similarly directed biochemical changes and alterations in ventricular mass of the contralateral ventricle (13, 22). Thus the present findings reveal an as yet unobserved and contradictory phenomenon in this respect. The results provide a further indication that the mechanisms responsible for biochemical changes and alterations in components of the ventricular wall are probably different in various "models" of cardiac hypertrophy.

References

1. Neal, W. M., L. L. Rusoff, C. F. Ahmann: The isolation and some properties of an alkaloid from Crotalaria spectabilis. Roth. J. Amer. chem. Soc. **57,** 2560–2561 (1953).
2. Thomas, E. F.: The toxicity of certain species of Crotalaria seed for the chicken, quail, turkey and dove. J. Amer. vet. med. Ass. **85,** 617–623 (1934).
3. Emmel, M. W., D. A. Sanders, W. W. Henley: Crotalaria spectabilis Roth. Seed poisoning in swine. J. Amer. vet. med. Ass. **86,** 43–55 (1935).
4. Sanders, D. A., A. L. Shealy, M. W. Emmel: The pathology of Crotalaria spectabilis Roth. Poisoning in cattle. J. Amer. vet. med. Ass. **89,** 150–159 (1936).
5. Hill, K. R., K. Rhodes, J. L. Stafford, R. Aub: Serous hepatosis: a pathogenesis of hepatic fibrosis in Jamaican children. Brit. med. J. **1953/I,** 117–122.
6. Kay, J. M., P. Harris, D. Heath: Pulmonary hypertension produced in rats by ingestion of Crotalaria spectabilis seeds. Thorax **22,** 176–179 (1967).
7. Kay, J. M., P. Smith, D. Heath: Electron microscopy of Crotalaria pulmonary hypertension. Thorax **24,** 511–526 (1969).
8. Chesney, C. F., J. R. Allen, I. C. Hsu: Right ventricular hypertrophy in monocrotaline pyrrole treated rats. Exp. Mol. Pathol. **20,** 257–268 (1974).
9. Chesney, C. F., J. R. Allen: Monocrotaline induced pulmonary vascular lesions in non-human primates. Cardiovasc. Res. **7,** 508–518 (1973).
10. Kajihara, H.: Electron microscopic observations of hypertrophied myocardium of rat produced by injection of monocrotaline. Acta Pathol. Japan **20,** 183–206 (1970).

11. Hislop, A., L. Reid: Arterial changes in Crotalaria spectabilis-induced pulmonary hypertension in rats. Brit. J. exp. Path. **55,** 153–163 (1974).
12. Meyrick, B., L. Reid: Development of pulmonary arterial changes in rats fed Crotalaria spectabilis. Amer. J. Pathol. **94,** 37–50 (1979).
13. Medugorac, I.: Collagen content in different areas of normal and hypertrophied rat myocardium. Cardiovasc. Res. **14,** 551–554 (1980).
14. Medugorac, I.: Myocardial collagen in different forms of heart hypertrophy in the rat. Res. exp. Med. (Berl.) **177,** 201–211 (1980).
15. Holubarsch, Ch., Th. Holubarsch, R. Jacob, I. Medugorac, K.-U. Thiedemann: Passive elastic properties in different models and stages of hypertrophy. A study comparing mechanical, chemical and morphometric parameters. Advanc. Myocardiol. (in press).
16. Jacob, R., G. Kissling, G. Ebrecht, Ch. Holubarsch, I. Medugorac, H. Rupp: Adaptive and pathological alterations in experimental cardiac hypertrophy. Advanc. Myocardiol. 55–77 (1983).
17. Lalich, J. J., W. D. Johnson, T. J. Raczniak, R. C. Shumaker: Fibrin thrombosis in monocrotaline pyrrole-induce cor pulmonale in rats. Arch. Pathol. Lb. Med. **101,** 69–73 (1977).
18. Heimburg, P., A. Bouchi, R. Schenk, E. Perings: Untersuchungen zum experimentellen pulmonalen Hochdruck durch Samen von Crotalaria spectabilis. Verh. dtsch. Ges. Kreisl.-Forsch. **38,** 201–205 (1972).
19. Stötzer, H., M. Herbst, R. Reichl, H. Köllmer: Zur Pathogenese der experimentellen pulmonalen Hypertonie. Virchows Arch. Abt. A Path. Anat. **356,** 331–342 (1972).
20. Bonnin, C. M., R. R. Taylor, M. P. Sparrow: Collagen synthesis during hypertrophy of the right ventricle of the dog heart. J. Mol. Cell. Cardiol. **12,** 21 (Suppl.) (1980).
21. Cutilletta, A. F., R. T. Dowell, M. Rudnik, R. A. Arcilla, R. Zak: Regression of myocardial hypertrophy. I. Experimental model, changes in heart weight, nucleic acids and collagen. J. Mol. Cell. Cardiol. **7,** 767–781 (1975).
22. Carey, R. A., G. Natarjan, A. A. Bove, W. P. Santamore, J. F. Spann: Elevated collagen content in volume overload induced cardiac hypertrophy. J. Mol. Cell. Cardiol. **12,** 929–926 (1980).

Authors' address:

Dr. I. Medugorac, Physiol. Institut II der Universität Tübingen, Gmelinstraße 5, 7400 Tübingen, FRG

Cardiac Adaptation to Hemodynamic Overload, Training and Stress
Dr. D. Steinkopff Verlag 349–353 (1983)

Heterogeneity of collagen in the normal and hypertrophied left ventricle of the rat

I. Medugorac and R. Jacob

Physiologisches Institut II, Universität Tübingen (FRG)

Summary

Polyacrylamide gel electrophoresis and densitometric analysis were employed in the present study to examine the influence of aging and various types of left ventricular hypertrophy on intramuscular collagen heterogeneity in the rat left ventricle. The relative proportion of type III collagen increased substantially with age.

Increased type III collagen was also observed in various types of left ventricular hypertrophy. It is conceivable that the conditions resulting from such changes may influence the mechanical properties of myocardium.

Key words: rat ventricular myocardium, collagen heterogeneity, age-dependent alterations, cardiac hypertrophy, swimming training, aortic stenosis, Goldblatt hypertension

Introduction

The rapid progress in the identification and chemical characterization of collagen molecules of various organisms in the past decade has not yet reached the heart. The application of previous analytical methods to cardiac collagen is limited by problems of amount, solubility and separation of available samples. Type I and III collagen molecules are known to occur, however, in ventricular connective tissue of man and various mammals (4, 8). Furthermore, the biochemistry, structure, and the chemical properties of both types of molecules differ distinctly. Since myocardial collagen content and composition influence passive elastic properties of myocardium, and thereby mechanical heart function, precise knowledge of collagen changes during heart growth, hypertrophy development or failure – or other pathogenetic processes – may provide useful insight into changes in mechanical heart function.

The present paper is a report on the influence of aging, as well as various types of left ventricular hypertrophy on collagen heterogeneity of intramuscular left ventricular connective tissue of the rat.

Materials

Rat breeds and induction of cardiac hypertrophy by swimming training, Goldblatt operation and aortic stenosis have been reported earlier (9). Animals from these experimental groups were ca. 4 months old when sacrificed – whereby swimming training lasted 10 weeks, aortic stenosis 8 weeks, and coarctation of one renal artery (Goldblatt) 8 weeks prior to sacrifice.

Methods

Preparation of tissue samples and soluble collagen has been outlined previously (8). Methods reported by Medugorac (9) were used for estimation of collagen content from the hydroxyproline concentration determined from aliquots of lyophilized tissue. The proportion of hydroxyproline in collagen was assumed to be 13.4 %.

0.4 M glycine buffer, pH 8.8, and 3.6 M urea (8) were used for SDS-polyacrylamide gel electrophoresis (SDS-PAGE) performed essentially as outlined by Hayashi and Nagai (5). Treatment of electrophoresis gels and densitometric analysis was conducted as described earlier (8).

Results and discussion

Electrophoresis patterns of nonreduced (A) and reduced (B) left ventricular collagen of (a) 1-month, (b) 4-month, (c) 8-month, and (d) 24-month-old rats are shown in figure 1. Only monomeric α_1 (I) and α_2 (I), dimeric β_{11} (I) and β_{12}(I), and trimeric γ components were revealed by electrophoretic analysis in the absence of reducing reagent (2-mercaptoethanol) (fig. 1A). However, collagen type III also appeared in electrophoresis gels when the pepsin-solubilized collagen was reduced (fig. 1B). The patterns reveal marked differences in the distribution of types I and III collagen in the left ventricles of rats of various ages. The ventricle of young rats contains considerably more α_1 (III) compared to ventricles of mature animals.

Densitometric analysis revealed that 33, 22, 12, and 10 % type III collagen (of total collagen) was contained in the pepsin-solubilized left ven-

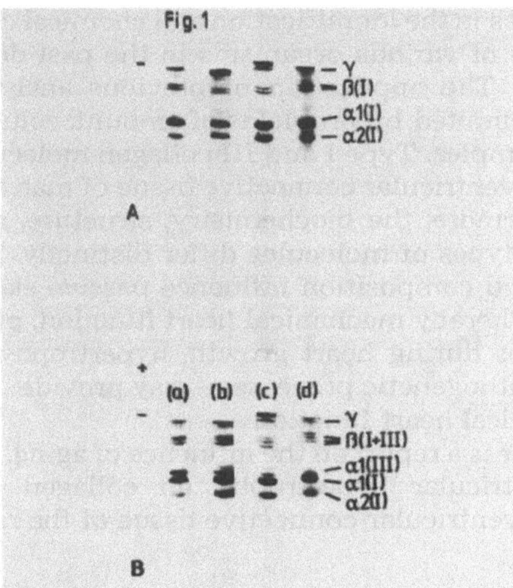

Fig. 1. SDS-polyacrylamide electrophoresis gels of left ventricular collagen obtained from rats of various ages. For detailed explanation, see the text.

Table 1. Relative proportion of α_1(I) to α_2(I), and collagen type I to III in pepsin-solubilized left ventricular collagen of rats of various ages. The relative proportions were calculated with the aid of densitometric analysis of the areas under each peak revealed by electrophoretic evaluation. The calculations took the α chains represented by β components into account.

Left ventricle of	a_1(I)/a_2(I)	collagen type I/type III
1-month-old rats	2.9/1	2.0/1
4-month-old rats	2.0/1	3.6/1
8-month-old rats	2.0/1	7.3/1
24-month-old rats	2.0/1	8.8/1

tricular collagen of 1, 4, 8, and 24-month-old rats, respectively. The proportion of α_1 (III) chains in ventricular tissue clearly decreased as a function of age, and the ratio of type I to type III increased accordingly (table 1). A similar age-related change in the distribution of both collagen types has been observed in human (3) and calf (2) skin.

The ratio of type I to type III ventricular collagen may not only be intimately related to growth and aging, but also to left ventricular hypertrophy induced by chronic hemodynamic overloading of cardiac muscle.

Figure 2 shows electrophoresis runs in the presence of 3.6 M urea, of nonreduced (A) and reduced (B) ventricular collagen of normal mature rats and those with various types of left ventricular hypertrophy: (a) 4-month-old rats, (b) Goldblatt rats, (c) rats with aortic stenosis, (d) 24-month-old rats, (e) 24-month-old spontaneously hypertensive rats (SHR).

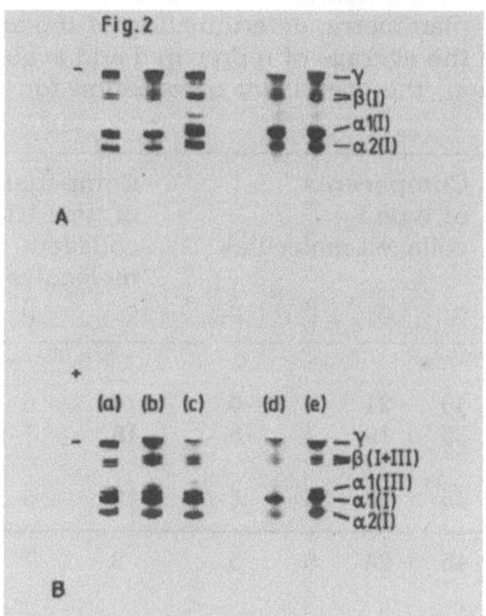

Fig. 2. SDS polyacrylamide electrophoresis gels of left ventricular collagen obtained from rats of various ages and from various models of left ventricular hypertrophy. For details, see the text.

Densitometric evaluation of protein patterns in electrophoresis gels revealed that the proportion of α_1 (III) is greater in the hypertrophied than in the normal left ventricle. This difference in ventricular collagen composition was particularly striking when comparing left ventricles from 24-month-old normotensive and spontaneously hypertensive rats of the same age.

Densitometric evaluation of protein patterns in electrophoresis gels, including the α chains in β components (table 2), revealed the relative content of type III collagen molecules in total ventricular collagen to be 18 % in SHR and 10 % in control ventricles. Increased synthesis and deposition of collagen type III has also been reported in early stages of wound healing, pathological scars, a number of inflammatory states, and in response to various injurious agents (1, 4, 11).

Earlier investigations of our group consistently revealed variable but considerably increased total collagen concentration in different areas of the hypertrophied ventricle of spontaneously hypertensive rats (10). Necrosis, subsequent healing, and thus greater increase in type III collagen synthesis than in normal ventricular tissue may result from substantially diminished blood flow (6) of the hypertrophied ventricle. Moreover, ventricular growth during cardiac hypertrophy may partly revert to an embryonic pattern of intramuscular collagen synthesis in the heart. The mechanism by which collagen type distribution is regulated during growth and aging, as well as during disease, though of considerable theoretical interest, is also unknown.

Table 2. Distribution*) of collagen components in pepsin-solubilized and heat-denatured left ventricular collagen of various models of left ventricular hypertrophy of the rat, calculated using densitometric analysis of electrophoresis runs in polyacrylamide gels and planimetric determination of the area under each peak. Each analysis represents the average of n prepared and evaluated electrophoresis gels from each preparation; the coefficient of variation for each component was 0.70–1.37.

Left ventricle of	n	Components of type I collagen molecules				Components of type III collagen molecules		γ components
		α_1	α_2	β_{11}	β_{12}	α	β	
4-month-old rats (control rats)	10	40	21	4	6	14	6	9
Goldblatt rats	12	39	19	4	5	18	7	8
aortic stenosis rats	12	35	20	5	6	19	6	9
24-month-old rats	10	45	24	5	5	2	7	12
24-month-old spontaneously hypertensive rats	10	41	23	4	5	10	6	11

*) Percentage of total content of collagen components which entered electrophoresis gels.

In any case, collagen polymorphism in the left ventricle of the rat, as well as changes in collagen type distribution in left ventricular hypertrophy are revealed by the present findings. Occasionally observed discrepancies between alterations in hydroxyproline concentration, on the one hand, and passive elastic properties of myocardium, on the other hand (7) may be explained in part by the substitution of one type of collagen for another, as well as changes in the anatomic distribution of collagen types. It is conceivable that conditions resulting from an altered pattern of collagen distribution may influence the mechanical properties of myocardium.

References

1. Adam, M., R. Vitasek, Z. Deyl, G. Felsch, J. Musilova, Z. Olsovska: Clin. Chim. Acta **70**, 61–69 (1976).
2. Bailey, A. J., T. J. Sims: Chemistry of the collagen cross-links (nature of the cross-links in the polymorphic forms of dermal collagen during development). Biochem. J. **153**, 211–215 (1975).
3. Epstein, E. H. Jr.: α_1 (III)/$_3$ human skin collagen. J. Biol. Chem. **249**, 3225–3231 (1974).
4. Epstein, E. H., N. H. Munderloh: Isolation and characterisation of CNBr peptides of human /α_1 (III)/$_3$ collagen and tissue distribution of /α_1 (I)/$_2$ α_2 and /α_1 (III)/$_3$ collagens. J. Biol. Chem. **250**, 9304–9312 (1975).
5. Hayashi, T., Y. Nagai: Separation of the α chains of type I and III collagens by SDS-polyacrylamide gel electrophoresis. J. Biochem. **86**, 453–459 (1979).
6. Holtz, J., W. Restorff, P. v. Bard, E. Bassenge: Transmural distribution of myocardial blood flow and of coronary reserve in canine left ventricular hypertrophy. Basic Res. Cardiol. **72**, 286–292 (1977).
7. Jacob, R., B. Brenner, G. Ebrecht, Ch. Holubarsch, I. Medugorac: Elastic and contractile properties of the myocardium in experimental cardiac hypertrophy of the rat. Methodological and pathophysiological considerations. Basic Res. Cardiol. **75**, 253–261 (1980).
8. Medugorac, I.: Characterization of intramuscular collagen in the mammalian left ventricle. Basic Res. Cardiol. **77**, 589–598 (1982).
9. Medugorac, I.: Collagen type distribution in the mammalian left ventricle during growth and aging. Res. Exp. Med. (Berl) **180**, 255–262 (1982).
10. Medugorac, I.: Collagen content in different areas of normal and hypertrophied rat myocardium. Cardiovasc. Res. **14**, 551–554 (1980).
11. Weiss, J. B., C. A. Shuttleworth, R. Brown, K. Sedowfia, A. Baildam, J. A. Hunter: Occurrence of type III collagen in inflamed synovial membranes: A comparison between non-rheumatoid, rheumatoid, and normal synovial collagen. Biochem. Biophys. Res. Commun. **65**, 907–912 (1975).

Authors' address:

Dr. I. Medugorac, Physiologisches Institut II, Universität Tübingen, Gmelinstr. 5, D-7400 Tübingen, FRG

Cardiac Adaptation to Hemodynamic Overload, Training and Stress
Dr. D. Steinkopff Verlag 354–363 (1983)

Determination of left ventricular diastolic wall stress and elasticity in situ. A methodological investigation*)

Ch. Brilla, R. Jacob, and G. Kissling

Physiologisches Institut II, Universität Tübingen (FRG)

Summary

A methodological study of the requirements for reliable determination of the left ventricular end-diastolic pressure-volume relationship, wall stress and wall elasticity was performed using angiocardiographic measurement of the inner volume and wall thickness, as well as simultaneous measurement of left ventricular pressure on closed-chest dogs. The reliability of the actual roentgenological volume determination was tested by comparing x-ray and direct volume measurement of ventricular casts.

The close correlation of angiocardiographic volume determination with direct volume measurement reveals that the area-length method of Sandler and Dodge permits reliable determination of left ventricular enddiastolic volume. During diastasis, the diastolic portion of the pressure-volume loop of an individual contraction coincides substantially with the static pressure-volume relationship, at low and medium heart rates. Only the pressure and volume changes during this period, corresponding to a short portion of the pressure-volume loop, should be used for an approximate determination of static wall elasticity, particularly in the volume-loaded heart. Under the conditions of the present experiments, ca. 50 % of the shift in the left ventricular diastolic pressure-volume relationship under hypoxia can be attributed to the influence of increased right ventricular filling. In an early phase of hypoxia, a contracture-like effect can be simulated by an increase in right ventricular pressure, although actual contracture does not yet occur. As in contracture, the decrease in ventricular distensibility due to geometric conditions neither changes the slope of the relation between reciprocal compliance $\left(\frac{dP}{dV} \cdot V\right)$ and ventricular pressure (P) nor the relation between tangent elastic modulus (E) and wall stress (σ).

Key words: angiocardiography, left ventricular casts, left ventricular wall stress and elasticity, myocardial stiffness, hypoxia, influence of right ventricular pressure

Introduction

Analysis and evaluation of the systolic parameters of cardiac action from the point of view of muscle physiology requires knowledge of the end-diastolic pressure-volume relationship and – strictly speaking – the elastic properties of myocardium. In addition to muscle mass increase, chronically increased hemodynamic loading of the left ventricle generally leads to a change in ventricular size and configuration with corresponding alteration of ventricular distensibility. Furthermore, tissue elasticity is frequently altered. Accurate characterization of the pressure-volume rela-

*) Supported by the Deutsche Forschungsgemeinschaft

tionship as well as determination of wall stress and elastic wall properties involve substantial methodological difficulties (3, 6, 7, 9, 10, 12, 13, 16, 18, 19, 20).

Of the large number of relevant methodological problems, the following subjects have been considered in the present study:

1. The reliability of angiocardiographic determination of left ventricular diastolic volume has been checked using direct volume measurements of casts.
2. The feasibility of constructing the "resting tension curve" using the diastolic portion of the phasic pressure-volume loop has been examined. This question is of particular significance to clinical cardiologists who attempt to characterize left ventricular compliance by deriving the static left ventricular pressure-volume relationship from the left ventricular pressure and volume values measured during the filling phase in a given cardiac cycle; some authors use merely the pressure values early and late in diastole together with the stroke volume (as a measure of diastolic influx) (2).
3. In closed-chest dogs, the influence of right ventricular volume on the left ventricular pressure-volume relationship and the relationship between left ventricular tangent modulus (E) and wall stress (σ) have been examined particularly with regard to the significance under hypoxic conditions.

Methods

1. Casts were made of the relaxed left ventricles of 5 dogs (body weight 8–14 kg, left ventricular weight 28.4–52.5 g) using Technovit 7143 (Kulzer, Bad Homburg). The volume of the casts was directly determined by water displacement and correlated with the angiocardiographic results (area-length method; single plane; a.p. projection).
2. Cineangiocardiographic volume determinations of the left ventricle were performed in 14 mongrel closed-chest dogs (10 ml Urografin 76 %, 5 ml/s; 90 frames/s, a.p. projection, 70 kV). The dogs were anesthetized (urethane, 1 g/kg body weight; succinylcholine, 5 mg/kg body weight) and artificially respirated with air using a Starling pump. Left ventricular (catheter tip manometer) as well as right ventricular, aortic, and inferior vena caval pressures were recorded simultaneously.
3. Right ventricular filling pressure was varied by intraventricular infusion of blood or Macrodex®. Hypoxia was induced by artificial respiration with pure N_2 for 3 minutes. Blood gases were monitored throughout the experiments.

Data analysis and calculations

Left ventricular volume was derived from single-plane angiocardiograms (a.p. projection) based on the area-length method (Sandler and Dodge, 1968): $V = \frac{8}{3\pi}\frac{A^2}{l}$; A = planimetered area of the a.p. projection; l = longest measured length of the area.

Average wall thickness was determined according to Rackley et al. (1964).

Midwall circumferential stress (σ) at the equator of the left ventricle was calculated assuming a thick-walled prolate spheroid (Mirsky, 1979):
$\sigma = \frac{pB}{h}\left(1 - \frac{B^2}{2A^2} - \frac{h}{2B} + \frac{h^2}{8A^2}\right)$; A, B = midwall semimajor and semiminor axis, respectively; p = left ventricular pressure; h = average wall thickness.

Midwall tangent (differential) elastic modulus (E) was calculated on the basis of the same model (Mirsky et al., 1974):

$$E = \delta \frac{\sigma}{p} V \frac{\Delta P}{\Delta V} + \frac{\sigma\,(1+\gamma)}{(1-h/2Bc_1)};$$

$$\gamma = \frac{\alpha_1 V_w - \beta_1 V}{\alpha_2 V_w + \beta_2 V};\ V = \text{left ventricular volume};\ V_w = \text{wall volume};$$

$$\delta = \left(2 + \frac{\gamma h}{B}\right)\left(1 + \frac{h}{2B} + \frac{h^2}{4B^2}\right) + \left(1 + \frac{\gamma h}{2A}\right)\left(1 + \frac{h}{2A}\right);$$

$$\alpha_1 = 3 - \frac{h}{B} - \frac{h}{2A} + \frac{h^2}{2B^2};\ \alpha_2 = \frac{h}{B}\left(1 - \frac{h}{2B} + \frac{h^2}{4B^2}\right) + \frac{h}{2A}\left(1 - \frac{h}{2A}\right);$$

$$\beta_1 = \frac{h}{A} + \frac{2h}{B};\ \beta_2 = \frac{h}{B}\left(2 + \frac{h^2}{2B^2}\right) + \frac{h}{A};$$

$$c_1 = 1 - \frac{B^2}{2A^2}.$$

Midwall circumference at the equator (l_{circ}) was calculated from the semiminor axis: $l_{circ} = 2\pi B$. Circumferential shortening velocity was taken as the first derivative (dl_{circ}/dt).

Results

Figures 1a and 1b show casts of the left ventricle of dog hearts in a.p. and lateral projection. A representative laevocardiogram in a.p. projection at the end of diastole is shown in figure 1c. Figure 1d reveals the close correlation of roentgenologically determined ventricular volume (V_{AP}) using the single plane area-length method (17), and the ventricular volume measured directly from water displacement of the casts (V_{Real}). The close correlation presented here only applies to the relaxed state, i.e. end-diastolic volume. Correlation was less exact in casts made under rigor. Thus in individual cases an error of up to 30 % was observed under conditions in which the volume corresponded approximately to the end-systolic value.

The most important measured and calculated parameters (intraventricular pressure and volume, wall thickness, midwall circumferential wall stress at the equator, midwall circumference, circumferential shortening velocity) are presented as a function of time in figures 2a and 2b. The data for these curves were obtained from a representative experiment with moderate volume loading subsequent to blood infusion. In the context of the present study, the diastolic portion of the curves is of primary interest. It is apparent that the rate of volume and circumferential increase attain a maximum before pressure and wall tension reach their minimums. Accordingly, the plot of the pressure-volume curve of an individual contraction, which is represented in the loop of figure 2c, only coincides substantially with the "static pressure-volume relationship" during a period of time which corresponds approximately to diastasis. The beginning and the end of the phase during which both curves coincide –

representing substantially the same physical states of the heart muscle – are indicated by the large symbols. The beginning of the filling period has also been labeled. In addition, the region of the length-stress loop which coincides with the "static" length-stress relationship is labelled in figure 2d. Figure 2b shows the corresponding period which is nearly,

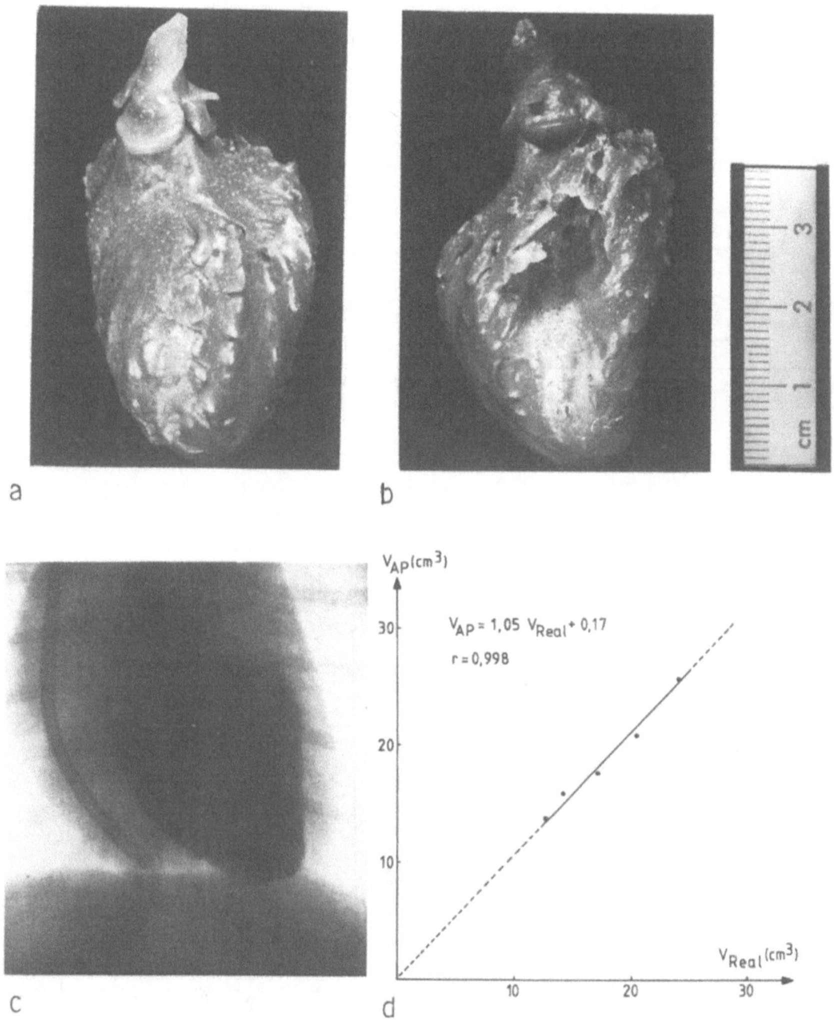

Fig. 1. Verification of the accuracy of left ventricular volume determination according to the area-length method of Sandler and Dodge (1968). Representative casts of the relaxed canine left ventricle as viewed in a.p. projection (fig. 1a) and lateral projection (fig. 1b). A close correlation was found between the angiocardiographic determinations (a.p. projection) (V_{AP}) and the directly measured (V_{Real}) volumes (fig. 1d). 5 dogs, body weight 8–14 kg; left ventricular weight 28.4–52.5 g. Fig. 1c shows a laevocardiogram of the canine heart in situ in a.p. projection at the end of diastole.

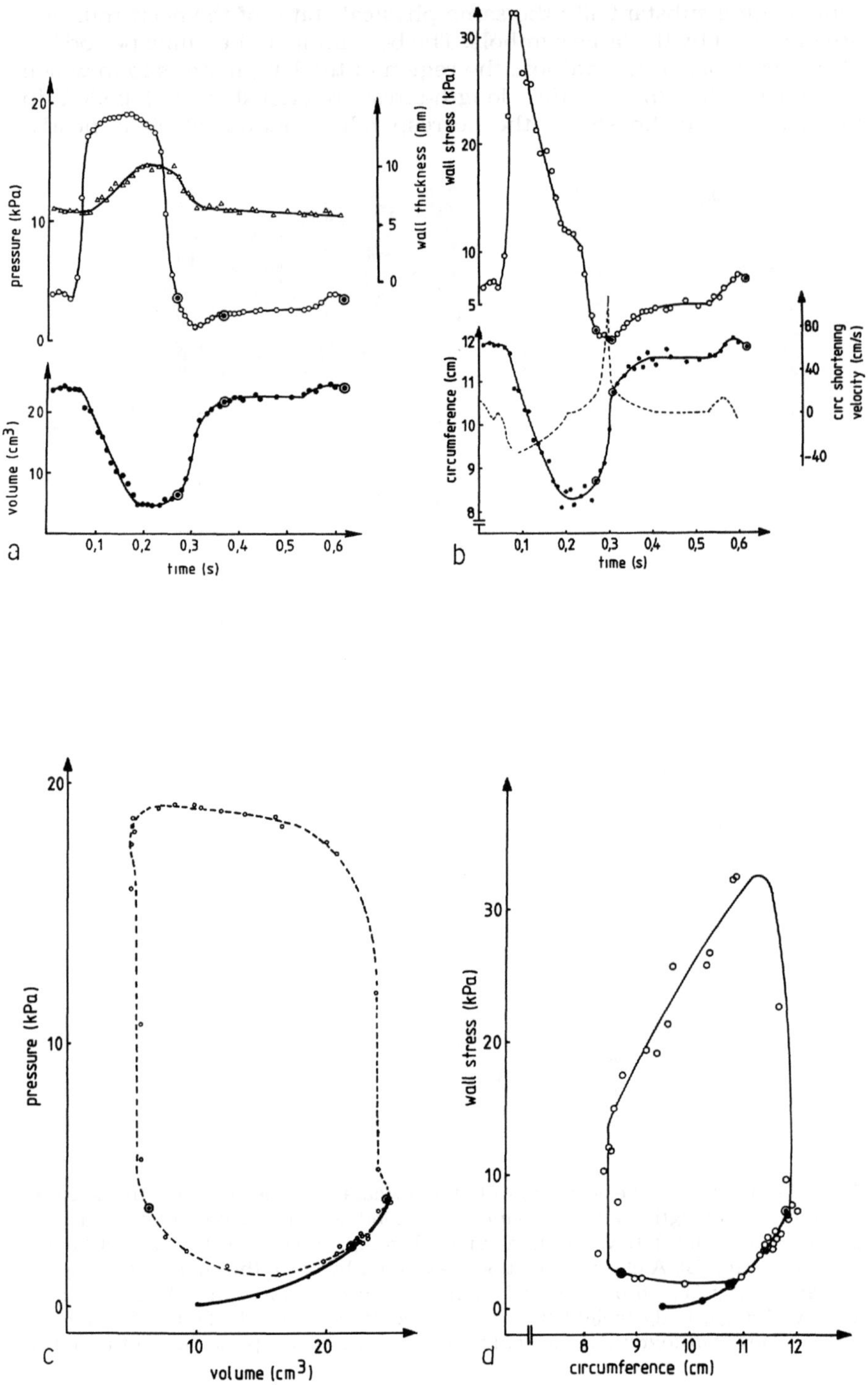
pressure (kPa)
wall thickness (mm)
volume (cm3)
time (s)
a
wall stress (kPa)
circumference (cm)
circ shortening velocity (cm/s)
time (s)
b
pressure (kPa)
volume (cm3)
c
wall stress (kPa)
circumference (cm)
d

though not exactly synchronous with the analogous period in figure 2a and figure 2c.

Under normal filling conditions, the coinciding portion of both curves is somewhat larger (no figure), but in no case does the P-V plot during the entire filling phase correspond to the static P-V relationship.

A representative example of the enddiastolic pressure-volume relationships and the curves derived therefrom under various experimental conditions is presented in figure 3. Substantial steepening of the enddiastolic pressure-volume curve (H) occurs as early as 3 min after ventilation with N_2, compared to the control curve obtained under air ventilation (C) (fig. 3a).

When rapid intraventricular infusion is used under normoxic conditions to raise right ventricular pressure to the same values which had been measured under hypoxia, the result is also a significant, though less pronounced shift of the enddiastolic pressure-volume curve (RV). Similar effects appear in the length-tension relationships calculated from the same data (fig. 3c). The slope of the relationship between the "volume-elasticity modulus" $\left(\frac{\Delta P}{\Delta V} \cdot V\right)$ and enddiastolic pressure (P) is the same under both sets of conditions (fig. 3b). When the tangent elastic modulus (E) is plotted as a function of the midwall circumferential stress (σ), neither the slope of the curves under hypoxia (H) nor under increased right ventricular volume (RV) differs from that of the control curve (fig. 3d).

Discussion

The volume measurements of the casts confirmed the reliability of the area-length method of Sandler and Dodge for determination of end-diastolic left ventricular volume. The accuracy of this method under the present experimental conditions is not perceivably less than that reported when using biplane angiocardiography (11). The method used in the present study is much less reliable, however, when determining end-systolic volume (1). Nevertheless, undue significance should not be

Fig. 2. Analysis of an individual heart cycle at a heart rate of 104/min. Representative graphs:

a) Left ventricular pressure (○), volume (●) and average wall thickness (Δ) as a function of time.

b) Calculated midwall circumferential stress (σ) (○), midwall circumference (●) and circumferential shortening velocity (– – –) as a function of time. Note the rapid relaxation during the early filling period.

c) Pressure-volume loop (○) according to the heart cycle of a) and static "resting tension curve" (●) obtained from the correlation of enddiastolic pressure and volume values.

d) Length-stress loop (○), obtained from the same contraction, and "static" length-stress relationship (●), obtained from the correlation of enddiastolic values.

Three given points are indicated in all graphs by large symbols (○): 1) The beginning of the filling period, 2) the point at which the pressure-volume loop (length-stress loop) begins to coincide with the curve of the "static" pressure-volume relationship (length-stress relationship), 3) the end of diastole. All data obtained from the same dog (body weight 8.7 kg, heart weight 55.8 g, left ventricular weight 32 g).

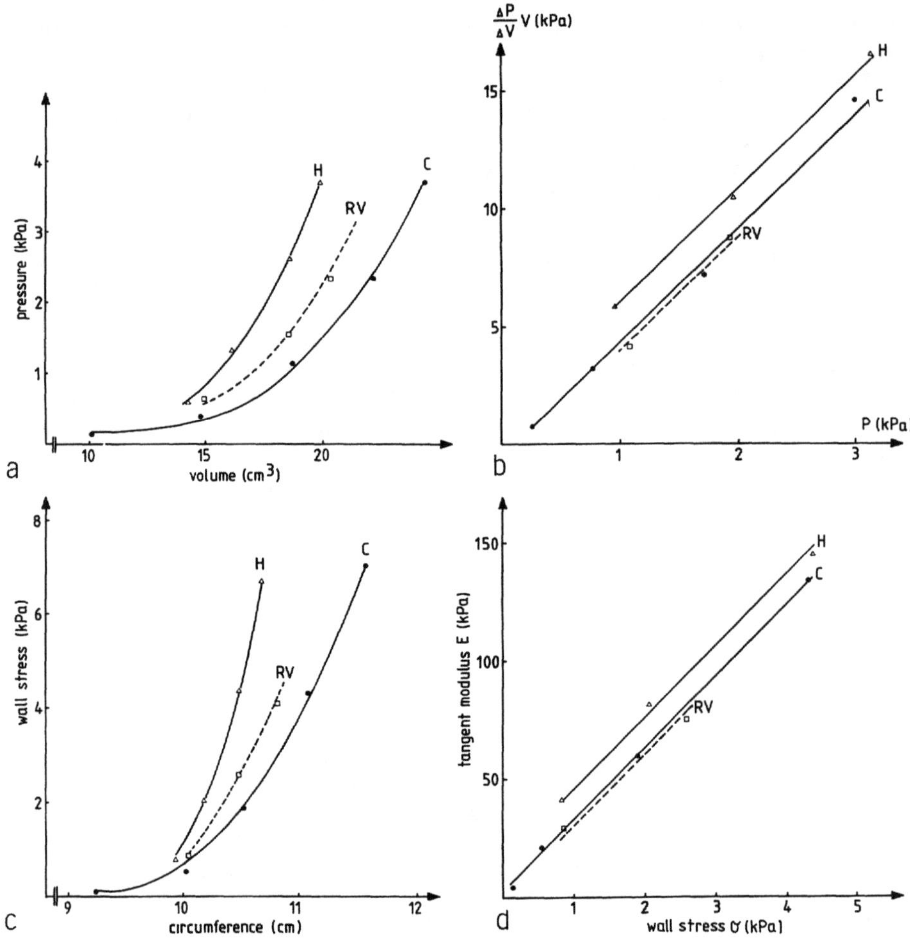

Fig. 3. Representative end-diastolic pressure-volume relationships and derived graphs. All data obtained from the same dog as in figure 2.

a) Correlation between end-diastolic left ventricular pressure and volume under different conditions. – ● – (C) control condition (ventilation with air); – Δ – (H) after 3 min of hypoxia (ventilation with N_2); □ (RV) left ventricular end-diastolic pressure-volume relationship under normoxia, but with artifically increased right ventricular pressure and volume. The right ventricular end-diastolic pressure was increased by intraventricular infusion to the same values which had been measured under hypoxia.

b) "Volume elasticity modulus" $\left(\frac{\Delta P}{\Delta V} \cdot V\right)$ as a function of the end-diastolic pressure (P). $\left(V = V_i + \frac{(V_{i+1} - V_i)}{2}\right)$.

c) Left ventricular midwall circumferential stress at the equator as a function of equatorial midwall circumference.

d) Midwall tangent (differential) elastic modulus (E) as a function of midwall circumferential stress (σ). Note the constancy of the slope of the curves under different conditions.

Symbols in figures 3b, 3c and 3d as in fig. 3a.

attached to such an error, because deviation of the determined endsystolic volume of even 20 % compared to the true value would not gravely change the formal shape of the pressure-volume loop (fig. 2c).

The second question which was considered in the present methodological study was the feasibility of deriving conclusions about the static pressure-volume relationship from the diastolic portion of the pressure-volume loop of a single contraction.

Of course, heart rate is of great significance in this context. In addition to the possibility of incomplete relaxation in tachycardia, one should also consider that diastasis is the phase which is shortened the most under increasing heart rate. At a high rate of blood inflow and initially still decreasing diastolic pressure, one cannot expect the diastolic portion of the individual pressure-volume loop to coincide with the "resting tension curve". There are also additional technical difficulties because the position of the tip of the catheter relative to the actual stream of blood can lead to variations which may have a noticeable effect on values obtained from the venous system or in ventricular diastole (4). Even at the medium and low heart rates which were used in the present experiments, substantial coincidence of the diastolic portion of the pressure-volume loop in a single contraction, and the curve derived from enddiastolic pressure-volume values, was limited to the phase of diastasis. This was particularly pronounced in the case of the volume-loaded ventricle.

Earlier reports noted a steepening of the end-diastolic left ventricular pressure-volume relationship very early in the course of oxygen-deficient ventilation of the rat (8, 14). The influence of extraventricular factors, particularly right ventricular filling, on left ventricular distensibility has been known in principle since the investigations of Ullrich et al. (1954) and has been confirmed in the meantime by many authors (e.g., 3, 10, 16). The present study shows that a substantial portion of the alteration in left ventricular distensibility of the dog heart revealed after 3 min of oxygen deficiency must be attributed to the effect of the contralateral ventricle. Experiments on open-chest rats indicate that only a small portion of the changes in ventricular distensibility in the first 8 min of oxygen deficiency is actually due to a change in tissue elasticity (Köhler, M., and Jacob, R., unpublished results). In addition to the effect of hemodynamic conditions, species differences also appear to play a role in the manifestation of rigor, e.g., species-dependent mobilization of glucose for anaerobic cardiac metabolism.

Earlier investigations revealed that contracture and fibrosis can be distinguished with the aid of the relationship between tangent elastic modulus (E) and stress (σ) (6, 8). Furthermore, it has also been shown that rigor increases the slope of this plot only in advanced stages (5). In the framework of the present study, a central question was whether analysis of the left ventricular diastolic pressure-volume curve can be used to distinguish between contracture-induced increase in myocardial stiffness, on the one hand, and a decrease in whole ventricular compliance due to enhanced contralateral ventricular volume, on the other hand. The present angiocardiographic study as well as the above-mentioned measurements conducted on the left ventricle of open-chest rats indicate that the slope of the E-σ relationship, i.e., the "stiffness constant", does not permit the latter differentiation in early stages of hypoxia.

References

1. Brilla, Ch.: Wandspannung und Elastizität des linken Ventrikelmyokards unter Rechtsherzbelastung und Hypoxie im akuten Versuch. Thesis, University of Tübingen, 1983.
2. Diamond, G., J. S. Forrester: Effect of coronary artery disease and acute myocardial infarction on left ventricular compliance in man. Circulation **45,** 11–19 (1972).
3. Glantz, S. A., W. W. Parmley: Factors which affect the diastolic pressure-volume curve. Circulat. Res. **42,** 171–180 (1978).
4. Hepp, A., D. Gradistanac, G. Kissling, R. Jacob: Influence of catheter position on blood pressure values in the pulmonary artery of the dog. Basic Res. Cardiol. **68,** 470–479 (1973).
5. Holubarsch, Ch., R. Jacob: Diastolic tension of rat cardiac muscle during deficiency of oxygen and glucose. Stress-strain relationships and reversibility. Basic Res. Cardiol. **76,** 690–703 (1981).
6. Holubarsch, Ch., R. Jacob: Die „Compliance“ des Herzens. Med. Welt **31,** 136–144 (1980).
7. Jacob, R.: Anpassung des Herzens an veränderte Anforderungen. Pacemaker Digest **13,** 83–116 (1977).
8. Jacob, R., Ch. Holubarsch, H. Moser, B. Brenner: Quantification of changes in myocardial elasticity under hypoxia. In: Heiss, H. W. (Ed.), Advances of Clinical Cardiology **1,** 211–228. G. Witzstrock (New York 1980).
9. Jacob, R., G. Kissling: Dynamik des intakten Herzens. In: Handbuch der Inneren Medizin, VEB G. Fischer, Berlin (in press).
10. Janicki, J. S., K. T. Weber: Factors influencing the diastolic pressure-volume relation of the cardiac ventricles. Fed. Proc. **39,** 133–140 (1980).
11. Lange, P. E., D. Onnasch, F. L. Farr, P. H. Heintzen: Angiocardiographic left ventricular volume determination. Accuracy, as determined from human casts, and clinical application. Europ. J. Cardiol. **8,** 449–476 (1978).
12. Mirsky, I., W. W. Parmley: Evaluation of passive elastic stiffness for left ventricle and isolated heart muscle. In: Mirsky, I., Ghista, D. N., Sandler, H., Cardiac Mechanics. John Wiley & Sons Inc. New York, London, Sydney, Toronto, 331–358 (1974).
13. Mirsky, I.: Elastic properties of the myocardium: A quantitative approach with physiological and clinical applications. Handbook of Physiology, Sect. 2, The Cardiovascular System, Berne, R. M., Washington, D.C., 497–531 (1979).
14. Moser, H., R. Jacob: Diastolic tension during the initial phase of hypoxia in isolated cardiac muscle preparations and in the left ventricular wall of rats. Pflügers Arch. **368,** Suppl. R1 (1977).
15. Rackley, Ch. E., H. T. Dodge, Y. D. Coble, R. E. Hay: A method for determining left ventricular mass in man. Circulation **29,** 666–671 (1964).
16. Ross, J. Jr.: Acute displacement of the diastolic pressure-volume curve of the left ventricle: Role of the pericardium and the right ventricle. Circulation **59,** 32–37 (1979).
17. Sandler, H., H. T. Dodge: The use of single plane angiocardiograms for the calculation of left ventricular volume in man. Amer. Heart J. **75,** 325–334 (1968).
18. Streeter, D. D., Jr., H. M. Spotnitz, D. P. Patel, J. Ross, Jr., E. H. Sonnenblick: Fiber orientation in the canine left ventricle during diastole and systole. Circulat. Res. **24,** 339–347 (1969).

19. Ullrich, K. J., G. Riecker, K. Kramer: Das Druckvolumendiagramm des Warmblüterherzens. Pflügers Arch. **259,** 481–498 (1954).
20. Yin, F. C. P.: Ventricular wall stress. Circulat. Res. **49,** 829–842 (1981).

Authors' address:

Physiologisches Institut II, Universität Tübingen, Gmelinstraße 5, 7400 Tübingen, FRG

Cardiac Adaptation to Hemodynamic Overload, Training and Stress
Dr. D. Steinkopff Verlag 364–368 (1983)

The influence of antihypertensive treatment on left ventricular compliance and myocardial stiffness

W. Motz, R. Ippisch, G. Ringsgwandl, and B. E. Strauer

Medizinische Klinik I, Klinikum Großhadern, Ludwig-Maximilians-Universität München (FRG)

Summary

To investigate whether an antihypertensive treatment with a vasodilatator and a betareceptor-blocker will affect left ventricular (LV) compliance ($\Delta V/\Delta P$) and myocardial stiffness, 4-week-old spontaneously hypertensive rats (SHR) were treated with hydralazine only (H) and with hydralazine and metoprolol (M+H) combined and compared with equally aged untreated ones. LV compliance and stiffness data were obtained by means of a passive pressure-volume relationship of the diastolically arrested left ventricle. An inverse relationship was found between LV hypertrophy, which was quantified by the LV muscle mass divided by the LV end-diastolic volume, i.e., mass-volume ratio, and LV compliance ($\Delta V/\Delta P$). After treatment with hydralazine and metoprolol, LV mass-volume ratio was considerably reduced (H: −21.8 %; M+H: −38.5 %), and LV compliance (H: +61.4 %; M+H: +111 %) enhanced in comparison to the untreated controls. Myocardial stiffness and LV collagen concentration were not different between treated and untreated animals.

Key words: left ventricular hypertrophy, left ventricular compliance, myocardial stiffness, antihypertensive treatment, hydralazine, metoprolol, myocardial collagen concentration, spontaneously hypertensive rats, arterial hypertension

Introduction

Hypertensive hypertrophy is usually associated with a reduced left ventricular (LV) compliance and an unaltered or an increased myocardial stiffness (1–12). Antihypertensive treatment may improve LV distensibility by a quantitative reduction in LV muscle mass as well as by direct effects on the elastic properties of the myocardium or by both. Consequently it was the objective of the study to investigate (I) whether an antihypertensive treatment with hydralazine and metoprolol will prevent the decrease in LV compliance as observed in sustained hypertension, and (II) whether possible changes in LV compliance are caused by a reduced LV muscle mass or by an altered myocardial stiffness.

Methods

Experiments were performed on 44–45-week-old spontaneously hypertensive rats (SHR) of the Okamoto strain after treatment with (I) hydralazine (15 mg/kg day, n =

8) and (II) metoprolol (50 mg/kg day) and hydralazine (15 mg/kg day) combined (n = 9). Untreated age-matched SHR (n = 25) were used as controls. Treatment was started at an age of 4–5 weeks and performed for a period of 40 weeks.

Terminology (17)

Compliance (or distensibility) refers to the changes in volume of a hollow object induced by changes in internal pressure ($\Delta V/\Delta P$).

Extensibility of a tissue expresses the ability of the material to extend (L) with the application of stress ($\Delta L/\Delta T$).

Stiffness describes the ratio of the increment in stress to the corresponding change in length in isolated muscle ($\Delta T/\Delta L$).

Passive pressure-volume curve

After completion of pressure (systolic and diastolic pressure in the left ventricle) and flow measurements (stroke volume, cardiac output, for details see ref. 13), the heart was arrested in diastole with adenosine solution to define the passive pressure-volume characteristics of the left ventricle. Then the atrioventricular groove was ligated, and the ventricle was compressed manually to expel blood and create a negative pressure, which was taken as zero volume. To avoid fluid accumulation and a compressing force on the septum, the right ventricular free wall was incised. Then a passive pressure-volume curve was performed by stepwise injecting saline in the left ventricle.

Left ventricular compliance ($\Delta V/\Delta P$)

To assess left ventricular compliance, a pressure-volume relationship encompassing a normal cardiac filling cycle was used. For that purpose stroke volume was taken as ΔV and divided by the difference between the end-diastolic pressure and the initial diastolic pressure ΔP.

Myocardial stiffness

By means of the passive pressure-volume curve myocardial stiffness was assessed using the formulas suggested by Mirsky and Parmley (14).

a) Midwall elastic stiffness:

$$E_m = 3\,[1+(V_{LV}/V)r_i^2 \,/\, (r_i^2+r_e^2)]\,[1+(V/P)\,(dP/dV)]\,\sigma_m - 3\,[r_e^2/(r_i^2+r_e^2)]\,[(r_e^3-r_i^3)\,/\,(2R^3+r_e^3)]\,\sigma_m$$

b) Midwall stress (spherical model):

$$\sigma_m = P\,(V/V_{LV})\,(1+r_e^3/2R^3)$$

V_{LV} = wall volume; r_i = internal radius; R = midwall radius
V = volume; r_e = external radius

The slope of the relationship between elastic stiffness and midwall stress, i.e., the stiffness constant Km was determined and used as an equivalent for myocardial stiffness (14).

Hydroxyproline

Hydroxyproline concentration was determined according to Woessner (15).

Results

The table lists left ventricular peak systolic pressure, LV muscle mass related to body weight, mass-volume ratio, left ventricular compliance $\Delta V/\Delta P$, myocardial elastic stiffness constant Km, and the hydroxyproline concentration of the treated and untreated animals.

Table 1.

		P_{LV} mm Hg	LV/BW mg/g	M/V mg/μl	ΔV/ΔP μl/mm Hg	Km –	[OH-proline] mg/g
SHR,	x̄	181	3.08	3.95	25.4	26.4	3.09
untreated	SD ±	18	0.29	0.49	5.0	4.4	0.38
	n	25	25	25	8	11	6
SHR, treated	x̄	129*	2.67*	3.09*	41.0*	22.0	3.45
with	SD ±	19	0.24	0.47	10.7	1.6	0.30
hydralazine	n	8	8	8	6	8	8
SHR, treated	x̄	124*	2.48*	2.43*	53.6*	29.3	3.08
with metoprolol	SD ±	17	0.17	0.59	19.0	7.0	0.50
and hydralazine	n	9	9	9	9	9	9

All values in the table are means (x̄) ± standard deviations (SD). * Significant difference from untreated SHR ($p < 0.05$).
Abbreviations used: P_{LV} = peak systolic LV pressure; LV/BW: LV muscle mass/body weight; M/V = mass-volume ratio (LV muscle mass/LV end-diastolic volume); ΔV/ΔP = LV compliance; Km = LV myocardial elastic stiffness constant; [OH-proline] = LV hydroxproline concentration.

Figure displays the inverse relationship between left ventricular compliance ΔV/ΔP and the degree of left ventricular hypertrophy expressed by the mass-volume ratio.

Discussion

This study revealed that an antihypertensive treatment with hydralazine and metoprolol improves LV compliance by a quantitative reduction in

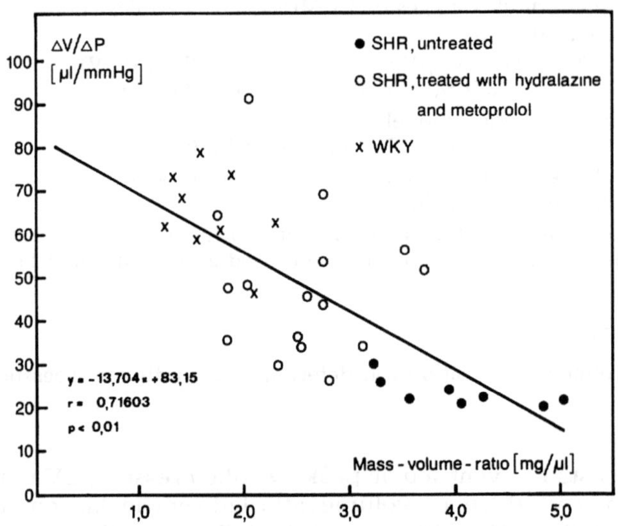

Fig. 1. An inverse relationship between the mass-volume ratio (LV muscle mass/end-diastolic volume) and LV compliance ΔV/ΔP was found.

left ventricular (LV) muscle mass rather than by altered elastic properties of the myocardium.

Due to a reduced LV distensibility, the hypertrophied left ventricle needs a higher filling pressure than a normal ventricle to exert the same average degree of end-diastolic fiber prestretch, thereby affecting stroke volume regulation and potentially the entire circulation in the forward direction. The increased LV filling pressure is transmitted backward to the lungs and the venous system, potentially leading to pulmonary congestion and the clinical symptoms of dyspnea even in the absence of heart failure (4).

LV distensibility is mainly determined by the relation between LV wall thickness and LV internal radius or the mass-volume ratio, i.e., LV geometry and by the elastic properties of the myocardium, i.e., myocardial stiffness (16). The extensibility of the myocardial fiber, which equals the reciprocal of myocardial stiffness, is mainly determined by the amount of non-contractile protein in the myocardial interstitial tissue, i.e., collagen concentration (16, 17).

The inverse relationship between LV compliance and the mass-volume ratio (figure) demonstrates that the improved LV distensibility following blood pressure normalization is due to altered LV dimensions. That conclusion is supported by the finding that the myocardial stiffness and one of its most important determinants, the LV hydroxyproline concentration, remained nearly unaltered after a medical control of LV hypertrophy.

The lack of any difference in myocardial stiffness and LV collagen concentration between treated and untreated animals in this study does not remove the importance of the elastic properties of the myocardium in general, because antihypertensive treatment was started at an age before LV hypertrophy was completely established (13). Since collagen fibers within the myocardial interstitial tissue cannot be removed as easily as intracellular components (18), a raised myocardial collagen concentration was found in spontaneously hypertensive rats after a late onset of antihypertensive treatment with alpha-methyldopa (19). In this event, LV distensibility is expected to remain impaired despite of the nearly complete reversal of cardiac hypertrophy. Therefore the age and the actual extent of LV hypertrophy at beginning an antihypertensive treatment may decide on its effectivness upon LV compliance and myocardial stiffness.

Acknowledgement

The work of M. Ploeger and S. Schulig is gratefully acknowledged.

References

1. Serizawa, T., J. Mirsky, B. Carabello, W. Grossman: Diastolic myocardial stiffness in gradually developing left ventricular hypertrophy in dog. Amer. J. Physiol. **224,** H633–H637 (1982).
2. Gaasch, W. H., W. E. Battle, A. A. Oboler, J. S. Banas, Jr., H. J. Levine: Left ventricular stress and compliance in man: with special reference to normalized ventricular function curves. Circulation **45,** 746–762 (1972).
3. Grossman, W., L. P. McLaurin: Diastolic properties of the left ventricle. Ann. Int. Med. **84,** 316–326 (1976).

4. Grossman, W., L. P. McLaurin, M. A. Stefadouros: Left ventricular stiffness associated with chronic pressure and volume overloads in man. Circulat. Res. **35,** 793–800 (1974).
5. Mirsky, I.: Assessment of passive elastic stiffness of cardiac muscle: Mathematical concepts, physiologic and clinical considerations, directions of future research. Progr. Cardiovasc. Dis. **18,** 277–308 (1976).
6. Peterson, K. L., J. Tsuji, A. Johnson, J. DiDonna, M. LeWinter: Diastolic left ventricular pressure-volume and stress-strain relations in patients with valvular aortic stenosis and left ventricular hypertrophy. Circulation **58,** 77–89 (1978).
7. Schwarz, F., W. Flameng, J. Schaper, F. Henrein: Correlation between myocardial structure and diastolic properties of the heart in chronic aortic valve disease: effects of corrective surgery. Amer. J. Cardiol. **42,** 895–903 (1978).
8. Alpert, N. R., B. B. Hamrell, W. Halpern: Mechanical and biochemical correlates of cardiac hypertrophy. Circulat. Res. **35,** Suppl. II, 71–82 (1974).
9. Bing, O. H. L., S. Matsushita, B. L. Fanburg, H. J. Levine: Mechanical properties of rat cardiac muscle during experimental hypertrophy. Circulat. Res. **28,** 234–244 (1971).
10. Spann, J. F., R. A. Buccino, E. H. Sonnenblick, E. Braunwald: Contractile state of cardiac muscle obtained from cats with experimentally-produced ventricular hypertrophy and heart failure. Circulat. Res. **21,** 341–354 (1967).
11. Grimm, A. F., R. Kubota, W. V. Whitehorn: Properties of the myocardium in cardiomegaly. Circulat. Res. **12,** 118–124 (1963).
12. Williams, J. F., R. D. Potter: Normal contractile state of hypertrophied myocardium after pulmonary artery constriction in the cat. J. Clin. Invest. **54,** 1266–1275 (1974).
13. Motz, W., M. Ploeger, G. Ringsgwandl, N. Goeldel, B. Garthoff, S. Kazda, B. E. Strauer: The influence of nifedipine on ventricular function and myocardial hypertrophy in spontaneously hypertensive rats. J. Cardiovasc. Pharmacol. **5,** 55–61 (1983).
14. Mirsky, J., W. Parmley: Assessment of passive elastic stiffness for isolated heart muscle and the intact heart. Circulat. Res. **33,** 233–243 (1973).
15. Woessner, J. F.: The determination of hydroxyproline in tissue and protein samples containing small proportions of this amino acid. Arch. Biochem. Biophys. **93,** 440–447 (1961).
16. Gaasch, W. H., H. J. Levine, M. A. Quinones, J. K. Alexander: Left ventricular compliance: mechanism and clinical implications. Amer. J. Cardiol. **38,** 645–653 (1976).
17. Covell, J., J. Ross, Jr.: Nature and significance of alterations in myocardial compliance. Amer. J. Cardiol. **32,** 449–445 (1973).
18. Cutiletta, A. F., R. T. Dowek, M. Rudnik, R. A. Arcilla, R. Zak: Regression of myocardial hypertrophy I. Experimental model, changes in heart weight, nucleic acids and collagen. J. Mol. Cell. Cardiol. **7,** 767–781 (1975).
19. Sen, S., R. C. Tarazi, F. M. Bumpus: Biochemical changes associated with development and reversal of cardiac hypertrophy in spontaneously hypertensive rats. Cardiovasc. Res. **10,** 254–261 (1976).

Authors' address:

Dr. med. Wolfgang Motz, Medizinische Klinik I der Universität München, Klinikum Großhadern, Marchioninistraße 15, D-8000 München 70, FRG

Acknowledgements

The authors would like to express their gratitude to the Erwin Riesch-Stiftung whose generous support has made this symposium possible.

A note of appreciation is all due for the Deutsche Gesellschaft für Herz- und Kreislaufforschung which provided generous organizational assistance.

We would also like to thank the following contributors for additional assistance:

Pharma Schwarz, Monheim
Byk Gulden, Konstanz
Universitätsbund Tübingen
Bayer AG, Leverkusen
Pfizer, Karlsruhe
Schering, Berlin
Cassella, Frankfurt
Bälz, Heilbronn
Verla-Pharma, Tutzing
HAG-Kaffee, Bremen

AUTHORS' INDEX

Alpert, N. R. ... 147, 158
Amaral, de E. . 69
Arkhipenko, Yu. V. 258
Aussedat, J. 228
Beyer, A. 204
Bing, O. H. L. 235
Boszkov, B. 78
Bouveret, P. 104
Brecht, K. 288
Brilla, Ch. 354
Brooks, W. W. 235
Bukhari, A. R. .. 59, 267
Charlemagne, D. .. 94
Cluzeaud, F. 69
Coffelt, R. J. 197
Conrad, Ch. H. 235
Dhalla, N. S. 189
Dhillon, K. S. 189
England, P. J. 139
Everett, A. W. 39
Felbier, H.-R. 274
Gergely, J. 27
Gorza, L. 101
Goulette, R. P. 158
Gregorova, I. 65
Gülch, R. W. 174
Hatt, P. Y. 69
Heisterkamp, M. .. 330
Hirzel, H. O. 123
Holubarsch, Ch. ... 158
Iimura, T. 182
Ippisch, R. 364
Jacob, R. 3, 46, 267, 274, 341, 349, 354
Javich, M. P. 83
Jeacocke, S. A. 139
Jespersen, L. T. ... 253
Kagan, V. E. 258
Kawamura, M. 182
Kawanishi, M. 182
Kissling, G. 166, 204, 354
Klepzig, M. 213
Kölbel, F. 65
Kolarova, R. 78
Korecky, B. 297
Kvetnansky, R. ... 265
Lakatta, E. G. 53
Lavanchy, N. 228
Lederballe Pedersen, O. 253
Lelievre, L. 94
Lindner, J. 314
Litten, R. Z. 147
Lompré, A. M. 104
Mabuchi, K. 129
Maeno, H. 134
Malloy, L. 167
Mansier, P. 94
Martin, J. 228
Medugorac, I. .. 341, 349
Meerson, F. Z. .. 83, 258
Mercadier, J. J. 104
Mikkelsen, E. 253
Mills, D. 139
Moalic, J. M. 94
Mohrmann, J. 174
Moravec, J. 245
Motz, W. 282, 364
Mulieri, L. A. .. 147, 158
Mulvany, M. J. 253
Nagano, M. 34, 182
Nagata, T. 182
Nguyen Duong, H. 288
Noma, K. 134
Nunotani, H. 70
Nyborg, N. 253
Nzonzi, J. 245
Ohkubo, T. 134, 182
Onishi, S. 70
Panagia, V. 189
Parmley, W. W. 197
Pask, H. T. 139
Pauletto, P. 101
Perennec, J. 69
Petkova, I. 78
Popova, N. 46, 78
Pott, G. 304
Pribyl, T. 65
Rabinowitz, M. 39
Radvany, P. 235
Rakusan, K. 297
Rappaport, L. ... 94, 104
Rauterberg, J. 304
Ray, A. 228
Ringsgwandl, G. .. 364
Rossi, A. 228
Rupp, H. 46, 59, 167, 267, 274
Samuel, J. L. ... 94, 104
Sartore, S. 101
Schaub, M. C. 123
Schiaffino, S. 101
Schmiebusch, H. .. 330
Schmiegelow, P. .. 314
Schreiber, V. 65
Schwartz, K. 94, 104
Sievers, R. 197
Singal, P. K. 189
Sinha, A. M. 39
Somogyi, E. 129
Sotonyi 219
Spadaro, K. B. 235
Sreter, F. A. 129
Srihari, T. 123
Staubesand, J. 330
Stepan, J. 65
Strauer, B. E. .. 213, 282, 364
Swynghedauw, B. 94, 104
Takeda, N. 134
Tochino, Y. 70
Torda, T. 265
Tuchschmid, C. R. . 123
Ueda, S. 113
Valfré, C. 101
Voss, B. 304
Vrbová, G. 33
Watari, S. 182
Weinstein, K. B. ... 235
Wikman-Coffelt, J. 197
Willemin, M. 69
Yazaki, Y. 113
Zak, R. 39
Ziegler, H. 330
Zimmer, H.-G. 220

SUBJECT INDEX

(Numbers refer to the first page of respective articles)

actin-myosin interaction 27
action potential 174
activation of connective tissue cells 304
activity 33
actomyosin 134
adaptation 3, 158
adenine nucleotide biosynthesis 220
adrenal weight 65
adrenergic receptors 266
adult aging 53
afterload 220
age-dependent alterations 349
angiocardiography 354
anti-hypertensive therapy 253
antihypertensive treatment 364
aorto-caval fistula 69, 245
aortic constriction 69
- stenosis 189, 349
arterial hypertension 364
ATPase 27
ATP depletion 228
ATP hydrolysis 197
atrophy 297

beta-adrenergic blockade 78
blood pressure 274

Ca^{++}-activated ATPase activity . 134
Ca^{2+} binding 182
Ca^{2+} regulation 27
calcium 253
- accumulation 258
- antagonism 288
- transport ATPase 258
cardiac ATP content 220
- contractility 220
- failure 134
- growth 69
- biopsy 129
- hypertrophy ... 53, 69, 101, 123, 174, 213, 228, 253, 341, 349
- myosin isozyme 113
-- isozymes 129
-- light chains 129
- overload 94
cardioprotection 220
cardiovascular aging 315
catecholamines 266
catecholamine-synthesizing and degrading enzymes 266
catechol-O-methyltransferase 59, 267
chromatin 69
chronical volume overload 245
chronic exercise 53
- concentration 341
- content 315
- heterogeneity 349
- pattern 315
collagen(s) 304
compensatory growth 83
congestive cardiomyopathy 129
connective tissue 304
-- aging 315
contractile and biochemical properties 33
contractile performance 197
coronary arteries 330
- reserve 213
- resistance 213
- spasms 288
C-protein 139
crossbridge 27, 158
- cycling 147
crotalaria 174
- spectabilis 46
-- intoxication 341
cyclic nucleotides 78
cytoplasmic factors 83

digitalis 94
dopamin-β-hydroxylase 266
D-thyroxine 39

economy 147
elasticity 27
electron microscopic 330
emotional excitation 267, 274
- painful 258
endocrine status 3
essential hypertension 213
exercise 267, 274
excitation-contraction coupling 158
experimental cardiac hypertrophy 65

fetal and adult cardiac V_1 and V_3 isomyosins 104

fibre orientation 297
fibrosis 304
foetal cardiac myosin 219
force generation 27
freeze clamp 197
force-frequency relationship 189
kinetics 27
'k'-myocytes 330

glycogen storage disease 129
glycosaminoglycan 315
Goldblatt hypertension 349
- rats 182

heart 39, 83, 297
- hypertrophy 189
- weight 65
heat 158
heavy chains 113
^{3}H-thymidine-labeling index 315
human heart 101, 123
- myocardium 134
hydralazine 213, 253, 364
hydroxylase 266
hypercapnia 204
hypertension 158, 253, 266, 330
hypertensive rats 181
hypertrophy 46, 147, 297
hypocapnia 204
hypoxia 354

immobilization stress 266
immunofluorescence 94, 101
immunological and electrophoretical analyses 104
increased afterload 189
influence of right ventricular pressure 354
interval-strength relation 174
intracellular pH 228
ischemia 228, 245
isolated cardiac muscle 53
- muscle preparation 235
- perfused rat heart 245
isometric contraction 53, 147
- relaxation 147
isomyosins 39
isoproterenol 69, 220, 267

left ventricular afterload 282
-- casts 354
-- compliance 364
-- function 282
-- hypertrophy 167, 282, 364
-- mechanics 204
-- systolic wall stress 282
----- reserve 282
-- wall stress and elasticity 354
light chains 113
lipid peroxidation 258
liver 83
long chain acyl-CoA 245
L-thyroxine 147

magnesium ions 288
membrane fluidity 258
messenger RNA 94
metropolol 213, 364
'm'-myocytes 330
monoamine oxidase 59, 267
morphological and morphometric investigation 330
myocardial buffer capacity 204
- collagen concentration 364
- contractility 282
- efficiency 167
- energetics 167
- hypertrophy 78
- infarction 235
- mechanics 235
- nucleus 69, 78
- oxygen consumption 167
- stiffness 354, 364
myocardium 266
myofibrillar ATPase 53
-- activity 3
myofibrillar function 3
myosin 59, 101
- flexibility 27
- heavy chains 39, 134
- isoenzymes 3, 46, 123, 147, 167, 197, 274
- light chain 139
- motion 27
- subunits 123
- synthesis 39
myothermal techniques 147

Na^{+}-Ca^{2+} exchange 182
Na-K ATPase 94
Na^{+}-K^{+} ATPase 182
nifedipine 282
noradrenaline 253

overload 297

phenyl-ethanolamine-N-methyltransferase 59, 267
phosphorus nuclear magnetic resonance spectroscopy 228

phosphorylation potential 197
pressure cardiac hypertrophy .. 104
- overload 3, 147, 167
- - hypertrophy 158
proliferation 304
propranolol 267
protein phosphorylation 139
proteoglycan 315
pulmonary hypertension 46, 341

rat 69, 266
- and human ventricles 104
- heart 94
- myocardium 53
- ventricular myocardium 349
reconstitution 113
resistance vessel abnormalities . 253
RNA polymerases 83

sarcolemma 94, 182
sarcoplasmic reticulum 258
serum digoxin-like reactivity ... 65
SHR-long-term antihypertensive therapy 213
SHR/WKY hybrids 253
skeletal muscle 33
spontaneously hypertensive rats 134, 182, 253, 364
steric blocking 27
stress 3, 258, 267, 274

subfragment-1 113
succinate 245
swimming 267, 274
- training 349
- - of rats 204
Syrian Hamster 197

tension-dependent heat 147
testicular arteries 330
thin filament 27
thyroid hormones 46, 59
thyrotoxicosis 174
thyroxine 39, 113
training 3
transcriptional control 39
translation 94
transmitters 3
transplanted heart 297
triiodothyronine 220
tropomyosin 27
troponin 27
troponin-I 139
tubulin 94
tunica media 253
tyrosin 266

vascular pacemaker cells 288
- smooth muscle 253, 288
ventricular hypertrophy 235
- myocardium 94

MIX
Papier aus verantwortungsvollen Quellen
Paper from responsible sources
FSC® C105338

If you have any concerns about our products,
you can contact us on
ProductSafety@springernature.com

In case Publisher is established outside the EU,
the EU authorized representative is:
Springer Nature Customer Service Center GmbH
Europaplatz 3, 69115 Heidelberg, Germany

Printed by Libri Plureos GmbH
in Hamburg, Germany